Hematopoietic Stem Cells

The Mulhouse Manual

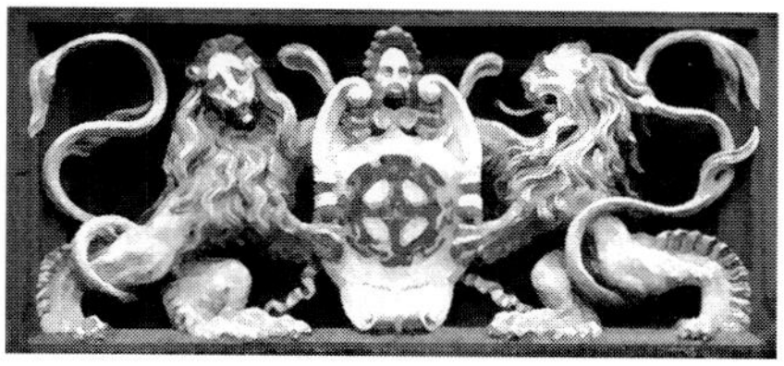

AlphaMed Press, 4100 South Kettering Boulevard, Dayton, Ohio 45439-2092 USA

Library of Congress Cataloging-in-Publication Data

Hematopoietic stem cells: the Mulhouse manual/edited by /Eckart Wunder ... [et al.].
p. cm.
Includes bibliographical references and index.
ISBN 1-880854-17-1
1. Hematopoietic stem cells—Laboratory manuals. I. Wunder, E. (Eckart). 1943- .
[DNLM: 1. Hematopoietic Stem Cells—chemistry—laboratory manuals.
2. Hematopoietic Stem Sells—transplantation—laboratory manuals.
3. Antigens, CD—analysis—laboratory manuals. 4. Cell Separation—methods—laboratory manuals. 5. Cell Separation—instrumentation—laboratory manuals.
WH 25 H487 1994]
QP92.H455 1994
612.4'1—dc20
DNLM/DLC
for Library of Congress

First Printing, 1994
Second Printing, 1995

93-42864
CIP

While every effort is made by the publisher and editorial office to see that no inaccurate or misleading data, opinion or statement appears in this publication, the data and opinions appearing in the chapters and advertisements herein are the responsibility of the contributor or advertiser concerned. Accordingly, the publisher, the editor and respective employees, officers and agents accept no liability whatsoever for the consequences of any such inaccurate or misleading data, opinion or statement. While every effort is made to ensure that drug doses and other quantities are presented accurately, readers are advised that new methods and techniques involving drug usage, and described within this publication, should only be followed in conjunction with the drug manufacturer's own published literature.

The Cover: **Bone Marrow Development**—graphics by Leon W.M.M. Terstappen, M.D., Becton Dickinson Fellow, San José, California. Cover design by Bil Myers, WSM Advertising & Graphics, Dayton, Ohio.

Printed in the United States of America on paper that adheres to the requirements for library/archival stability.

Hematopoietic Stem Cells

The Mulhouse Manual

Editors

Eckart Wunder, M.D.
Hôpital du Hasenrain
Mulhouse, France

Hanna Sovalat, M.D.
Hôpital du Hasenrain
Mulhouse, France

Philippe Hénon, M.D.
Hôpital du Hasenrain
Mulhouse, France

Stefan Serke, M.D.
Freie Universität Berlin
Berlin, Germany

About the cover. . .

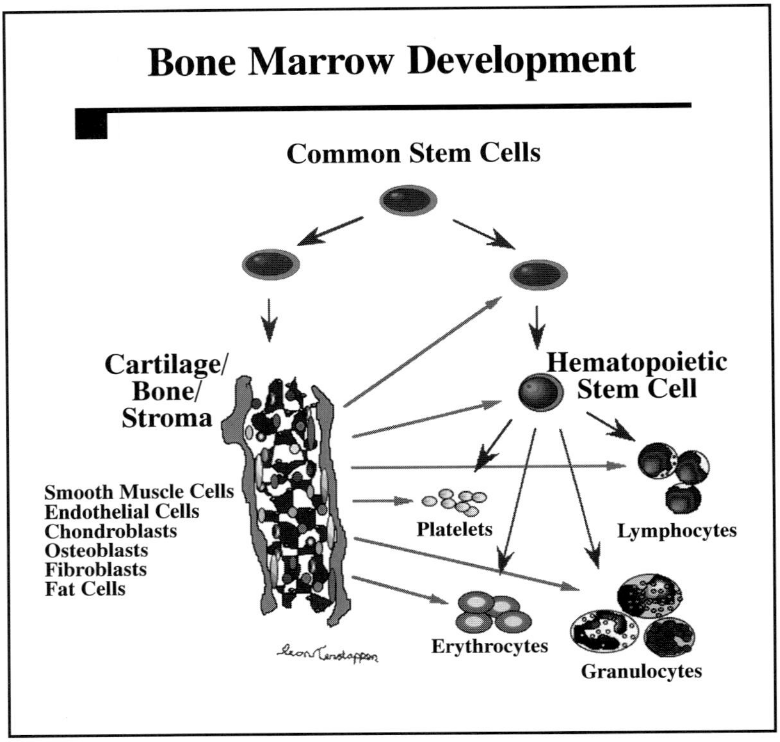

Putative development of fetal human bone marrow. Created in MacDraw® by Leon W.M.M. Terstappen.

Hematopoietic Stem Cells

The Mulhouse Manual

Table of Contents

Contributors

James G. Bender
Baxter Healthcare Corporation
Round Lake, Illinois USA

Ronald J. Berenson
CellPro, Inc.
Bothell, Washington USA

Bruno Brando
Ospedale Niguarda
Milan, Italy

Marco Bregni
Istituto Nazionale Tumori
Milan, Italy

Wolfgang Brehm
Children's Hospital
University of Tübingen
Tübingen, Germany

Wolfram Brugger
Albert-Ludwigs-University
Medical Center
Freiburg, Germany

Hans-Jörg Bühring
University of Tübingen
Tübingen, Germany

Julie Burgess
Baxter Healthcare Corporation
Santa Ana, California USA

Michaela Burkhardt
University of Tübingen
Tübingen, Germany

Christophe Camilla
Immunotech SA
Marseille, France

Gianluigi Castoldi
University of Ferrara
Ferrara, Italy

Pierre Charbord
INSERM/C.R.T.S.
Besançon, France

Curt I. Civin
Johns Hopkins Hospital
Baltimore, Maryland USA

Lucia H. Coutinho
Christie Hospital NHS Trust
Manchester, United Kingdom

Erika de Wynter
Christie Hospital NHS Trust
and University of Manchester
Paterson Institute for
Cancer Research
Manchester, United Kingdom

Magda De Smedt
University of Ghent
Ghent, Belgium

Nathalie Debernardi
Immunotech SA
Marseille, France

Massimo Di Nicola
Istituto Nazionale Tumori
Milan, Italy

Tracey L. Dowse
Institute of Medical and
Veterinary Science
Adelaide, South Australia

Pamela G. Dyson
Institute of Medical and
Veterinary Science
Adelaide, South Australia

Torstein Egeland
The National Hospital
Oslo, Norway

Stefan Fruehauf
University of Heidelberg
Heidelberg, Germany

Gustav Gaudernack
The National Hospital
Oslo, Norway

Adrian P. Gee
Richland Memorial Hospital
University of South Carolina
Columbia, South Carolina USA

A. Massimo Gianni
Istituto Nazionale Tumori and
Università degli Studi
Milan, Italy

Simone Guth
Miltenyi Biotec GmbH
Bergisch Gladbach, Germany

Rainer J. Haas
University of Heidelberg
Heidelberg, Germany

Mike Haberkorn
German Cancer Research
Center
Heidelberg, Germany

Rupert Handgretinger
Children's Hospital
University of Tübingen
Tübingen, Germany

Giao Hangoc
Baxter Healthcare Corporation
Santa Ana, California USA

Alan Hardwick
Baxter Healthcare Corporation
Santa Ana, California USA

Mark Harvey
Applied Immune Sciences, Inc.
Santa Clara, California USA

David N. Haylock
Institute of Medical and
Veterinary Science
Adelaide, South Australia

Shelly Heimfeld
CellPro, Inc.
Bothell, Washington USA

Philippe R. Hénon
Hôpital du Hasenrain
Mulhouse, France

R. Henschler
Albert-Ludwigs-University
Medical Center
Freiburg, Germany

Georges Herbein
Sir William Dunn School
of Pathology
Oxford, United Kingdom

Bjørn V. Herikstad
Dynal A.S.
Oslo, Norway

Joëlle Hirn
Immunotech SA
Marseille, France

Raimund Hoeft
German Cancer Research
Center
Heidelberg, Germany

Werner Hunstein
University of Heidelberg
Heidelberg, Germany

Lori Ishizawa
Baxter Healthcare Corporation
Santa Ana, California USA

Christopher A. Juttner
Institute of Medical and
Veterinary Science
Adelaide, South Australia

Lothar Kanz
Albert-Ludwigs-University
Medical Center
Freiburg, Germany

André Kirn
Institut de Virologie et
Unité INSERM
Strasbourg, France

Andreas Kirsch
Freie Universität Berlin
Berlin, Germany

Lawrence S. Lamb, Jr.
Richland Memorial Hospital
University of South Carolina
Columbia, South Carolina USA

Francesco Lanza
University of Ferrara
Ferrara, Italy

Jørgen K. Larsen
University Hospital
Copenhagen, Denmark

Ping Law
Baxter Healthcare Corporation
Santa Ana, California USA

Jane Lebkowski
Applied Immune Sciences, Inc.
Santa Clara, California USA

Georges Leclercq
University of Ghent
Ghent, Belgium

Eli Lien
Dynal A.S.
Oslo, Norway

Michele Magni
Istituto Nazionale Tumori
Milan, Italy

Shigeyoshi Makino
Institute of Medical and
Veterinary Science
Adelaide, South Australia

Roland Mertelsmann
Albert-Ludwigs-University
Medical Center
Freiburg, Germany

Stefan Miltenyi
Miltenyi Biotec GmbH
Bergisch Gladbach, Germany

Robert Möhle
University of Heidelberg
Heidelberg, Germany

Annemarie Moseley
Applied Immune Sciences, Inc.
Santa Clara, California USA

Claudia A. Müller
University of Tübingen
Tübingen, Germany

Martin J. Murphy, Jr.
Hipple Cancer Research Center
Dayton, Ohio USA

Sylvana Niutta
Institute of Medical and
Veterinary Science
Adelaide, South Australia

Thomas B. Okarma
Applied Immune Sciences, Inc.
Santa Clara, California USA

Fedro Peccatori
Istituto Nazionale Tumori
Milan, Italy

Eckhard Pflüger
Miltenyi Biotec GmbH
Bergisch Gladbach, Germany

Margit Pförsich
University of Heidelberg
Heidelberg, Germany

Jean Plum
University of Ghent
Ghent, Belgium

Andreas Radbruch
University of Cologne
Cologne, Germany

Ferdinando Ravagnani
Istituto Nazionale Tumori
Milan, Italy

Trevor P. Rawling
Institute of Medical and
Veterinary Science
Adelaide, South Australia

Caroline M. Rawling
Institute of Medical and
Veterinary Science
Adelaide, South Australia

Marion M. Roberts
Institute of Medical and
Veterinary Science
Adelaide, South Australia

Phillip A. Rowlings
Institute of Medical and
Veterinary Science
Adelaide, South Australia

Sabine Säuberlich
Freie Universität Berlin
Berlin, Germany

Lisa Schain
Applied Immune Sciences, Inc.
Santa Clara, California USA

Stefan Serke
Freie Universität Berlin
Berlin, Germany

Salvatore Siena
Istituto Nazionale Tumori
Milan, Italy

Federico Silvestri
Udine University School
of Medicine
Udine, Italy

Paul J. Simmons
Institute of Medical and
Veterinary Science
Adelaide, South Australia

Hanna Sovalat
Hôpital du Hasenrain
Mulhouse, France

Nydia G. Testa
Christie Hospital NHS Trust
Paterson Institute for
Cancer Research
Manchester, United Kingdom

Andreas Thiel
University of Cologne
Cologne, Germany

L. Bik To
Institute of Medical and
Veterinary Science
Adelaide, South Australia

Yves Traore
Immunotech SA
Marseille, France

Sandra Trimboli
Institute of Medical and
Veterinary Science
Adelaide, South Australia

Kristen Unverzagt
Baxter Healthcare Corporation
Round Lake, Illinois USA

Bart Vandekerckhove
University of Ghent
Ghent, Belgium

Donald Walker
Baxter Healthcare Corporation
Round Lake, Illinois USA

Barbara Witt
University of Heidelberg
Heidelberg, Germany

Eckart Wunder
Hôpital du Hasenrain
Mulhouse, France

Walter Jens Zeller
German Cancer Research
Center
Heidelberg, Germany

Robert Zimmermann
Freie Universität Berlin
Berlin, Germany

Publisher's Foreword

This volume, **Hematopoietic Stem Cells,** evolved from a need expressed by the participants of two recent workshops in Mulhouse, France, on stem cell methodologies. These workshops were designed to introduce standardized methods of cell preparation and to compare major hematopoietic stem cell purification methods for fresh human cells. Organized by Mulhouse's Institut de Recherche en Hématologie-Transfusion (*Ph. Hénon,* Director), these workshops were guided by an internationally recognized faculty of stem cell aficionados. The meetings proved encyclopedic, since they were directed at both the theory and practice of hematopoietic stem cell characterization, mobilization, purification and transplantation. They were, in fact, so excellent that the participants agreed to extend these benefits to a much wider audience through the publication of a manual.

Because the book was conceived in Mulhouse and has been principally authored by the invited faculty who conducted the most recent workshop (May 1993), it is fitting that it be subtitled "The Mulhouse Manual." Mulhouse, located along the beautiful Route du Vin of the Alsatian region of France, has historically been an international intersection, situated as it is at the corners of France, Switzerland and Germany. The lions on its coat of arms (see below) represent the nobility who once protected the city, and the mill wheel they hold reminds us of the water mills which dotted the countryside and from which the name Mulhouse (German "Mülhausen" or "mill") was derived. This coat of arms became the Manual's icon, for which we are grateful to *Madame Agnes Hénon,* who photographed it on the facade of the ancient City Hall.

AlphaMed Press is pleased to publish this first-ever laboratory manual recording state-of-the-science stem cell methodologies, cytofluorimetry and stem cell purification. Encompassing both the theory and the practice of stem cell mobilization, separation and transplantation, it addresses the needs of both clinical transplanters and stem cell biologists.

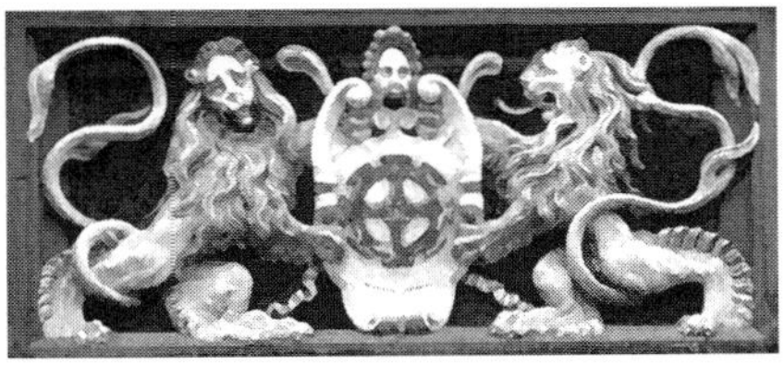

Preface

Since the advent of anti-CD34 monoclonal antibodies (MAbs), transplantation centers worldwide have been applying cytofluorimetric determination of hematopoietic cells as an important grafting index of cells from bone marrow and from mobilized adult or umbilical cord blood. A novel perspective of paramount importance was introduced with the pioneering work of the Milan group led by *Salvatore Siena* [1, 2]. This team demonstrated that by applying red cell lysis, instead of density fractionation, the absolute number of $CD34^+$ cells per volume of blood could be rapidly determined and conveniently used for "on line monitoring" to optimize leukapheresis harvest after induction of stem cell mobilization. In addition, conjugated fluorescent anti-CD34 MAbs, which became commercially available in 1992, improved these determinations.

In recent meetings on "Bone Marrow Processing and Purging" (Orlando; September 1993) and "International Symposium on Peripheral Blood Stem Cell Autografts" (Bordeaux; October 1993), many contributors presented data concerning the size of hematopoietic cell compartments in terms of $CD34^+$ cell numbers, usually accompanied by conventionally determined in vitro-derived progenitor cell numbers. In view of the widespread use of new in vitro parameters aimed at predicting recovery of hematopoiesis after grafting, it became apparent that inter-laboratory standardization of the measurement would be of value. Two methodology workshops were held in Mulhouse, France, in 1992 [3] and 1993 [4, 5]. Experts from the world over focused on this subject, and in 1993 we made an attempt to introduce standardized methods of cell preparation with "hands-on" training. We also demonstrated and compared current major hematopoietic stem cell purification methods for fresh human cells.

It was at the most recent of these workshops where the suggestion was made that the benefits of this expertise from major European and American laboratories be captured in the form of a published manual which would address not only the practical "bench-oriented" aspects of these developing technologies, but also record the theocratical bases of these advances. Another workshop was directed by *Leon Terstappen* on "Multidimensional Flow Cytometric Analysis of Bone Marrow and Peripheral Blood Stem Cells" (San Jose, 1993). We are grateful to *Adrian Gee* for his summary of this meeting, included within this manual.

The intention of this manual is to present the current methodologies used by leading laboratories. Included are technical details, explanations and advice to solve frequently encountered practical problems. For the scientist wishing to repeat these same methods, materials, reagents and addresses of commercial distributors are also given along with the relevant literature references. The topics are grouped according to their relationship to one another; in instances where a technical element is covered elsewhere in more detail, cross references are provided.

As part of the Mulhouse workshop, cell samples from a fresh leukapheresis were distributed to the participants, along with CD34 antibodies. The results of this inter-laboratory attempt at standardization are also recorded.

This manual is intended to serve as a useful resource to: (1) provide detailed "recipes" as a lab bench reference, and (2) simultaneously sharpen the critical interpretation of one's own data. In this way it is hoped that the manual will support the advancement of this promising field.

The authors are grateful to *Martin J. Murphy, Jr.,* whose enthusiasm for this subject initiated and sustained the manual's preparation. Once the project was launched, all our authors engaged without hesitation in preparing and completing their contributions within tight time limits. Our thanks go to each of them. Special thanks are due to the following companies, who generously supplied their instruments (even prototypes) and materials for the workshop demonstrations: Applied Immune Sciences, Baxter Healthcare, Beckman Instruments, Becton Dickinson, CellPro, Dynal, Immunotech, and Miltenyi.

The speed and professionalism of the manual's publication owes a great debt of gratitude to the intense and sustained efforts by *Ann Murphy, Edie McBride* and *Vanessa Blaylock* at our publisher, AlphaMed Press. We are also most thankful for our secretary, *Francine Morgenthaler.*

Eckart Wunder for the Editors

References

1 Siena S, Bregni M, Brando B, Ravagnani F, Bonadonna G, Gianni AM. Circulation of CD34+ hematopoietic stem cells in the peripheral blood of high dose cyclophosphamide-treated patients: enhancement by intraveneous recombinant human granulocyte-macrophage colony stimulating factor. Blood 1989;74:1905-1914.

2 Siena S, Belli N, Ravagnani F, Grandola L, Stern AC, Lansdorp PM, Bonadonna G, Gianni AM. Flow cytometry for clinical estimation of circulating hematopoietic progenitors for autologous transplantation in cancer patients. Blood 1991;77:400-409.

3 Wunder E, Sovalat H, Fritsch G, Silvestri F, Hénon P, Serke S. Report on the European Workshop on Peripheral Blood Stem Cell Determination and Standardization–Mulhouse, France. J of Hematotherapy 1992;1:131-142.

4 Silvestri F, Wunder E, Sovalat H, Hénon P, Serke S. Positive Selection of CD34+ Cells: A Short Review of the Immunoadsorption Methods Currently Available for Experimental and Clinical Use. (Report on the "2nd European Workshop on Stem Cells Methodology"). J of Hematotherapy (in press).

5 Sovalat H, Wunder E, Tienhaara A, Olofsson T, Fritsch G, Silvestri F, Serke S. Commentary. Prospects for Standardization of Stem Cell Determination within Europe. J of Hematotherapy 1993;2:293-295.

uction

Standardization was the theme of the second European Workshop on Stem Cell Methodology. Standardization efforts are much needed to support the burgeoning worldwide explorations of hematopoietic stem cell transplantation for cancer and related diseases. Much was accomplished by the collective efforts summarized in this volume. I will open this manual by posing a series of relevant questions relating to methodology in this field and then speculating on the answers.

Can we count stem/progenitor cells?

Estimation of the total size of the stem/progenitor cell compartment can be quantified, in theory, by total flow cytometric counts of immunolabeled $CD34^+$ cells. Intense labeling of CD34 is needed to clearly distinguish the $CD34^+$ cells from nonspecific background fluorescence, and available phycoerythrin-conjugated monoclonal antibodies accomplish this quite well. Staining could be further enhanced, if necessary, by use of cocktails of CD34 monoclonal antibodies recognizing distinct epitopes. CD34 determination is aided by simultaneously staining the cell preparation with CD45, since the $CD34^+$ cells fall in a fairly characteristic region of the CD34 versus CD45 bivariate plot. Computer programs for automated gating of flow cytometric light scatter and fluorescence data will soon be available to help standardize these measurements.

The major $CD34^+$ cell subset in peripheral blood mobilized by chemotherapy and/or colony stimulating factors (GM-CSF or G-CSF) is the $CD34^+/(CD33^+/CD13^+)$ monogranulocytic progenitor. CD13 labels these cells more intensely and distinctly than CD33. Because of the rapid platelet recoveries which have been noted in patients after transfusion of mobilized peripheral blood, platelet progenitors may also be in this cell subset. Since this appears always to be such a dominant subset (~90%) in mobilized peripheral blood, it is not clear that any $CD34^+$ subsets must be measured in blood cells mobilized by G-CSF or GM-CSF. However, measurement of subsets may be useful in assessing marrow and other collections. Erythroid progenitors can be quantified as $CD34^+/(CD36^+/CD71^+)$. In marrow, the frequency of $CD34^+/(CD19^+/CD10^+)$ B lymphoid progenitors varies from ~10-40% of the $CD34^+$ compartment. Since these committed lymphoid cells do not contribute to recovery of red cells, granulocytes or platelets (the cell types where prompt reconstitution is clinically most important), it may be useful to quantify this subset to eliminate this fraction from the assessment of a preparation's capacity to restore blood cell counts (short-term). It is probably not necessary (or feasible) to consider the routine quantitation of the extremely rare T lymphoid and natural killer (NK) cell progenitors. It would be of great interest to have a measure of the content of "true" stem cells, i.e., those rare cells (<1%)

Correspondence: Dr. Curt I. Civin, The Johns Hopkins Oncology Center & Department of Pediatrics, The Johns Hopkins University School of Medicine, 600 N. Wolfe St., Baltimore, MD 21287-5001, USA.

©AlphaMed Press ISBN 1-880854 17-1

within the CD34$^+$ cell compartment capable of restoring lymphohematopoiesis for (at least) the life of the patient. These cells would be the most interesting to quantitate, and recent work suggests that the CD34$^+$/CD38$^-$ subset is an enriched source of stem cells. However, accurate measurement of this tiny subset (<0.1% of marrow mononuclear cells) is not yet routinely feasible.

Might the enumerated stem/progenitor cells be dead or injured?

In addition to antibody-based quantitation of numbers of progenitor/stem cells, we need at least a semi-quantitative determination of their viability and growth capacity. Probably a standardized method (i.e., a commercial "kit") for colony forming unit-granulocyte macrophage (CFU-GM) determination is the best available possibility to ascertain that at least some progenitors are capable of growth. In the future, a rapid flow cytometric proliferation assay should be substituted. For example, the growth fraction of CD34$^+$ cells after overnight culture in hematopoietic growth factors could be measured using DNA dyes (e.g., propidium iodide) or proliferation-related antigens (e.g., Ki67).

Can we optimize stem cell mobilization?

The combination of assessments of CD34$^+$ cell subsets and growth assays should help in optimization of peripheral blood stem cell mobilization strategies. Nevertheless, until the stem cell is rigorously defined, this will need to be combined with in vivo measurements of long-term engrafting capacity. It is intriguing to speculate that use of growth factor combinations could allow harvest of sufficient stem cells for repeated transplants in a single leukapheresis. Repeated transplants might lead to higher cancer cure rates. In addition, a single leukapheresis would make processing/purging more feasible.

Can we effectively purify and purge stem/progenitor cells?

High yields and high purities of stem/progenitor cells are obvious goals. A robust, fast, easy procedure would be a plus. Negative selection methods are widely available, and several means for CD34$^+$ cell selection are in clinical trials for feasibility. Each method offers potential and actual advantages and disadvantages. The research and clinical goals in a given patient population may determine the best method to use. Likely, combined positive/negative selection approaches will be used for maximal cell purification and purging. On the other hand, if sufficient enhancement of stem cell mobilization could be achieved, almost any available means of CD34$^+$ cell selection might be adequate.

Can we expand stem cells?

The currently known hematopoietic growth factors strongly favor proliferation with differentiation, as opposed to purely proliferative self-renewal of stem cells. Several groups have expanded the progenitor cell compartment ex vivo. Such preparations may further accelerate short-term blood count recovery. However, it certainly appears that we need novel growth factors and probably additional fundamental information on stem cell biology before we can achieve extensive self-renewal of normal lymphohematopoietic stem cells. This topic should provide several years of exciting translational laboratory and clinical research.

Of course, the above speculations provide many more questions than answers. We will have to read on in this manual and future volumes to pose the next questions and to find all the answers. Nevertheless, I look forward with confidence to the near future when endogenous stem and progenitor cells will no longer limit, but will instead enable our therapies.

Curt I. Civin

Role of Stem and Progenitor Cells in Reconstitution of Hematopoiesis

Stem Cells, Microenvironment and Grafting

Establishment of a Clinical Threshold Cell Dose: Correlation Between CFU-GM and Duration of Aplasia

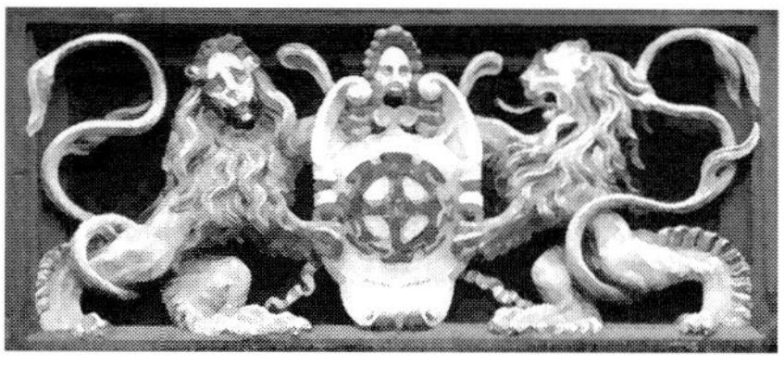

Stem Cells, Microenvironment and Grafting

P. Charbord
INSERM/C.R.T.S., Besançon, France

Key Words. Stem cells • Bone marrow transplantation • Marrow cultures • Stromal cells • Hemopoiesis

Hemopoietic stem cells (HSC) may be defined as cells with hemopoietic reconstitutive ability when administered to aplastic recipients (the aplastic pancytopenia resulting from disease or myeloablative therapy). HSC may be considered as a set of immature cells located after birth in bone marrow, whose different subsets are distinguished by their stage of maturity or their potential for reconstitution. The most immature subset is endowed with two essential properties; cells from this subset a) are multipotential, i.e., able to reconstitute the different lymphoid (T, B, NK) and myeloid (granulomonocytic, erythroblastic, megakaryocytic, eosinophilic and basophilic) lineages and b) are able to self-renew, i.e., generate daughter cells identical to mother ones. At the level of individual cells, self-renewal implies asymmetrical division; however, at the level of a population of cells, it implies that while n cells divide and differentiate (generating 2^n cells without self-renewal capacity), n distinct cells divide and self-renew (generating 2^n cells still able to self-renew).

There are different assays for HSC in mice and humans. These assays have made it possible to categorize stem cells according to discrete criteria. Presently, assays in mice are the most refined and have helped greatly to understand the murine stem cell hierarchy, which may serve as a model for human HSC.

Murine HSC

Murine HSC assays have made it possible to classify stem cells into three broad categories: spleen pre-colony forming units (pre-CFU-S), CFU-S and progenitors. Cells from these three classes show distinct properties.

Many assays define cells with properties of pre-CFU-S. *Ploemacher* and *Brons* [1] devised an assay modified from that of *Hodgson et al.* [2] to evaluate marrow cells able to generate CFU-S. Lethally irradiated primary recipients were grafted with marrow cells from syngeneic donors. Thirteen days later, the primary recipients were sacrificed, and femoral bone marrow cells were collected. Cells from the bone marrows were then injected into secondary recipients, and CFU-S were evaluated 12 days later by counting spleen nodules. CFU-S detected in the secondary recipients necessarily

Correspondence: Dr. P. Charbord, C.R.T.S., 1 Blvd. A. Fleming, Besançon 25000, France.

 ISBN 1-880854 17-1

derived from cells seeding into the femoral bone marrow of the primary recipients within the time frame of 13 days lapsing from injection to sacrifice. *Ploemacher* and *Brons* showed that marrow cells generating CFU-S in secondary recipients were distinguishable from CFU-S in primary recipients on the basis of cell size [1], binding to WGA [1] and staining by rhodamine 123 (Rh 123) [3]. Other assays define cells at a similar stage of maturity. *Harrison* [4] devised an assay where two types of histocompatible cells were competing to repopulate a lethally irradiated recipient. For example [5], one may inject cells from a female mouse with those of a male one. Female donors already underwent marrow transplantation; their cells therefore show restricted repopulating capacity. Male donors, on the contrary, had no history of previous transplantation; their cells, even if at a low level in the graft (most cells being provided by the "compromised" female donor), take over after several weeks and repopulate the host.

Pre-CFU-S are cells in G_0 and therefore resistant to S-specific drugs [6]. When assessed by flow cytometry or separated by elutriation, they appear to be lymphocyte-like [1, 7]. These cells have low mitochondrial activity [3]. The multidrug resistance (*mdr*) gene, coding for a membrane pump glycoprotein (P-gp) [8], is expressed at a high level. Since the P-gp pumps out the supravital dye Rh 123, these cells will be stained weakly by Rh 123 and are therefore designated as "Rh 123 dim" [3, 9]. Study of the pre-CFU-S membrane proteins or sugar moieties has made it possible to purify the subset. On the pre-CFU-S membrane there are a) high amounts of the stem cell antigen (Sca or Ly-6A/E antigen) [9], b) low amounts of the Thy-1 antigen [9], and c) moderate amounts of sugar moieties binding to the lectin wheat germ agglutinin (WGA) [1]. Pre-CFU-S may consequently be described as Ly-6A/E^+, Thy-1^{low} and WGA^+ cells.

Some in vitro assays may provide an estimate for pre-CFU-S: cells which form cobblestone areas 28 days after seeding onto an irradiated layer of long-term marrow culture [10], or cells which generate very large colonies in the presence of several cytokines, such as interleukin 1 (IL-1) + IL-3 + macrophage colony stimulating factor (M-CSF): high proliferative potential CFU (HPP-CFU) [11].

In 1961 *Till* and *McCulloch* devised the first assay demonstrating cells with stem cell properties [12]. Lethally irradiated mice are rescued by injection with marrow cells from syngeneic donors. Examination of spleens of grafted mice which are sacrificed 12 days after transplantation shows the presence of nodules. Each nodule is a clone (as shown by studies using chromosomal markers) [13]. Most of the nodules are mixed, comprising cells of the myeloid lineages, erythroblasts, granulocytes and megakaryocytes. When nodules are excised and cells of each are injected into secondary recipients, most of these, sacrificed

12 days later, show secondary splenic nodules [14]. CFU-S are multipotential (day 12 nodules are mixed) and able to self-renew (secondary nodules).

Most CFU-S are in G_0 [15, 16]. Most CFU-S appear as more granular [1] and larger cells [1, 7] than pre-CFU-S. They contain many mitochondria. The activity of the *mdr* gene is low; the uptake of Rh 123 is high [3, 9]. They are Ly-6A/E$^+$ and Thy-1^{low} [16]. They present high amounts of sugar moieties binding to WGA; they are WGA^{++} [1]. CFU-S are therefore distinct from pre-CFU-S by a number of properties: they are elutriated with cells larger than lymphocytes, they are Rh 123 bright instead of dim, and they are WGA^{++} instead of WGA$^+$.

Some in vitro assays may provide an estimation for CFU-S: cells which form cobblestone areas 10 days after seeding onto an adherent layer of long-term marrow culture [10], or cells which generate large colonies in the presence of a single cytokine (IL-1, IL-3 or M-CSF) [11].

The last class of the most mature stem cells in the mouse is that of cells giving rise to nodules in the spleen eight days after grafting. These day-8 CFU-S are largely unipotential; most nodules are made of erythroblasts only [17]. Progenitor cells (or CFU), as defined by in vitro assays [18-20], have properties similar to those of day-8 CFU-S. Cells in this category are in cycle [15]. They appear as blast-like cells [7]. They are Rh 123 bright [21, 22]. They are Ly-6A/E$^-$ [23] and Thy-1^{low} [23].

It must be emphasized that the classification of murine stem cells as described above, although providing a useful pattern to understand most of the properties of the cells with reconstitutive ability, must not be adopted without caveats. For example, it has been shown by *Spangrude et al.* that CFU-S belonged to the population of cells which are Ly-6A/E$^+$ and Thy-1^{low}, cells devoid of membrane antigens specific for different myeloid cells (Lin$^-$ cells) [16]. Fifty to one hundred cells with this phenotype were able to repopulate irradiated mice [16] but only 1 in 10 or 1 in 40 in the long-term [24].

However, recent studies have shown that this phenotype for CFU-S was found only for Thy-1.1 (and not Thy-1.2) mouse strains with the Ly-6b haplotype. In Thy 1.2 strains, CFU-S can also be found among the Thy-1 negative subset [25]; and for strains with the Ly-6a haplotype, Ly-6A/E antigens are not expressed to any great extent on HSC membrane [25].

Human HSC

In humans, HSC may be assessed by in vivo assays. One may use immunodeficient mice presenting with a severe combined immunodeficiency syndrome

(SCID). SCID mice may harbor human tissues such as thymic lobes or bone fragments. Such mice, called SCID-human (SCID-hu) by *McCune et al.* [26], are able to sustain human hematopoiesis for several months when human HSC are injected into the human implants. SCID mice may also be used without being submitted to any previous human tissue transplantation [27]. Human cell expansion from human HSC is then insured by systemic injection of human-specific growth factor (human Steel factor, granulocyte-macrophage CSF [GM-CSF] or IL-3 or the fusion GM-CSF/IL-3 molecule, pixy 123). One may also use sheep fetuses [28]. Human HSC are injected in utero into the fetus at a time when they are not yet immunocompetent, i.e., at approximately 60 days of gestation. These HSC will expand and their progeny will be detected before and after birth.

These in vivo assays for human HSC suffer from a major drawback: they are not quantitative. Quantitative assays are in vitro assays. Pre-CFU can be detected when marrow cells devoid of CFU are cultured on stroma [29] or in liquid medium containing cytokines [30]. Under these conditions, pre-CFU give rise to CFU within weeks following culture inception. It is possible to quantify the amount of pre-CFU seeded by culturing them at limiting dilution on irradiated stroma; by this method *Sutherland et al.* [31] described the "long-term culture initiating cells" (LTC-IC). Cultures of CFU-blasts (CFU-Bl) by *Leary* and *Ogawa* [32] are cultures of cells consisting of undifferentiated blasts with replating ability. Eventually, in humans as in mice, the different types of progenitor cells have been described [20]: multipotential progenitors, the CFU granulocyte/erythroid/macrophage/megakaryocyte (CFU-GEMM) containing granulocytes, erythroblasts, monocytes/macrophages and megakaryocytes, unipotential progenitors, the CFU-GM, burst forming units erythroid (BFU-E), CFU megakaryocyte (CFU-Meg) and CFU eosinophil (CFU-Eo).

Cells described as pre-CFU, LTC-IC or CFU-Bl have the following properties: They are in G_0 [33, 34]. They appear as lymphocyte-like cells [35]. They are Rh 123 dim [36]. Finally, they present on their membrane high amounts of CD34 antigens [35], moderate to barely detectable amounts of HLA-DR [30, 35, 36], lack of membrane antigens specific for different myeloid cells [29, 30, 36-38] and moderate amounts of the Thy-1 antigen [37]. They are described as $CD34^{++}$, HLA-$DR^{\pm}$, Lin^{-} and Thy-1^{+} cells.

Progenitors have the following properties: They are in cycle. They appear as blast-like cells [33]. They are Rh 123 dim [8]. On their membrane are also found moderate amounts of CD34 antigens [35], moderate to high amounts of HLA-DR [35], the CD38 activation antigen [38] and antigens specific for the myeloid lineages [35, 36]. They are therefore described as $CD34^{+}$, HLA-DR^{+}, $CD38^{+}$ and Lin^{+} cells.

Progenitor cells are therefore distinct from more immature cells by a number of features, and it now appears possible to establish a human stem cell hierarchy somewhat similar to that described for mice. One may oppose the set of pre-CFU (or LTC-IC or CFU-Bl) presenting with some of the characters of the pre-CFU-S to the set of progenitors very similar to the day-8 CFU-S or murine progenitors.

HSC Frequency

Whatever the species, one may expect a low frequency for the most immature cells, as opposed to a higher frequency for more mature cells. In mice the frequency of pre-CFU-S may be deduced from studies of animals grafted with cells with long-term (several months) repopulating ability. The frequency of these cells is within the range 0.2-10 per 10^5 marrow cells [39-43]. The frequency of CFU-S is higher, 50-300 per 10^5 cells [39], and the cloning efficiency of progenitors is within the range 50-500 [20]. In Thy-1.1 mouse strain with Ly-6b haplotype, the frequency of Sca^+, Thy^{low}, Lin^- cells is 20-50 per 10^5 marrow cells [16]. In humans, the frequency of LTC-IC [31] or CFU-Bl [33] is approximately 1 per 10^5 cells; the cloning efficiency for CFU-GEMM is 5-20 and that of committed progenitors is within the range 50-300 [20]. $CD34^+$ cells comprise approximately 1% of the marrow cells (1) [44]. $CD34^+$, 38^- cell frequency is approximately 0.1% [38] and that of $CD34^+$, 38^-, $HLA\text{-}DR^-$ cells is approximately 0.01% [45]. (1)

Strategy for Transplantation

Until recently, transplantation of HSC in humans implied the graft of unseparated marrow cells from histocompatible donors (allografts) or collected from the host himself at a previous time (autografts). Progress made by analyzing the stem cell compartment makes it now possible to devise the transplantation of HSC of different sources (peripheral blood [46] or cord blood [47]) and more or less purified according to different criteria such as the presence of CD34 antigens [48]. There are two major points of debate concerning a) the quality of the stem cells that should engraft the host, and b) the required quantity of stem cells with a distinct phenotype that may be considered as "safe" for the recipient. To answer both questions, lessons from experiments in mice are informative.

From the very description of the stem cell hierarchy one may predict that different types of stem cells should be engrafted. It has been shown indeed that pre-CFU-S were responsible for late phase (several weeks to months) and durable grafting, while progenitors were responsible for early, but transitory engraftment [49, 7]. Cells with long-term repopulating ability are fragile cells; previous transplantations impair the cell number and the repopulating ability of each cell [50]; repeated serial transplantations render the cells inefficient [49]. Culture before transplantation usually decreases the cell

(1) Since the frequency of LTC-IC (closest thing so far to the HSC) in humans is 10^{-5} (0.001%), only ~10% of $CD34^+$, $CD38^-$ HLA DR⁻ cells would be LTC-IC.

number, although single clones may proliferate and repopulate distinct hosts [51]. Cells with short-term populating ability are resistant cells. They are maintained even in the case of repeated and serial transplantations [49]. Culture (in the presence of cytokines) before transplantation may increase the cell number, which may be beneficial for graft-take [52].

Many experiments show that engraftment in mice comprises two different phases [40, 41, 53]. Early grafting is insured by 20-200 clones whose life-span is usually short (months), although they may not die after this period of time but merely be "extinct," i.e., able to reactivate when a second transplantation is performed [54]. On the contrary, late engraftment is insured by a small number of clones (<10) with long life span (>1.5 years) [55, 56].

Other significant data provided by mouse studies concern the role of the cell dose. It has been shown that repopulating cells do not behave in the same way when many or few cells are injected [40]. When few cells are injected (10^5 nucleated cells per mouse) repopulating cells behave like immature stem cells, i.e., a small number of clones develop at different locations in bone, thymus and spleen. When many cells are injected (10^7 nucleated cells per mouse) repopulating cells behave more like mature stem cells; many independent clones develop at different locations in bone, and usually different clones are found in thymus and spleen. Repopulation results from the proliferation of these different clones.

These studies in mice provide a word of caution for studies in humans. Cells with a very well defined phenotype may not insure engraftment at different time points. It has indeed been shown that $CD34^+$ cells (comprising pre-CFU as well as all kinds of progenitors) were able to engraft hosts with a pattern of peripheral cell recovery similar to that of conventional autografts [48]. On the contrary, it has been observed that, in patients engrafted with $CD33^-$ marrow cells (devoid of CFU-GM), the pattern of neutrophil recovery was slower than in conventional autografts [57]. When cell numbers are considered, it appears cautious to assume that the more HSC injected, the better the recovery should be. It has in fact been calculated that one year after conventional allografts in humans (when large numbers of cells were injected) the number of repopulating clones was approximately 100 [58]. Some oligoclonal reconstitution has been observed when less than 10 clones were actively contributing to hemopoiesis [59]. These observations are rare and may be related to small numbers of HSC injected. However, they suggest that few clones with repopulating activity may be functional in humans as well as in mice, which validates gene transfer for therapy using these cells.

The Role of the Marrow Microenvironment

Once transfused, HSC arrive via circulating blood into bone marrow sinuses. They have then to bind to homing receptors on the endothelial cell membrane

[60], pass through the endothelial wall and seed into hemopoietic logettes. In these logettes HSC are in the vicinity of fixed cells from the marrow microenvironment. Studies in vivo by *Wolf* and *Trentin* [17] have suggested that microenvironmental (m.e.) cells play a role in HSC differentiation and proliferation. *Dexter et al.* in 1976 [61] have described a culture system where microenvironmental adherent cells were crucial for HSC maintenance (survival) and function (proliferation and differentiation). The culture system was adapted to human marrow in 1980 [62]. It has not only shown that m.e. cells were essential for HSC maintenance but has also been instrumental in defining HSC hierarchy. Pre-CFU-S and CFU-S numbers are correlated to those of cells forming cobblestone areas 28 and 10 days, respectively, after seeding onto an irradiated adherent layer [10]. Pre-CFU in humans have been defined by their property to generate CFU when plated onto adherent layers [29], and LTC-IC have been quantitated using this culture system [31].

One may infer from these studies that successful engraftment will depend not only on the quality and quantity of HSC (which has been until recently the major concern) but also on the quality of the microenvironment. Were HSC unable to home (due to endothelial cell damage) or to seed (due to damage of fixed cells within the logettes), the engraftment would be endangered.

Using long-term marrow cultures it has been possible to define the phenotype of m.e. cells and to evaluate their regulatory role on HSC. Microenvironmental cells comprise three cell types: a) macrophages similar to tissue macrophages [63], b) stromal cells which are mesenchymal cells that differentiate following different pathways, the major one being that of immature vascular smooth muscle cells [64, 65] and c) endothelial-like cells [65, 66]. These different cell types control HSC function by producing cytokines and expressing adhesion molecules. Cytokines may be growth factors [63] or inhibitors which are secreted or remain bound to the m.e. cell membrane (or its extracellular matrix). Adhesion molecules may either exist as membrane molecules or be secreted and incorporated into the extracellular matrix (the most conspicuous example being that of fibronectin [67]). Cytokine and adhesion molecules interact, making possible a tight paracrine control of HSC function at very close range by m.e. cells.

This recently acquired knowledge on m.e. cells makes it now conceivable to transplant autologous stromal cells along with HSC. Stromal cell transplantation would allow the regeneration of the marrow microenvironment (whose function may be altered by radio- or chemotherapy). It would also provide membrane-bound cytokines and essential adhesion molecules and likely target these functional molecules at critical sites for HSC. This issue remains speculative but appears to be feasible [68] and may be of considerable interest.

It is not excluded that stromal cells are indeed transplanted with HSC, since a common ancestor to both stromal and hemopoietic lineages may exist. This issue was first raised by *Singer et al.* [69], studying stromal cells in selected cases of myeloproliferative disorders. It has been substantiated by data on SV40 transformed stromal cell clones which are able to differentiate into stromal cells and HSC [70]. Eventually, it was shown by *Huang* and *Terstappen* that $CD34^{+}$, $CD38^{-}$ and HLA-DR^{-} cells were able to differentiate into hemopoietic cells or stromal cells depending on the culture conditions [45].

Whether a common ancestor to stromal and hemopoietic cells exists seems presently doubtless. However, the major question is whether this cell is reconstitutive after a usual transplantation procedure. The answer is likely to be negative since stromal cells (as grown in long-term cultures from marrow recipients) are in most cases not provided by donor cells. *Keating et al.* [71] reported in 1982 that stromal cells were transplantable. Numerous subsequent studies in humans [72-74] and in mice [75] have disavowed this initial report. It appears therefore reasonable to suggest that stromal cell transplantation will require either enrichment of selected cell subsets or culture of stromal cell lineages before grafting.

In conclusion, it must be emphasized that, although it is now possible to engraft selected cell subsets, which may be beneficial in many cases (for example by downgrading graft-versus-host (GvH) disease in allografts or by discarding tumor cells in autografts), new protocols should be devised cautiously since our knowledge of the hemopoietic system and its microenvironment has disclosed its extreme complexity due to the variety of reconstituting cells and the interrelationships between the different cell types.

References

1 Ploemacher RE, Brons NHC. Isolation of hemopoietic stem cell subsets from murine bone marrow: II. Evidence for an early precursor of day-12 CFU-S and cells associated with radioprotective ability. Exp Hematol 1988;16:27-32.

2 Hodgson GS, Bradley TR, Radley JM. The organization of hemopoietic tissues as inferred from the effects of 5-fluorouracil. Exp Hematol 1982;10:26-35.

3 Ploemacher RE, Brons NHC. Separation of CFU-S from primitive cells responsible for reconstitution of the bone marrow hemopoietic stem cell compartment following irradiation: evidence for a pre-CFU-S cell. Exp Hematol 1989;17:263-266.

4 Harrison DE. Competitive repopulation: a new assay for long-term functional capacity. Blood 1980;55:77-81.

5 Szilvassy SJ, Lansdorp PM, Humphries RK, Eaves AC, Eaves CJ. Isolation in a single step of a highly enriched murine hematopoietic stem cell population with competitive long-term repopulating ability. Blood 1989;74:930-939.

6 Hodgson GS, Bradley JR. Properties of haematopoietic stem cells surviving 5-fluorouracil treatment: evidence for a pre-CFU-S. Nature 1979;281:381-382.

7 Jones RJ, Wagner JE, Celano P, Zicha MS, Sharkis SJ. Separation of pluripotent haematopoietic stem cells from spleen colony-forming cells. Nature 1990;347:188-189.

8 Chaudhary PM, Roninson IG. Expression and activity of p-glycoprotein, a multidrug efflux pump, in human hematopoietic stem cells. Cell 1991;66:85-94.

9 Spangrude GJ, Johnson GR. Resting and activated subsets of mouse multipotent hematopoietic stem cells. Proc Natl Acad Sci USA 1990;87:7433-7437.

10 Ploemacher RE, van der Sluijs JP, van Beurden CAJ, Baert MJM, Cham PL. Use of limiting-dilution type long-term marrow cultures in frequency analysis of marrow-repopulating and spleen colony-forming hematopoietic stem cells in the mouse. Blood 1991;78:2527-2533.

11 Bertoncello I, Bradley TR, Hodgson GS, Dunlop JM. The resolution, enrichment, and organization of normal bone marrow high proliferative potential colony-forming cell subsets on the basis of rhodamine-123 fluorescence. Exp Hematol 1991;19:174-178.

12 Till JE, McCulloch EA. A direct measurement of the radiation sensitivity of normal mouse bone marrow cells. Rad Res 1961;14:213-222.

13 Becker AJ, McCulloch EA, Till JE. Cytological demonstration of the clonal nature of spleen colonies derived from transplanted mouse marrow cells. Nature 1963;197:452-454.

14 Till JE, McCulloch EA, Siminovitch L. A stochastic model of stem cell proliferation, based on the growth of spleen colony-forming cells. Proc Natl Acad Sci USA 1963:29-36.

15 Lajtha LG, Pozzi LV, Schofield R, Fox M. Kinetic properties of haematopoietic stem cells. Cell Tissue Kinet 1969;2:39-49.

16 Spangrude GJ, Heimfeld S, Weissman IL. Purification and characterization of mouse hematopoietic stem cells. Science 1988;241:58-62.

17 Trentin JJ. Hematopoietic microenvironments. Historical perspective, status and projections. In: Tavassoli M, ed. Handbook of the Hematopoietic Microenvironment. Clifton, NJ: Humana Press, 1989:1-87.

18 Pluznik DH, Sachs L. The cloning of normal mast cells in agar gel. J Cell Comp Physiol 1966;66:319-324.

19 Metcalf D. Potentiation of bone marrow colony growth in vitro by the addition of lymphoid or bone marrow cells. J Cell Physiol 1968;72:9-20.

20 Metcalf D. The Hematopoietic Colony-Stimulating Factors. Amsterdam: Elsevier 1984.

21 van der Sluijs JP, de Jong JP, Brons NHC, Ploemacher RE. Marrow repopulating cells, but not CFU-S establish long-term in vitro hemopoiesis on a marrow-derived stromal layer. Exp Hematol 1990;18:893-896.

22 Phillips RL, Reinhart AJ, Van Zant G. Genetic control of murine hematopoietic stem cell pool sizes and cycling kinetics. Proc Natl Acad Sci USA 1992;89:11607-11611.

23 Heimfeld S, Hudak S, Weissman I, Rennick D. The in vitro response of phenotypically defined mouse stem cells and myeloerythroid progenitors to single or multiple growth factors. Proc Natl Acad Sci USA 1991;88:9902-9906.

24 Smith LG, Weissman IL, Heimfeld S. Clonal analysis of hematopoietic stem-cell differentiation in vitro. Proc Natl Acad Sci USA 1991;88:2788-2792.

25 Spangrude GJ, Brooks DM. Phenotypic analysis of mouse hematopoietic stem cells shows a Thy-1-negative subset. Blood 1991;80:1957-1964.

26 McCune JM, Namikawa R, Kaneshima H, Shultz LD, Lieberman M, Weissman IL. The SCID-hu mouse: murine model for the analysis of human hematolymphoid differentiation and function. Science 1988;241:1632-1635.

27 Lapidot T, Pflumio F, Doedens M, Murdoch B, Williams DE, Dick JE. Cytokine stimulation of multilineage hematopoiesis for immature human cells engrafted in SCID mice. Science 1992;255:1137-1141.

28 Zanjani ED, Ascensao JL, Tavassoli M. Liver-derived fetal hematopoietic stem cells selectively and preferentially home to the fetal bone marrow. Blood 1993;81:399-404.

29 Andrews RG, Singer JW, Berstein ID. Precursors of colony-forming cells in humans can be distinguished from colony-forming cells by expression of the CD33 and CD34 antigens and light scatter properties. J Exp Med 1989;169:1721-1731.

30 Brandt J, Srour EF, van Besien K, Briddell RA, Hoffman R. Cytokine-dependent long-term culture of highly enriched precursors of hematopoietic progenitor cells from human bone marrow. J Clin Invest 1990;86:932-941.

31 Sutherland HJ, Lansdorp PM, Henkelman DH, Eaves AC, Eaves CJ. Functional characterization of individual human hematopoietic stem cells cultured at limiting dilution on supportive marrow stromal layers. Proc Natl Acad Sci USA 1990;87:3584-3588.

32 Leary AG, Ogawa M. Blast cell colony assay for umbilical cord blood and adult marrow progenitors. Blood 1967;69:953.

33 Brandt J, Baird N, Lu L, Srour E, Hoffman R. Characterization of a human hematopoietic progenitor cell capable of forming blast cell containing colonies in vitro. J Clin Invest 1988;82:1017-1027.

34 Siena S, Castro-Malaspina H, Gulati SC, Lu L, Colvin MO, Clarkson BD, O'Reilly RJ, Moore MAS. Effects of in vitro purging with 4-hydroperoxycyclophosphamide on the hematopoietic and microenvironmental elements of human bone marrow. Blood 1985;65:655-662.

35 Sutherland HJ, Eaves CJ, Eaves AC, Dragowska W, Lansdorp PM. Characterization and partial purification of human marrow cells capable of initiating long-term hematopoiesis in vitro. Blood 1989;74:1563-1570.

36 Srour EF, Leemhuis T, Brandt JE, van Besien K, Hoffman R. Simultaneous use of rhodamine 123, phycoerythrin, Texas red, and allophycocyanin for the isolation of human hematopoietic progenitor cells. Cytometry 1991;12:179-183.

37 Baum CM, Weissman IL, Tsukamoto AS, Buckle AM, Peault B. Isolation of a candidate human hematopoietic stem-cell population. Proc Natl Acad Sci USA 1992;89:2804-2808.

38 Terstappen L, Huang S, Safford M, Lansdorp PM, Locken MR. Sequential generation of hematopoietic colonies derived from single non lineage-committed $CD34^{+}$ $CD38^{-}$ progenitor cells. Blood 1991;77:1218-1227.

39 Boggs DR, Boggs SS, Saxe DF, Gress LA, Canfield DR. Hematopoietic stem cells with high proliferative potential. J Clin Invest 1982;70:242-253.

40 Micklem HS, Lennon JE, Ansell JD, Gray RA. Numbers and dispersion of repopulating hematopoietic cell clones in radiation chimeras as functions of injected cell dose. Exp Hematol 1987;15:251-257.

41 Harrison DE, Astle CM, Lerner C. Number and continuous proliferative pattern of transplanted primitive immunohematopoietic stem cells. Proc Natl Acad Sci USA 1988;85:822-826.

42 Harrison DE, Astle CM, Stone M. Numbers and functions of transplantable primitive immunohematopoietic stem cells. J Immunol 1989;142:3833-3840.

43 Szilvassy SJ, Humphries RK, Lansdorp PM, Eaves AC, Eaves CJ. Quantitative assay for totipotent reconstituting hematopoietic stem cells by a competitive repopulation strategy. Proc Natl Acad Sci USA 1990;87:8736-8740.

44 Strauss LC, Rowley SD, La Russa VF, Sharkis SJ, Stuart RK, Civin CI. Antigenic analysis of hematopoiesis. V. Characterization of My-10 antigen expression by normal lymphohematopoietic progenitor cells. Exp Hematol 1986;14:876-886.

45 Huang S, Terstappen L. Formation of haematopoietic microenvironment and haematopoietic stem cells from single human bone marrow stem cells. Nature 1992;360:745-749.

46 Juttner CA, To LB, Haylock DN, Branford A, Kimber RJ. Circulating autologous stem cells collected in very early remission from acute non-lymphoblastic leukaemia produce prompt but incomplete haematopoietic reconstitution after high dose melphalan or supralethal chemoradiotherapy. Br J Haematol 1985;61:739-745.

47 Broxmeyer HE, Douglas GW, Hangoc G, Cooper S, Bard J, English D, Arny M, Thomas L, Boyse EA. Human umbilical cord blood as a potential source of transplantable hematopoietic stem/progenitor cells. Proc Natl Acad Sci USA 1989;86:3828-3832.

48 Berenson RJ, Bensinger WI, Hill RS, Andrews RG, Garcia-Lopez J, Kalamasz DF, Still BJ, Spitzer G, Buckner CD, Bernstein ID, Thomas ED. Engraftment after infusion of $CD34^+$ marrow cells in patients with breast cancer or neuroblastoma. Blood 1991;77:1717-1722.

49 Jones RJ, Celano P, Sharkis SJ, Sensenbrenner LL. Two phases of engraftment established by serial bone marrow transplantation in mice. Blood 1989;73:397-401.

50 Harrison DE, Stone M, Astle CM. Effects of transplantation on the primitive immunohematopoietic stem cell. J Exp Med 1990;172:431-437.

51 Fraser CC, Szilvassy SJ, Eaves CJ, Humphries RK. Proliferation of totipotent hematopoietic stem cells in vitro with retention of long-term competitive in vivo reconstituting ability. Proc Natl Acad Sci USA 1992;89:1968-1972.

52 Muench MO, Moore MAS. Accelerated recovery of peripheral blood cell counts in mice transplanted with in vitro cytokine-expanded hematopoietic progenitors. Exp Hematol 1992;20:611-618.

53 Jordan CT, Lemischka IR. Clonal and systemic analysis of long-term hematopoiesis in the mouse. Genes Dev 1990;4:220-232.

54 Lemischka IR, Raulet DH, Mulligan RC. Developmental potential and dynamic behavior of hematopoietic stem cells. Cell 1986;45:917-921.

55 Keller G, Snodgrass R. Life span of multipotential hematopoietic stem cells in vivo. J Exp Med 1990;171:1407-1418.

56 Capel B, Hawley RG, Mintz B. Long- and short-lived murine hematopoietic stem cell clones individually identified with retroviral integration markers. Blood 1990;75:2267-2270.

57 Robertson MJ, Soiffer RJ, Freedman AS, Rabinowe SL, Anderson KC, Ervin TJ, Murray C, Dear K, Griffin JD, Nadler LM, Ritz J. Human bone marrow depleted of CD33-positive cells mediates delayed but durable reconstitution of hematopoiesis: clinical trial of MY9 mononuclear antibody-purged autografts for the treatment of acute myeloid leukemia. Blood 1992;79:2229-2236.

58 Nash R, Storb R, Neiman P. Polyclonal reconstitution of human marrow after allogeneic bone marrow transplantation. Blood 1988;72:2031-2037.

59 Turhan AG, Humphries RK, Philipps GL, Eaves AC, Eaves CJ. Clonal hematopoiesis demonstrated by X-linked DNA polymorphisms after allogeneic bone marrow transplantation. N Eng J Med 1989;320:1655-1661.

60 Tavassoli M, Hardy CL. Molecular basis of homing of intravenously transplanted stem cells to the marrow. Blood 1990;76:1059-1070.

61 Dexter TM, Allen TD, Lajtha LG. Conditions controlling the proliferation of haematopoietic stem cells in vitro. J Cell Physiol 1976;91:335-344.

62 Gartner S, Kaplan HS. Long-term culture of human bone marrow cells. Proc Natl Acad Sci USA 1980;77:4756-4759.

63 Charbord P, Tamayo E, Saeland S, Duvert V, Poulet J, Gown AM, Hervé P. Granulocyte-macrophage colony-stimulating factor (GM-CSF) in human long-term bone marrow cultures: endogenous production in the adherent layer and effect of exogenous GM-CSF on granulomonopoiesis. Blood 1991;78:1230-1236.

64 Galmiche MC, Koteliansky VE, Brière J, Hervé P, Charbord P. Stromal cells from human long-term marrow cultures are mesenchymal cells that differentiate following a vascular smooth muscle differentiation pathway. Blood 1993;82:66-76.

65 Penn PE, Jiang DZ, Fei RG, Sitnicka E, Wolf NS. Dissecting the hematopoietic microenvironment. IX. Further characterization of murine bone marrow stromal cells. Blood 1993;81:1205-1213.

66 Hasthorpe S, Bogdanovski M, Rogerson J, Radley JM. Characterization of endothelial cells in murine long-term marrow culture. Implication of hematopoietic regulations. Exp Hematol 1992;20:476-481.

67 Lerat H, Lissitski JC, Singer JW, Keating A, Hervé P, Charbord P. The role of stromal cells and macrophages in fibronectin biosynthesis and matrix assembly in human long-term marrow cultures. Blood 1993 (in press).

68 Lazarus HL, Haynesworth SE, Gerson SL, Caplan AL. Marrow-derived stromal progenitors (mesenchymal stem cells): a phase I clinical trial (Abot). Blood 1992;80(suppl 1):236a.

69 Singer JW, Keating A, Cuttner J, Gown AM, Jacobson R, Killen PD, Moohr JW, Najfeld V, Powell J, Sander J, Striker GE, Fialkow PJ. Evidence for a stem cell common to hematopoiesis and its in vitro microenvironment: studies of patients with clonal hematopoietic neoplasia. Leuk Res 1984;8:535-545.

70 Singer JW, Charbord P, Keating A, Nemunaitis J, Raugi G, Wight TN, Lopez AJ, Roth GJ, Dow LW, Fialkow PJ. Simian virus 40-transformed adherent cells from human long-term marrow cultures: cloned cell lines produce cells with stromal and hematopoietic characteristics. Blood 1987;70:1464-1474.

71 Keating A, Singer JW, Killen PD, Striker GE, Salo AC, Sanders J, Thomas ED, Thorning D, Fialkow PJ. Donor origin of the in vitro haematopoietic microenvironment after marrow transplantation in man. Nature 1982;298:280-283.

72 Simmons PJ, Przepiorka D, Thomas ED, Torok-Storb B. Host origin of marrow stromal cells following allogeneic bone marrow transplantation. Nature 1987;328:429-432.

73 Laver J, Jhanwar SC, O'Reilly RJ, Castro-Malaspina H. Host origin of the human hematopoietic microenvironment following allogeneic bone marrow transplantation. Blood 1987;70:1966-1968.

74 Agematsu K, Nakahori Y. Recipient origin of bone marrow-derived fibroblastic stromal cells during all periods following bone marrow transplantation in humans. Br J Haematol 1991;79:359-365.

75 Perkins S, Fleischman RA. Hematopoietic microenvironment. Origin, lineage, and transplantability of the stromal cells in long-term bone marrow cultures from chimeric mice. J Clin Invest 1988;81:620-625.

Establishment of a Clinical Threshold Cell Dose: Correlation Between CFU-GM and Duration of Aplasia

L. B. To, M. M. Roberts, C. M. Rawling, P. A. Rowlings, P. G. Dyson, T. P. Rawling, D. N. Haylock, C. A. Juttner

Hanson Centre for Cancer Research, Institute of Medical and Veterinary Science, Adelaide, South Australia

Key Words. Progenitor cell dose • Hemopoietic reconstitution • Autologous transplantation • Progenitor cell assay

Introduction

Correlation between Progenitor Cell Dose and Hemopoietic Reconstitution

Mounting evidences suggest that the number of hemopoietic progenitors infused in stem cell transplantation correlates with the rate of hemopoietic reconstitution. This was first suggested by *Spitzer et al.* [1] in a study of autologous bone marrow transplantation. *Rowley et al.* [2] reported a significant correlation in 4-hydroperoxycyclophosphamide purged autologous bone marrow transplantation. *Reiffers et al.* [3] reported a similar correlation in mobilized autologous peripheral blood transplantation. In the same report it was suggested that only patients receiving ≥15 × 10^4 colony forming units-granulocyte-macrophage (CFU-GM)/kg body weight (BW) experienced rapid reconstitution. This concept of a threshold CFU-GM dose for achieving rapid hemopoietic reconstitution echoed an earlier report [4] although a threshold of 50 × 10^4 CFU-GM/kg BW was suggested then. *Spitzer et al.* [1] also recommended giving 1 × 10^4 CFU-GM/kg BW in autologous bone marrow transplantation for sustained hemopoietic reconstitution. More recent reports show quite convincingly that mobilized autologous peripheral blood transplantation with CFU-GM doses higher than those in bone marrow transplantation lead to more rapid reconstitution, or conversely, shorter aplasia [5-7]. Furthermore, rapid hemopoietic reconstitution has contributed to the increasing safety, widening indications and lower resource utilization of high dose therapy.

There has not always been general agreement that such a correlation exists. It seems logical that infusing cells containing large numbers of CFU-GM which are capable of producing neutrophils and monocytes within two weeks in vitro would lead to generation of circulating cells in vivo in a similar time. However the number of nucleated cells given seems just as predictive in allogeneic bone marrow transplantation, autologous bone marrow and steady phase peripheral blood transplantation [5]. On the other hand *Jones et al.*

Correspondence: Dr. L. B. To, Director, Leukaemia Research Unit, Hanson Centre for Cancer Research, Institute of Medical & Veterinary Science, Frome Road, Adelaide, South Australia, 5000.

 ISBN 1-880854 17-1

demonstrated quite clearly in a murine model that hemopoietic reconstitution post transplant is polyphasic [8], and that the number of mature progenitors given predicts the rate of reconstitution [9]. Recent reports of enhanced hemopoietic reconstitution using cells that have been incubated with hemopoietic growth factors ex vivo provide further supportive evidence that the more mature progenitors and post-progenitors are the cells that mediate the early phases of reconstitution [10, 11].

Factors Affecting the Cell Dose: Reconstitution Correlation

One major reason for the conflicting views on the CFU-GM:reconstitution correlation is the inter- and intra-laboratory variability in the CFU-GM assay. Beyond personality and allegiance to established practices, the CFU-GM assay is a complex biological assay with a large number of components for which no standard or commonly agreed guidelines exist. Such factors include:

1 The growth supporting abilities of different batches of fetal calf serum may vary many folds, so the choice of a particular batch requires testing many batches and standardizing against the current batch. Serum free or serum deprived media would be an improvement but a generally accepted medium is not yet available.

2 The types of colony stimulating activity used vary from mixed native cytokines such as human placental conditioned medium (HPCM) and phytohaemagglutinin stimulated leukocyte conditioned medium (PHA-LCM) to recombinant hemopoietic cytokines such as granulocyte-macrophage colony stimulating factor (GM-CSF), granulocyte (G)-CSF, interleukin-3 (IL-3), IL-1, IL-6 and stem cell factor (SCF) used singly or in different combinations and at different concentrations. It is generally believed that single recombinant cytokines stimulate fewer colonies than optimally prepared mixed cytokines while multiple cytokine combinations, especially those incorporating SCF, probably stimulate more colonies although direct comparative data are not yet available.

   The biological significance of the higher number of colonies seen with multiple cytokine combinations remains unanswered. Whether the increase in colony number is due to a stronger proliferative stimulus so that even the more mature cluster forming cells are now capable of forming colonies or whether it is due to recruitment of more primitive cells that are normally not responsive to native mixed cytokines, or both, needs to be clarified. Hence the numbers of clonogenic progenitors measured using different sources of colony stimulating factors are not necessarily comparable to one another.

3 The effect of accessory cells such as T lymphocytes and monocytes on the in vitro proliferation of CFU-GM is complex because both stimulatory and inhibitory effects have been demonstrated [12]. Furthermore, mononuclear cells harvested during hemopoietic recovery secrete more cytokines than those harvested during steady phase hemopoiesis [13]. In a peripheral blood (PB) CFU-GM culture the number of T lymphocytes and monocytes may be 10 times or more than that in a bone marrow (BM) CFU-GM culture and this may explain that PB CFU-GM assay culturing PB mononuclear cells does not have a linear colony growth pattern at plating concentrations above 1 to 3 × 10^5 cells/ml. A number of laboratories would culture cells at several plating concentrations in the range of 0.1 to 1 × 10^5/ml to ensure that the optimal plating concentration range is covered.

4 The growth conditions such as the gaseous environment, scoring criteria and the consistency between different scorers as to what constitute a colony all contribute to variability.

5 The lack of a standard reagent to calibrate the culture remains a major hurdle. The use of cryopreserved cells is no substitute because the freeze/thaw process adds additional variables.

A number of measures may circumvent some of these problems. The major laboratories usually have a stringent in-house quality-control program including batch-testing various culture components and regular testing of specimens from normal subjects to ensure a stable culture system, frequent review of culture results and an established staff training program with validation of scoring. For smaller laboratories, the amount of work to carry out such a program is somewhat prohibitive and it may be more cost-effective to use pre-tested reagents from a major laboratory. Another measure which has considerable merit is for every laboratory to establish a reference range based on normal subjects. If all authors cite the reference range from their laboratory, it would be easier to assess how comparable the various assays are.

Culture issues aside, high dose therapy and stem cell rescue is a complex setting in which multiple events often take place concurrently. Accessory cells such as T cells and monocytes are known to secrete both stimulatory and inhibitory cytokines; stem cell and stromal damage by previous chemoradiotherapy, age and disease type all may influence hemopoietic reconstitution. In allogeneic transplants the effects of graft versus host disease and the associated therapy may further influence the rate of reconstitution. In a single institution study of 65 patients, even though the CFU-GM dose was identified to be the only significant variable influencing the rate of neutrophil and platelet reconstitution by multiple regression, it accounted for only 20 to 60% of the variance [5]. Hence a large number of patients is required for this type of analysis even when the laboratory issues are properly controlled.

$CD34^+$ Cell Measurement

Siena et al. were the first group to describe CD34 measurement by flow cytometry as a measurement of hemopoietic stem/progenitor cells in mobilized peripheral blood [14]. CD34 measurement has the obvious advantages of same day results instead of a 14 day wait and of requiring fewer reagents that require standardization. Numerous groups have now confirmed *Siena's* report that there is a significant correlation between the number of $CD34^+$ cells and CFU-GM in a specimen. However the measurement of rare events by flow cytometry also requires a vigorous and stringent protocol.

Progenitor Cell Dose Threshold for Rapid and Sustained Hemopoietic Reconstitution

Using the 50×10^4 CFU-GM/kg BW as a threshold dose and a significant correlation between the numbers of $CD34^+$ cells and CFU-GM, *Siena et al.* projected that 7.8×10^6 $CD34^+$ cells/kg BW would lead to rapid hemopoietic reconstitution [15]. *Berenson et al.* recommended 1×10^6 $CD34^+$ cells/kg BW when using bone marrow [16]. Based on a review of published data

Bender et al. [17] proposed that stem cell rescue with more than 20-50 × 10^4 CFU-GM/kg BW or 2 × 10^6 $CD34^+$ cells/kg BW is likely to lead to rapid reconstitution and that a lower progenitor cell dose such as 5-20 × 10^4 CFU-GM/kg BW or 0.5-2 × 10^6 $CD34^+$ cells/kg BW may still give rise to durable though not rapid reconstitution. The authors have analyzed the hemopoietic reconstitution data on a total of 106 transplants (62 chemotherapy mobilized PB-stem cells (PBSC), 21 allogeneic BM-transplants (BMT) and 13 autologous BMT, and including the 65 patients previously reported in [5]). We found that in 34 patients receiving <20 × 10^4 CFU-GM/kg BW, only 2 patients (6%) recovered 0.5 × 10^9 neutrophils/l by day 13 and only 1 patient (3%) recovered 50 × 10^9 by day 15. In contrast 65% and 54% of patients receiving ≥20 × 10^4 CFU-GM/kg BW achieved those respective milestones (Fisher's

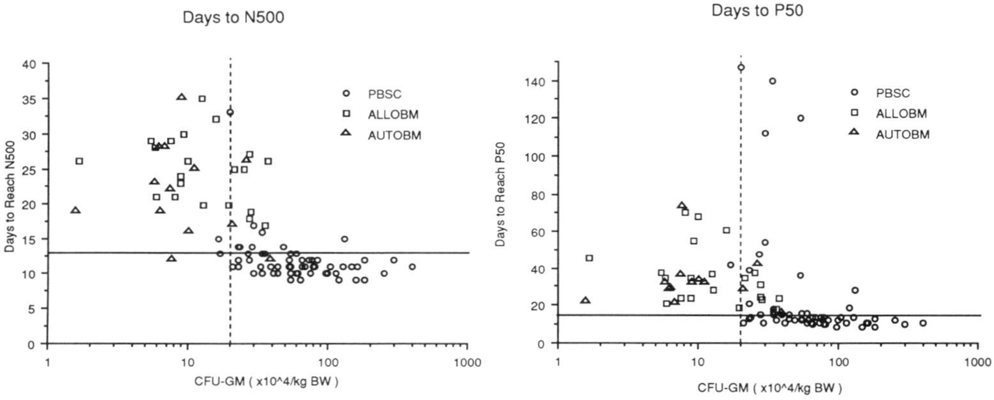

Fig. 1. The above diagrams show the CFU-GM threshold effect in achieving rapid neutrophil and platelet reconstitution. As referred to in the text, a CFU-GM threshold of 20 × 10^4/kg BW was chosen based on the number of days to reach 0.5 × 10^9 neutrophils/l (N500) and the number of days to reach 50 × 10^9 platelets/l (P50). The diagrams also show the threshold of the rate of hemopoietic reconstitution in spite of increasing CFU-GM doses infused. PBSC = mobilized peripheral blood transplantation; ALLOBM = allogeneic bone marrow transplantation; AUTOBM = autologous bone marrow transplantation.

exact test $p < 0.0001$ for both). These findings support the concept of a threshold for rapid reconstitution (Fig. 1).

The importance for each laboratory to establish its own threshold was emphasized by *Bender et al.* (pp. 31-43). This is particularly relevant because many different mobilization protocols are now used and there are as yet no published data showing whether the quality and the spectrum of hemopoietic cells mobilized by different methods are equivalent. It is also worth noting that CFU-GM is probably less accurate an indicator of long term marrow repopulating capacity than of rapid hemopoietic reconstitution because it is only a surrogate measure of the former. Other biological assays such as the long-term culture initiating cell assay or the pre-progenitor assay or flow cytometric measurements of primitive subsets of $CD34^+$ cells may be more appropriate.

Obligatory Delay Threshold for Hemopoietic Stem Cell Transplantation

There is another form of threshold in hemopoietic stem cell transplantation besides the progenitor cell dose threshold for rapid and sustained reconstitution. In spite of infusing very high numbers of progenitors, there remains an obligatory period of cytopenia. Even in patients who received mobilized PBSC as well as G-CSF post-transplant, the median time to neutrophil engraftment (0.5×10^9/l) is still nine days and platelet engraftment (50×10^9/l) is 15 days [17]. This is little better than that seen in mobilized PBSC alone, 11 and 14 days respectively [18]. Hence there seems to be a threshold of rapid hemopoietic reconstitution which cannot be lowered further by giving more progenitors and cytokines. This is probably due to the time required for the infused progenitors to mature to functional end-cells [19].

Conclusion

Notwithstanding that CFU-GM assay only measures a relatively mature hemopoietic progenitor and that there are probably numerous factors influencing hemopoietic reconstitution, there are three types of threshold in hemopoietic stem cell transplantation. Firstly, there is a progenitor cell dose threshold for rapid reconstitution. Secondly, there seems to be a dose threshold for sustained reconstitution. Thirdly, there is a threshold of rapid reconstitution which cannot be lowered even with very high progenitor cell dose and cytokine administration. The clinical implications are that transplant centers should focus on stem cell harvesting protocols that give high progenitor cell yields and that we have to look to additional maneuvers such as ex vivo processing of harvested cells to further shorten the duration of cytopenia.

Acknowledgments

Secretarial assistance was provided by *Mandy Huxtable*. This research was partly supported by grants from the National Health and Medical Research Council and the Anti-Cancer Foundation of the Universities of South Australia.

References

1 Spitzer G, Verma DS, Fisher R, Zander A, Vellekoop L, Litam J, McCredie KB, Dicke KA. The myeloid progenitor cell—its value in predicting hematopoietic recovery after autologous bone marrow transplantation. Blood 1980;55:317-323.

2 Rowley SD, Piantadosi S, Santos GW. Comparison of hematologic recovery with CFU-GM content of autologous bone marrow grafts treated with 4-hydroperoxycyclophosphamide. Culture after cryopreservation. Bone Marrow Transplant 1989;4:553-558.

3 Reiffers J, Leverger G, Marit G, Castaigne S, Tilly H, Lepage E, Hénon P, Douay L, Troussard X. Hematopoietic reconstitution after autologous blood stem cell transplantation. In: Gale RP, Champlin RE, eds. Bone Marrow Transplant: Current Controversies. Proceedings of Sandoz-UCLA symposium, New York: Alan R Liss, 1988:313.

4 To LB, Dyson PG, Juttner CA. Cell dose effect in circulating stem cell autografting. Lancet 1986;ii:404.

5 To LB, Roberts M, Haylock DN, Dyson PG, Branford AL, Thorp D, Ho JQK, Dart GW, Horvath N, Davy MLJ, Olweny CLM, Abdi E, Juttner CA. Comparison of hematological recovery times and supportive care requirements of autologous recovery phase peripheral blood stem cell transplants, autologous bone marrow transplants and allogeneic bone marrow transplants. Bone Marrow Transplant 1992;9:277-284.

6 Sheridan WP, Begley CG, Juttner CA, Szer J, To LB, Maher D, McGrath KM, Morstyn G, Fox RM. Effect of peripheral-blood progenitor cells mobilized by filgrastim (G-CSF) on platelet recovery after high-dose chemotherapy. Lancet 1992;339:640-644.

7 Elias AD, Ayash L, Anderson KC, Hunt M, Wheeler C, Schwartz G, Tepler I, Mazanet R, Lynch C, Pap S, Pelaez J, Reich E, Critchlow J, Demetri G, Bibbo J, Schnipper L, Griffin JD, Frei III E, Antman KG. Mobilization of peripheral blood progenitor cells by chemotherapy and granulocyte-macrophage colony-stimulating factor for hematologic support after high-dose intensification for breast cancer. Blood 1992;79:3036-3044.

8 Jones RJ, Celano P, Sharkis SJ, Sensenbrenner LL. Two phases of engraftment established by serial bone marrow transplantation in mice. Blood 1989;73:397-401.

9 Jones RJ, Sharkis SJ, Celano P, Colvin OM, Rowley SD, Sensenbrenner LL. Progenitor cell assays predict hematopoietic reconstruction after syngeneic transplantation in mice. Blood 1987;70:1186-1192.

10 Muench MO, Moore MA. Accelerated recovery of peripheral blood cell counts in mice transplanted with in vitro cytokine-expanded hematopoietic progenitors. Exp Hematol 1992;20:611-618.

11 Naparestek E, Hardan Y, Ben-Shahar M, Nagler A, Or R, Mumcuoglu M, Weiss L, Samuel S, Slavin S. Enhanced marrow recovery by short preincubation of marrow allografts with human recombinant interleukin-3 and granulocyte-macrophage colony-stimulating factor. Blood 1992;80:1673-1678.

12 To LB, Haylock DN, Juttner CA, Kimber RJ. The effect of monocytes on the peripheral blood CFU-c assay system. Blood 1983;62:112-117.

13 Takamatsu Y, Akashi K, Harada M, Teshima T, Inaba S, Shimoda K, Eto T, Shibuya T, Okamura S, Niho Y. Cytokine production by peripheral blood monocytes and T cells during hemopoietic recovery after intensive chemotherapy. Br J Haem 1993;83:21-27.

14 Siena S, Bregni M, Brando M, Ravagnani F, Bonadonna G, Gianni AM. Circulation of $CD34^+$ hematopoietic stem cells in the peripheral blood of high-dose cyclophosphamide-treated patients: enhancement by intravenous recombinant human granulocyte macrophage colony-stimulating factor. Blood 1989;74:1905-1914.

15 Siena S, Bregni M, Brando B, Belli N, Ravagnani F, Gandola L, Stern AC, Lansdorp PM, Bonadonna G, Gianni AM. Flow cytometry for clinical estimation of circulating hematopoietic progenitors for autologous transplantation in cancer patients. Blood 1991;77:400-409.

16 Berenson RJ, Bensinger WI, Hill RS, Andrews RG, Garcia-Lopez J, Kalamasz DF, Still BJ, Spitzer G, Buckner CD, Bernstein ID, Thomas ED. Engraftment after infusion of $CD34^+$ marrow cells in patients with breast cancer or neuroblastoma. Blood 1991;77:1717-1722.

17 Bender JG, To LB, Williams S, Schwartzberg LS. Defining a therapeutic dose of peripheral blood stem cells. J Hematotherapy 1992;1:329-342.

18 Grigg A, Begley CG, Juttner CA, Szer J, To LB, Maher D, McGrath KM, Morstyn G, Fox RM, Sheridan WP. Effect of peripheral blood progenitor cells mobilized by filgrastim (G-CSF) on platelet recovery after high-dose chemotherapy. Bone Marrow Transplant 1993;11(Suppl 2):23-29.

19 Haylock DN, To LB, Dowse TL, Juttner CA, Simmons PJ. Ex vivo expansion and maturation of peripheral blood $CD34^+$ cells into the myeloid lineage. Blood 1992;89:1405-1412.

Cytofluorimetric Determination of CD34$^+$ Cells

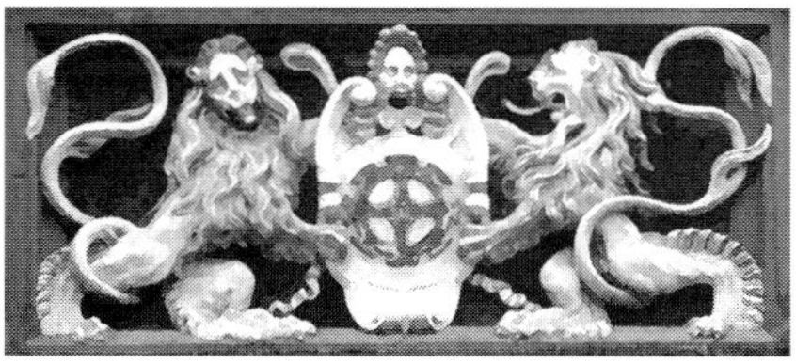

Milan Protocol for Clinical CD34⁺ Cell Estimation in Peripheral Blood for Autografting in Patients with Cancer

Salvatore Siena,[a] *Marco Bregni,*[a] *Massimo Di Nicola,*[a] *Fedro Peccatori,*[a] *Michele Magni,*[a] *Bruno Brando,*[b] *Ferdinando Ravagnani,*[a] *A. Massimo Gianni*[a,c]

[a]The Cristina Gandini Transplantation Unit, Division of Medical Oncology, Istituto Nazionale Tumori, Milan, Italy; [b]Renal Transplantation Unit, Ospedale Niguarda, Cà Granda, Milan, Italy; [c]Institute of Medical Sciences, Università degli Studi, Milan, Italy

Key Words. $CD34^+$ cell • Flow cytometry • Hematopoietic stem cell • Hematopoietic progenitor cell • Clinical estimation of $CD34^+$ cells

Introduction

Reasons for Developing a Flow Cytometry Assay for $CD34^+$ Cell Estimation

Cancer patients treated with intensive chemotherapy may or may not experience an expansion of the circulating hematopoietic progenitor cell (CPC) compartment of sufficient magnitude to justify large-scale collection of these cells for subsequent autologous transplantation after further myeloablative cancer therapy. In past years, the lack of a clinical assay for real-time determination of the number of CPCs has exposed patients with scarce or without overshoot of CPCs to insufficient or useless leukapheresis procedures [1].

To overcome this problem, based on our initial observation that CPCs, similarly to their marrow counterpart, express the CD34 differentiation antigen ($CD34^+$ cells) [2], we have developed a direct immunofluorescence flow cytometry assay to estimate $CD34^+$ cells in the peripheral blood of cancer patients recovering from intensive chemotherapy-induced pancytopenia [3]. This flow cytometry assay, replacing advantageously the colony forming unit granulocyte macrophage (CFU-GM) colony assay, has allowed us to define criteria to decide on a real-time basis and in a clinical setting: a) *which* patients experience an overshoot of CPCs of relevant magnitude for considering large-scale collection of these cells by leukapheresis(es); b) *when* leukapheresis(es) should be performed; and c) *how* many consecutive leukapheresis procedures are necessary to harvest quantities of CPCs sufficient for successful transplantation [3].

In comparison with the traditional CFU-GM colony assay, the estimation of CPCs for autologous transplantation as $CD34^+$ cells with *direct fluorescence by flow cytometry offers three relevant advantages:* a) same-day results for quick clinical decision-making; b) high intralaboratory and interlaboratory reproducibility; and c) permanent documentation of $CD34^+$ cell subpopulations.

Correspondence: Dr. Salvatore Siena, Istituto Nazionale Tumori, Via Venezian 1, 20133 Milan, Italy.

 ISBN 1-880854 17-1

Necessity of Direct Immunofluorescence to Detect Peripheral Blood CD34+ Cells for Clinical Decision-Making

Direct immunofluorescence with the fluorescein isothiocyanate (FITC)-conjugated 8G12 antibody [4], also commercially referred to as anti-HPCA-2 (Becton Dickinson, San Jose, CA), detected CD34+ CPCs with the same bright fluorescence of indirect fluorescence with anti-HPCA-1 antibody (Becton Dickinson) plus $F(ab')_2$ Ig second antibody [3, 5]. In comparison with the indirect technique that has been used in earlier studies [2], direct immunofluorescence provides the following advantages: a) considerably lower autofluorescence of the negative cell fraction; b) the need for one instead of two reagents, one of which is not monoclonal and thus variable with each preparation; and c) simpler, faster and more accurate sample processing that allows estimation of CD34+ cells without bias due to cell fractionation procedures.

Therefore, for clinical assessment of CD34+ CPCs *direct, and not indirect, immunofluorescence flow cytometry analysis should be used.*

Choice of Appropriate Fluorochrome-Conjugated CD34 Antibody to Detect Circulating CD34+ Cells for Clinical Decision-Making

Direct CD34 immunofluorescence was permitted by the development (*Dr. Peter Lansdorp,* Vancouver, BC) of the 8G12 monoclonal antibody also commercially referred to as anti-HPCA-2 (Becton Dickinson) that, unlike previously described CD34 antibodies, can be directly labeled with fluorochromes without loss of high-affinity binding properties [4].

The commercial availability of another FITC-conjugated CD34 monoclonal antibody referred to as FITC-QBEND10 prompted us to compare the latter reagent with FITC-anti-HPCA-2. Comparative experiments showed that FITC-QBEND10 detects CD34+ cells with a resolution index considerably lower than that of FITC-anti-HPCA-2 antibody [5]. Consequently, some experiments also indicated that the use of FITC-QBEND10 instead of FITC-anti-HPCA-2 exposes clinicians to the risk of either overestimating (false positive) or underestimating (false negative) these cells in peripheral blood [5]. The recent availability of phycoerythrin (PE)-conjugated anti-HPCA-2 monoclonal antibody has further increased the resolution between cytometrically CD34+ and CD34− cells with an even higher sensitivity and specificity of this assay.

Therefore, for clinical assessment of CD34+ CPCs, *direct immunofluorescence should be carried out with fluorochrome-conjugated anti-HPCA-2 CD34 monoclonal antibody.*

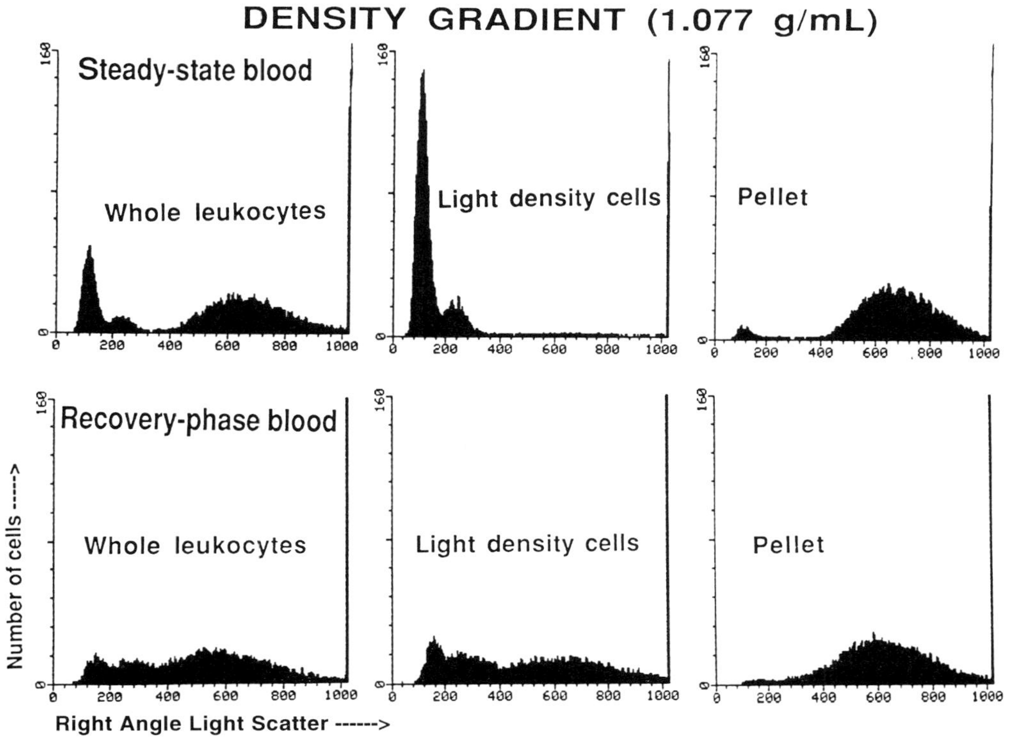

Fig. 1. Flow-cytometry scattergram analysis after centrifugation over density-gradient (1.077 g/ml) of two samples of peripheral blood obtained before chemotherapy in steady-state (upper panel) and during recovery-phase after high-dose chemotherapy and cytokine(s) (lower panel). Number of cells is on vertical axis; right angle light scatter is on horizontal axis. Steady-state leukocytes fractionated by centrifugation over 1.077 g/ml density gradient, are divided in two clear-cut populations: low-density cells comprising mononuclear cells and high-density cells comprising polymorphonuclear cells (upper panel). Fractionation of *recovery-phase leukocytes* by centrifugation over 1.077 g/ml density gradient does not allow a clear-cut separation between mononuclear and polymorphonuclear cells (lower panel).

Why Recovery-Phase Blood Leukocytes for CD34⁺ Cell Analysis Should Not Be Fractionated on a Density-Gradient

During hematopoietic recovery after myelotoxic cancer chemotherapy, peripheral blood leukocytes differ substantially from those in the steady-state (before chemotherapy).

In particular, it is well established that *steady-state leukocytes* can be fractionated by centrifugation over a 1.077 g/ml density gradient (Lymphoprep, Immuno, Italy) into low-density and high-density cells corresponding to mononuclear and polymorphonuclear cells, respectively (Fig. 1, upper panels).

Table I. Materials utilized at Istituto Nazionale Tumori, Milan, Italy, for peripheral blood $CD34^+$ cell estimation

Monoclonal Antibodies
- Anti-HPCA-2 (CD34), purchased from Becton Dickinson (FITC-conjugated, catalog 348053);
- Anti-Leu-M9 (CD33), purchased from Becton Dickinson (PE-conjugated, catalog 347787);
- Anti-Leu-5b (CD2), purchased from Becton Dickinson (PE-conjugated, catalog 347593), control reagent;
- Anti-Leu-12 (CD19), purchased from Becton Dickinson (PE-conjugated, catalog 349209), control reagent;

Red Blood Cell Lysis Buffer[a]
- Ammonium chloride (NH_4Cl), purchased from Sigma, Italy (catalog A4514);
- Ethylenediaminotetracetic (EDTA) tetrasodium salt ($C_{10}H_{12}N_2O_8Na_4$), purchased from Sigma, Italy (catalog ED4SS);
- Potassium bicarbonate ($KHCO_3$), purchased from Sigma, Italy (catalog P4913);
- Double distilled water;

Cell Washing Medium[b]
- Phosphate buffered saline (PBS) without Ca^{++}, Mg^{++} purchased from Seromed (catalog L1825);
- Sodium azide 20% purchased from Sigma (catalog S2002);

Miscellaneous
- FACScan Cell Analyzer, purchased from Becton Dickinson;
- Falcon tubes, purchased from Becton Dickinson (catalog 352052)

[a]Preparation of 100 ml of red blood cell lysis buffer: NH_4Cl 829 mg, EDTA 3.7 mg, $KHCO_3$ 100 mg, distilled water 100 ml. The solution pH should be adjusted with addition of NaOH 1N or HCl 1N. This solution expires after seven days.
[b]Preparation of 100 ml of cell washing medium: sodium azide 20% 1 ml (final concentration 0.2% v/c), PBS (without Ca^{++}, Mg^{++}) 100 ml.

In contrast, fractionation of *recovery-phase leukocytes* by centrifugation over a 1.077 g/ml density gradient does not allow a clear-cut separation between mononuclear and polymorphonuclear cells. Recovery-phase low-density cells fractionated with the same method comprise mononuclear as well as polymorphonuclear cells (Fig. 1, lower panels). Consequent to these findings, fractionation of recovery-phase leukocytes over a 1.077 g/ml density gradient not only fails to get rid of polymorphonuclear cells, but also it represents a remarkable bias for the interpretation of data concerning $CD34^+$ cell estimation.

Fractionation of recovery-phase leukocytes over a 1.077 density gradient and also visual, instead of flow cytometry, analysis are most likely the reason why some authors have not found a correlation between determinations of CPCs as $CD34^+$ cells and CFU-GM [6].

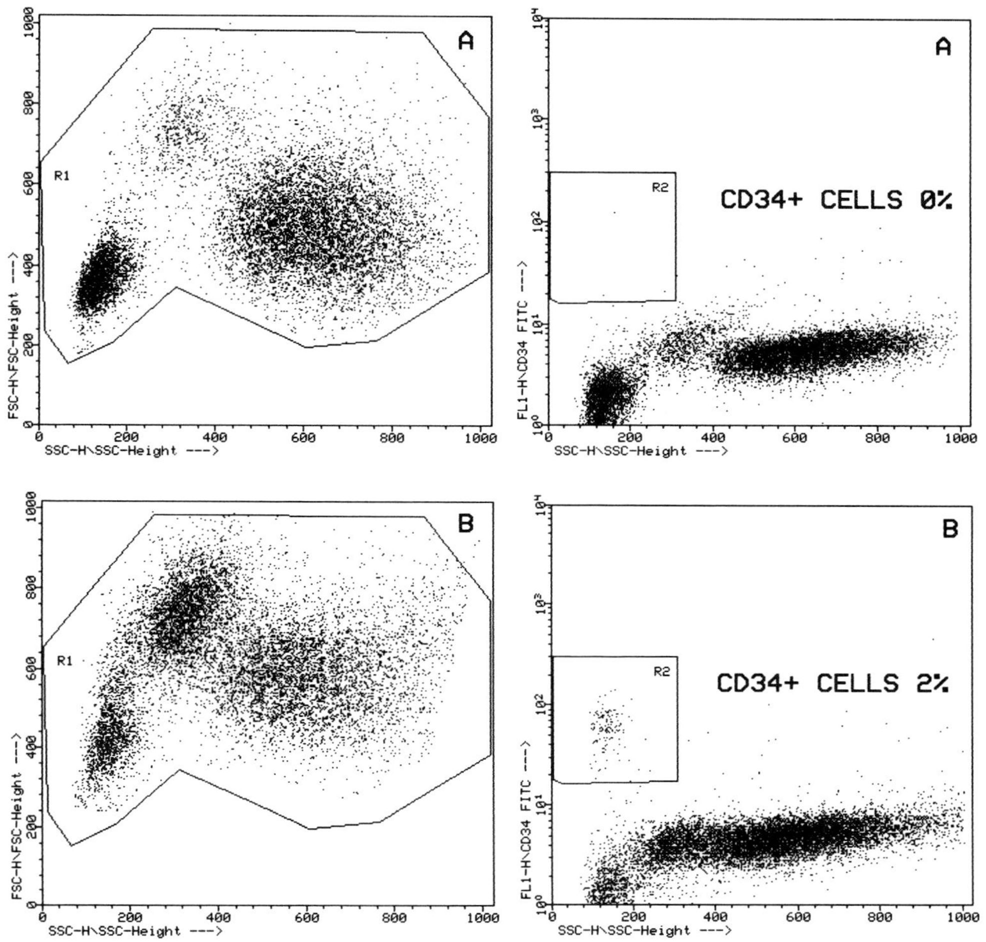

Fig. 2. Flow cytometry scattergrams of two samples of peripheral blood in the steady state (upper panels A) and during recovery-phase after high-dose chemotherapy and cytokine(s) (lower panels B). In the left panels, cells are acquired with dot plot, forward scatter (vertical axis) versus side (90°) light scatter (horizontal axis), by gating whole viable cells. In the right panels, green fluorescence (FITC-conjugated CD34) is on vertical axis while right angle side scatter is on horizontal axis.

Therefore, for the purpose of CPCs estimation, density-gradient fractionated recovery-phase leukocytes are not strictly representative of the whole leukocyte populations and should not be utilized for $CD34^+$ cell estimation for clinical decision-making. The only limitation of the whole blood assay may reside in the very low total WBC number usually found in the early recovery phase. This can be overcome by increasing the blood aliquot to be stained (i.e., 100 μl instead of 50 μl). *The whole recovery-phase leukocytes should be analyzed by flow cytometry after simple red blood cell lysis without any cell fractionation procedure, as described below.*

Materials and Methodology

The Milan Protocol for Peripheral Blood CD34+ Cell Estimation

Materials and equipment utilized at Istituto Nazionale Tumori, Milan, Italy, for peripheral blood CD34+ cell estimation are listed in Table I.

We suggest assaying at least three aliquots of the same sample: one unlabeled, one labeled with FITC-conjugated (green) CD34 antibody plus PE-conjugated (red) CD33 antibody for direct immunofluorescence analysis of CD34/CD33 surface antigens, and a third sample for control analysis of CD2/CD19 surface antigens (T and B cell markers, respectively).

1 Place three 50 μl aliquots of whole blood (in the case of leukocytes <150/μl, the quantity of blood and antibodies must be doubled) or leukapheresis cell suspension in Falcon tubes, i.e., one tube for unlabeled control, one for CD34/CD33, and one for CD2/CD19 analysis.

2 Add 15 μl of each commercial antibody to respective samples.

3 Incubate at 4°C for 25 min, in the dark.

4 At the end of incubation, add 2 ml of red blood cell lysis buffer medium to each tube and incubate at room temperature for 15 min, in the dark.

5 At the end of red blood cell lysis, add 1 ml of cell washing medium to each tube and centrifuge at 1,200 revolutions per minute (rpm) (300 *g*) for 7 min. Visual evaluation of the bottom of the tubes will show a white cell pellet (effective red blood cell lysis). If this is not the case, repeat the lysis procedure once. If after the latter the cell pellet shows gross presence of red blood cells (ineffective red blood cell lysis), change the lysis buffer medium.

6 By manual dumping (rapid placement of each tube upside-down) remove supernatant and add 2 ml of cell washing medium to each tube and centrifuge at 1,200 rpm for 7 min. Do not resuspend cells until flow cytometry analysis. Samples can be stored for up to 1 h at 4°C, in the dark.

7 Employing a FACScan (Becton Dickinson) cell analyzer, acquire cells with dot plot, forward scatter (vertical axis) versus side (90°) light scatter (horizontal axis) and run set up mode the unlabeled sample by gating whole viable cells, as shown in Figure 2.

8 Set up autofluorescent cells at a 10^1 level as shown in Figure 2. This procedure run with set-up mode the unlabeled sample by gating only viable cells and setting up autofluorescent cells at a 10^1 level as shown in Figure 2. This procedure eliminates from computer analysis cellular debris and nonspecific background fluorescence.

9 Analyze by dual color fluorescence by setting horizontal axis as green fluorescence (FITC-conjugated CD34 or control CD2) and vertical axis as red fluorescence (PE-conjugated CD33 or control CD19), with the appropriate fluorescence compensation.

10 Run with set up mode the double-conjugated (green/red) sample. Adjust the fluorescence level for each fluorochrome and compensate, i.e., eliminate the superimposed signals (see your FACscan manual for further details). Acquire ≥10,000 cells.

11 After having acquired and stored data on computer memory, analyze with dot plot or contour diagrams. Set up horizontal axis as side (90°) light scatter and vertical axis as fluorescence (red or green). CD34 analysis is *evaluable* (Fig. 2, right lower panel B) when the fluorescent upper dot cluster is well defined and separated from the negative autofluorescent cells. CD34 analysis is *not evaluable* (Fig. 2, right upper panel A) when the dot cluster is not well defined. Since CD34$^+$ cells usually display a sharp cluster of bright elements, along with a variable amount of dimly stained cells, the acceptance of the final number of CD34$^+$ cells must include criteria to manage CD34$^+$ dim cells. We usually exclude from analysis CD34$^+$ dim cells, gating only bright cells, as already described [3, 5].

12 To visualize the concomitant double fluorescence, analyze by contour plot diagrams. Set vertical axis as green fluorescence (FITC-conjugated CD34 or control FITC-conjugated CD2) and horizontal axis as red fluorescence (PE-conjugated CD33 or control PE-conjugated CD19). Analyze percentages of single or double labeled cells, i.e., CD34$^+$/CD33$^-$, CD34$^+$/CD33$^+$, CD34$^-$/CD33$^+$, CD19$^+$/CD2$^-$, and CD19$^-$/CD2$^+$ subpopulations.

The counts of circulating CD34$^+$/CD33$^-$, CD34$^+$/CD33$^+$, and CD34$^-$/CD33$^+$, CD19$^+$/CD2$^-$, and CD19$^-$/CD2$^+$ cells can be determined by multiplying their frequency (number of positive cells/number of analyzed leukocytes) for the leukocytes count in the same blood or leukapheresis sample. Results are expressed as CD34$^+$ cells per μl.

Concluding Remarks

The estimation of CPCs by flow cytometry has most probably resolved some of the current difficulties involved with collection and transplantation of CPCs. First, the ability to detect a meaningful expansion of the CPC population on the day of occurrence rather than two weeks later by colony assays offers a distinct advantage, because not only can the successful expansion attempt be identified, thus avoiding undesirable collections, but also the most effective time to initiate the leukapheresis procedure becomes obvious as well. Second, the Milan method of detecting CPCs as CD34$^+$ cells appears to be more reproducible than traditional CFU-GM progenitor culture assays. Third, the definition of an adequate collection of expanded CPCs is likely to become clear if, as we have proposed [3], collection of a specific number of circulating CD34$^+$ cells (8×10^6/kg patient body weight) indicates a very safe and most likely effective transplant product has been procured.

Acknowledgments

We are grateful to *Dr. Laura Zorzino* for constructive collaboration and to *Nadia Belli* and *Francesco Vitello* for skillful technical assistance in CD34$^+$ cell analyses. This article was partly supported by Italian National Research Council Grant 92-02329-PF39 to A.M.G.

References

1 Gianni AM, Siena S, Bregni M, Tarella C, Stern AC, Pileri A, Bonadonna G. Granulocyte-macrophage colony stimulating factor to harvest circulating haemopoietic stem cells for autotransplantation. Lancet 1989;2:580-585.

2 Siena S, Bregni M, Brando B, Ravagnani F, Bonadonna G, Gianni AM. Circulation of $CD34^+$ hematopoietic stem cells in the peripheral blood of high-dose cyclophosphamide treated patients: enhancement by intravenous recombinant human granulocyte-macrophage colony-stimulating factor. Blood 1989;74:1905-1914.

3 Siena S, Bregni M, Brando B, Belli N, Ravagnani F, Gandola L, Stern AC, Lansdorp PM, Bonadonna G, Gianni AM. Flow cytometry for clinical estimation of circulating hematopoietic progenitors for autologous transplantation in cancer patients. Blood 1991;77:400-409.

4 Lansdorp PM, Sutherland HJ, Eaves CJ. Selective expression of CD45 isoforms on functional subpopulations of $CD34^+$ hemopoietic cells from human bone marrow. J Exp Med 1990;172:363-366.

5 Siena S, Bregni M, Brando B, Belli N, Lansdorp PM, Bonadonna G, Gianni AM. Flow cytometry to estimate circulating hematopoietic progenitors for autologous transplantation: comparative analysis of different CD34 monoclonal antibodies. Haematologica 1991;76:330-333.

6 Siena S, Bregni M, Gianni AM. Estimation of peripheral blood $CD34^+$ cells for autologous transplantation in cancer patients. Exp Hematol 1993;21:203-205.

Guidelines for Determination of CD34+ Cells by Flow Cytometry: Application to the Harvesting and Transplantation of Peripheral Blood Stem Cells

James G. Bender, Kristen Unverzagt, Donald Walker
Immunotherapy Division, Biotech Group, Baxter Healthcare Corporation, Round Lake, Illinois, USA

Key Words. CD34 • Flow cytometry • Bone marrow transplantation • Leukapheresis • Progenitor cells • Mononuclear cells

Introduction

Autologous mobilized peripheral blood stem cells (PBSC) have now been used extensively for augmenting hematopoietic reconstitution after high dose chemoradiotherapy for neoplasias [1-4]. This process involves the harvesting of peripheral blood mononuclear cells (MNC) during a period when the numbers of stem cells are increased in the blood, the cryopreservation of these products and their subsequent thawing and reinfusion after myeloablative chemotherapy. The harvesting of MNC from patients receiving growth factors and/or recovering from chemotherapy presents a special challenge as a patient may have very low or very high leukocyte counts that are predominantly granulocytes. MNC are harvested by leukapheresis using continuous flow separators (e.g., Fenwal CS3000 or COBE spectra) or batch processing (e.g., Haemonetics) [5]. Generally 10 liters of blood, or about two blood volumes, are passed through the separator at a rate of 40-80 ml per minute resulting in the capture of about 1-3 $\times$ 10^{10} mononuclear cells [6, 7]. The anticoagulant acid citrate dextrose-A (ACD-A) is used to prevent clotting of the blood and is introduced into the blood as it enters the separator. Quality control of this process is important in validating the performance of the instrument and in defining the quality of the product. Flow cytometry offers a simple and robust method for monitoring this process.

Although a variety of methods have been used to increase the levels of progenitors in the blood, the mechanism(s) of PBSC mobilization is still unknown and information on the phenotypic and biological characterization of mobilized PBSC are still limited. Transplants using enriched populations of CD34+ cells have demonstrated that only a minor population of the cells reinfused are responsible for reconstitution [8, 9]. Hence a major clinical issue is to quantitate that minor population of MNC which is responsible for rapid and sustained hematopoietic reconstitution. Thus far the best documented surrogate measurement of the reconstituting population has been the number of colony

Correspondence: Dr. James G. Bender, Immunotherapy Division, Biotech Group, Baxter Healthcare Corporation, WG2-2S Baxter Technology Park, Round Lake, IL 60073, USA.

©AlphaMed Press ISBN 1-880854 17-1

forming units-granulocyte-macrophage (CFU-GM) infused which shows a correlation to the rate of hematopoietic reconstitution, degree of supportive care and duration of hospitalization [10-12]. However, considerable inter-laboratory variation in the CFU-GM assay exists and problems of turnaround time will remain insurmountable since this assay requires approximately two weeks. CD34 measurements may provide a faster and more reproducible indicator of the hematopoietic reconstitutive capacity than CFU-GM. Currently, however, there is not a standardized method for quantitating this population. We present here our method for performing this measurement and discuss some of the related issues.

Materials and Methods

Sample Preparation

The measurement of $CD34^+$ cells in clinical samples adheres to the principle of "garbage in, garbage out". The quality of the sample, the type of sample and the age will contribute to the accuracy and sensitivity of the measurement. As a sample gets older, separation becomes more difficult, granulocytes lose viability, debris accumulates, and antibodies tend to bind non-specifically. It is therefore optimum to stain and analyze a fresh sample within 24 hours or less. If circumstances do not allow for this, there are several alternatives. The sample can be stained, fixed and then stored for up to a week before analyzing. Alternatively, samples can be frozen, and thawed up to years later, before staining and analyzing.

One major issue is fractionation of the starting sample. Historically blood and marrow samples have been fractionated using Ficoll/hypaque to separate MNC from red cells and granulocytes. With normal peripheral blood this is an efficient way of obtaining a clean preparation of MNC. With patient samples, however, this separation may be unpredictable and compromise the quantitation of the CD34 population. The best strategy is to minimize, as much as possible, the manipulation of the sample. At present, the use of ammonium chloride to lyse the red cells provides the most reproducible manipulation that allows for efficient measurement of the leukocyte population. In the future, fractionation of the sample may be eliminated by using flow cytometry methodology to exclude red cells electronically [13].

Sample Preparation—Ammonium Chloride Lysis

Antibodies are added to the bottom of 12 × 75 polypropylene tubes and kept on ice. These tubes can be prepared in advance. The sample of peripheral blood (~ one ml) or leukapheresis product is diluted 10:1 with heparinized phosphate buffered saline (PBS) in a 15 ml conical polypropylene centrifuge tube, and centrifuged at room temperature for three minutes at 1500 rpm

(400*g*). This step removes contaminating platelets and plasma. The supernatant is discarded leaving a red pellet which includes all red and white cells. This pellet is vortexed and 50-100μl is added into each tube containing the antibodies. Samples which contain very low leukocyte number or when very low levels of CD34$^+$ cells are being estimated may require that several sample tubes are prepared to insure adequate cells for analysis. These tubes are vortexed and put on ice for 10-30 minutes. To each tube is added 3.5 ml NH_4Cl lysing solution (8.26 grams in one liter water) and the tubes are capped. The tubes are inverted 10 times to mix well and centrifuged at room temperature for three minutes at 1500 rpm. The caps are removed, and the supernate poured off and residual liquid is blotted on paper towels three times, (three times is very important). The pellets are vortexed and washed by adding two ml PAB (PBS containing bovine serum albumin (BSA) and azide), vortexing and then centrifuging in a Serofuge® for two minutes at high speed. Decant and repeat wash procedure. Resuspend final pellet in PAB and the samples may be run immediately. If samples cannot be run within 2-3 hours, add one ml of 1% paraformaldehyde rather than one ml PAB. The fixed samples can then be kept refrigerated and run within one week.

Sample Preparation—Using Thawed Samples

In studying many aspects of PBSC transplantation it is desirable to evaluate thawed cell preparations from cryopreserved pheresis product samples. The samples can be batched and the processing, staining and analysis scheduled. This approach also offers the opportunity to do retrospective studies as new antibodies and techniques become available. There are often difficulties encountered in processing and analyzing cell preparations after they are thawed. The quality of thawed cell preparations is often related to the manner in which they have been cryopreserved. The quality of the mononuclear cell harvest and the level of granulocyte contamination during the apheresis is also a consideration. Samples frozen using a controlled rate freezer and stored in the liquid phase of liquid nitrogen have shown the best viability [14]. Manipulation of the thawed cells can result in clumping and loss of viability and should be kept to a minimum to achieve the best results. After rapidly thawing the samples in a 37°C water bath, there appears to be no advantage to a prolonged dilution of the cryopreservation media at room temperature beyond 10 minutes [15, 16]. It may also be useful to include anticoagulant and DNAase in the dilution medium to prevent clumping. The cells can be put on ice, washed in staining buffer, stained with monoclonal antibodies, and analyzed. Again, the least amount of manipulation gives the best results so using directly tagged monoclonals will give the best staining patterns with second antibody reagents binding more non-specifically to thawed cells than fresh cells. It is also important to evaluate viability with propidium iodide to exclude dead cells. When performing calculations on thawed samples the loss of granulocytes during the preparation must be taken into account when correlating with measurements made on fresh samples. The denominator used for calculations with thawed samples should be MNC rather than total leukocytes.

Recipes:

NH_4Cl Lysing Solution

1 To one liter of sterile distilled water, add the following:

8.26 grams NH_4Cl (Mallinckrodt, Paris, KY)

1.0 grams potassium bicarbonate (Mallinckrodt)

.0037 grams tetra sodium ethylenediaminetetraacetate (EDTA) (Sigma, St. Louis, MO).

2 Mix all until dissolved. Store at room temperature. Expires in one month.

Heparinized PBS

Add heparin (Elkins-Sinn, Inc., Cherry Hill, NJ) to achieve a final concentration of 10 Units/ml. It comes at 1,000 Units/ml, sodium injection for i.v. or s.c. use. PBS can be obtained from many sources. For example, a 500 ml bottle of PBS would require five ml heparin.

PAB (PBS with Azide and Bovine Serum Albumin)

1 Mix together the following until dissolved:

four liters sterile distilled water

0.8 grams potassium chloride (Sigma)

0.8 grams KH_2PO_4 (Mallinckrodt)

32 grams NaCl (Mallinckrodt)

8.64 grams $Na_2HPO_4.7H_20$ (Mallinckrodt).

2 Adjust pH to 7.35.

3 Add:

20 grams bovine serum albumin (Sigma)

4 grams sodium azide (Sigma).

4 Stir until dissolved, filter (.22 micron, Corning, Corning, NY). Store refrigerated; expires in six months.

1% Paraformaldehyde

1 Dissolve 21.4 grams sodium cacodylate (cacodylate acid sodium salt, Mallinckrodt) in two liters sterile distilled water.

2 Adjust pH to 7.20.

3 Add 20 grams paraformaldehyde (Mallinckrodt), stirring on a hot plate in a fume hood until completely dissolved.

4 Add 15 grams sodium chloride (Sigma) and dissolve again.

5 Filter with .22 micron filter and keep refrigerated. Expires in 12 months.

Staining Tubes for CD34 Measurement

Two Color Stain

1 Phycoerythrin (PE)-CD34 (Becton Dickinson, San José, CA, HPCA-2) + fluorescein isothiocyanate (FITC)-CD45 (B-D, HLE-1)

2 PE-Mouse IgG1 (B-D) + FITC-CD45 (HLE-1)

3 PE-CD14 + FITC-CD45 (B-D, Leukogate)

Single Color Stain

1 PE-CD34 (HPCA-2)

2 PE- Mouse IgG1 (B-D)

3 FITC-CD45 (HLE-1)

The common strategy of these stains is to provide a measurement of $CD34^+$ cells (the numerator) that can be compared to an isotype control stain as well as a measurement of the leukocyte population with an antibody to CD45 that provides the denominator. The two color stain that includes CD14/CD45 provides a cell differential that will quantitate MNC purity. The examples and data presented here use antibodies marketed by Becton Dickinson. Other sources of antibodies may give similar results. Recent studies [17] of antibodies to the CD34 antigen, however, indicate that the 8G12 antibody (HPCA-2) to CD34, which is available directly tagged with PE or FITC, gives superior resolution of the $CD34^+$ population.

Data Acquisition and Analysis

Instrument Set-up and Compensation

The flow cytometer needs to be calibrated and set up correctly each time samples are analyzed. Calibration beads are commercially available to initially calibrate the instrument. The correct compensation settings for doing two color analysis can be determined by the following method, using cells from the sample being studied or another fresh sample of normal peripheral blood:

1 Stain the following three tubes to use as "compensation set-up" tubes:

a FITC-Mouse Ig (B-D control reagent)

Phycoerythrin-Mouse Ig (B-D control reagent)

b FITC-CD45 (B-D, HLE-1)

c PE-CD45 (Coulter Immunology, Hialeah, FL, KC56 (T200)-RD1)

2 Put tube #1 on and adjust linear forward and side scatter until the dot plot clearly distinguishes between granulocytes, monocytes, and lymphocytes while eliminating debris and RBCs using the electronic threshold on forward scatter (Fig. 1A). Put a gate around the lymphocyte population as shown.

3 With this lymphocyte gate on, display log FL1 vs. log FL2, as in Figure 1B. Adjust the FL1 and FL2 voltages until the gated lymphocyte population sits in quadrant three (lower left). Using quadrants, or histograms, determine the mean channel fluorescence in the X and Y direction.

4 With the lymphocyte gate still on, put tube #2 on and display FL1 vs. FL2, as in Figure 1C. The FITC-CD45 should move only in the FL1 direction , and therefore the Y mean

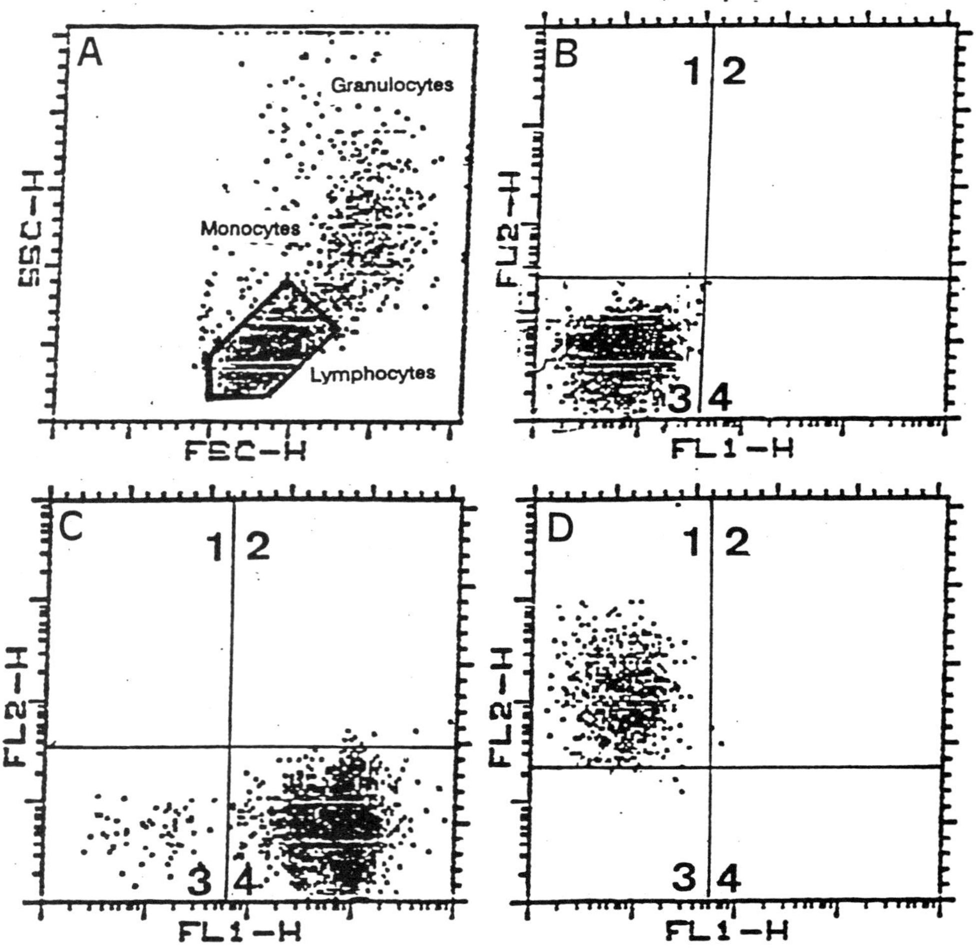

Fig. 1. Instrument set-up—establishing appropriate compensation setting. Shown is a dot plot of fresh ficoll/hypaque prepared peripheral blood containing predominantly lymphocytes and monocytes.

channel fluorescence in quadrant four (lower right) should be the same as the Y mean channel fluorescence from quadrant three (lower left) in tube #1. Adjust the compensation and/or voltages until they are very close.

5 Put tube #3 on, and with the lymphocyte gate still on, display FL1 vs. FL2, as in Figure 1D. The PE-CD45 should move into quadrant one (upper left), and therefore the X mean channel fluorescence in quadrant one should be the same as the X mean channel fluorescence from quadrant three in tube #1. Adjust the compensation and/or voltages until they are very close.

Because compensation was adjusted with lymphocytes, which are very bright, any other tubes run should all be dimmer, and thus compensated correctly. As a general rule, compensation should always be adjusted with the brightest stain to be used for a particular experiment.

Acquisition

Once the flow cytometer is calibrated and compensated correctly, samples can be analyzed for CD34$^+$ cells. An adequate sample of cells must be studied to assure a low coefficient of variation between identical measurements of the same preparation. For samples with higher levels of CD34 which are easily resolvable (>2%), a 20,000 event file will likely be enough. For low level samples, (<0.5%) larger files of 50,000 or greater may be collected to display a resolvable CD34 population.

Analysis

The most common method for resolving the CD34$^+$ population is to display CD34 fluorescence and side scatter. As shown in Figure 2 where a peripheral blood sample is compared to its corresponding leukapheresis product, a discrete population of fluorescent cells is observed in a region of low side scatter (Fig. 2, top panels) and can be compared to an isotype control sample (Fig. 2, middle panels). One gate is then applied to the CD45$^+$ population in a display of FITC-CD45 vs PE-CD34 fluorescence taking special care to include the CD34$^+$ cells that are dim (Fig. 2, bottom panels) and determine the percent CD34 of the CD45$^+$ population using a quadrant statistical marker or a window on the fluorescence vs side scatter display. This provides an objective approach by defining a discrete population of CD34$^+$ cells and has resulted in the best correlations with CFU-GM [18, 19]. It should be noted that there is not a one to one correlation of the CD34 with CFU-GM, but rather the CD34$^+$ population is always at a 5-10 × higher frequency than the CFU-GM [18, 20-22] representing a cloning efficiency of about 10% for the CD34$^+$ population. Recent studies [18, 22, 23] indicate that the cloning efficiency of the CD34$^+$ population may vary with the type of mobilization protocol and the growth factors used.

A key to accurate measurement of CD34$^+$ cells is a consistent definition of the denominator used for calculation. The proportion of leukocytes observed by

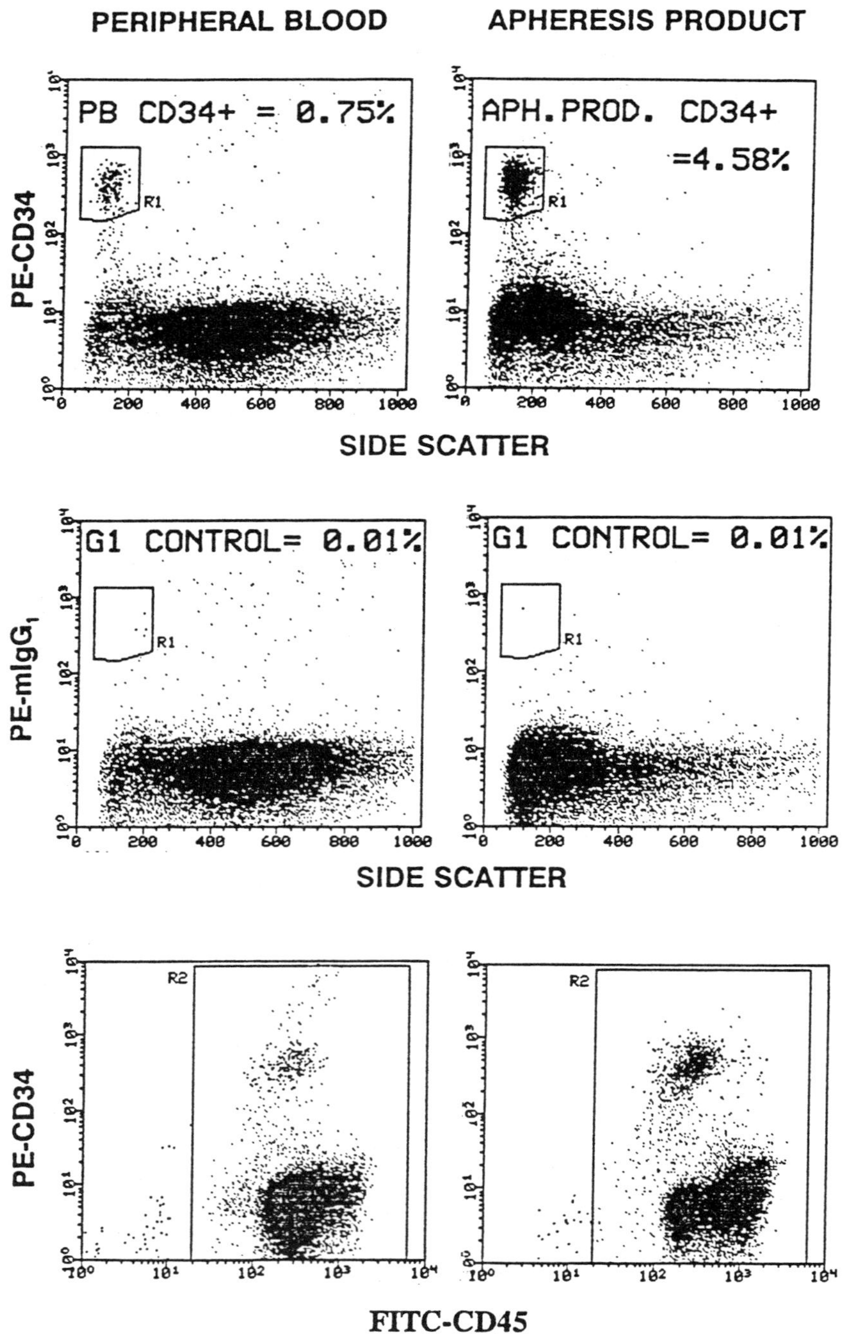

Fig. 2. Two color analysis of $CD34^+$ cells: comparison of peripheral blood and leukapheresis product from the same patient showing enrichment of $CD34^+$ cells and mononuclear cells. $CD34^+$ cells shown in the low side scatter region (top panels) are measured as a percent of $CD45^+$ cells (bottom panels) and compared to isotype control stains (middle panels).

light scatter may vary considerably between samples because of RBC contamination, and debris. A CD34 value expressed as a percent of $CD45^+$ leukocytes rather than just light scatter events provides for direct calculation of total numbers of CD34 using available hematology measurements of white blood cell counts. The assumptions in these calculations is that a $CD45^+$ leukocyte event is equivalent to a white blood cell counted by a hematology counter. The total numbers of CD34 that are reinfused can be used to estimate the therapeutic dose of cells obtained by a given mobilization protocol.

Flow cytometry also provides a simple straight forward measurement of the harvesting process by quantitating the enrichment of MNC from the peripheral blood to the leukapheresis product using light scatter (single color strategy) or a CD14 vs side scatter display when gating on $CD45^+$ cells (two color strategy) (Fig. 3) to estimate lymphocytes, monocytes and granulocytes.

Discussion

The Threshold of Detection

One issue that always comes up with this type of analysis is the question of how few $CD34^+$ cells can be detected in a sample, i.e., what is the limit of detection using this method? An illustration of this analysis is shown in Figure 4. Applying a gate around the low side scatter, $CD34^+$ region (Fig. 4,

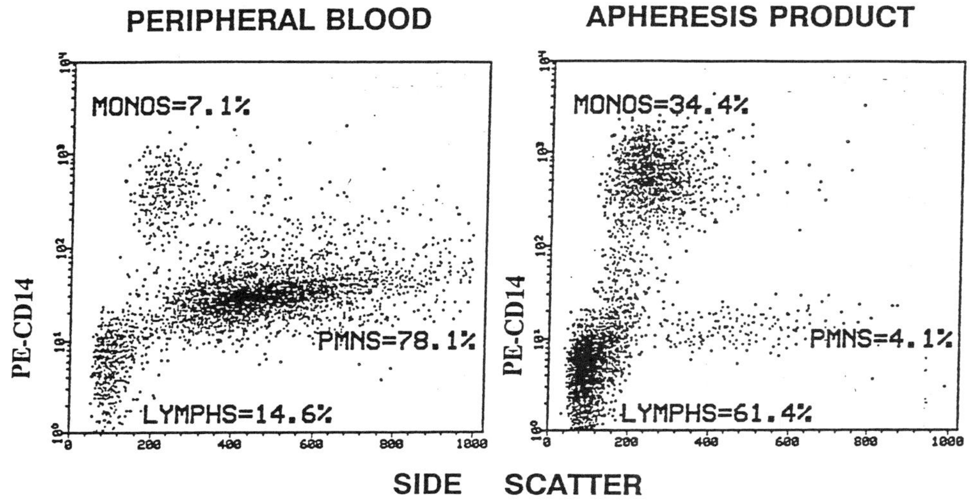

Fig. 3. Mononuclear cell differential using flow cytometry: comparison of peripheral blood and leukapheresis product. $CD45^+$ cells were gated on using a two color stain with CD14 and CD45. Displaying CD14 vs side scatter distinct populations of lymphocytes, monocytes and granulocytes can be identified.

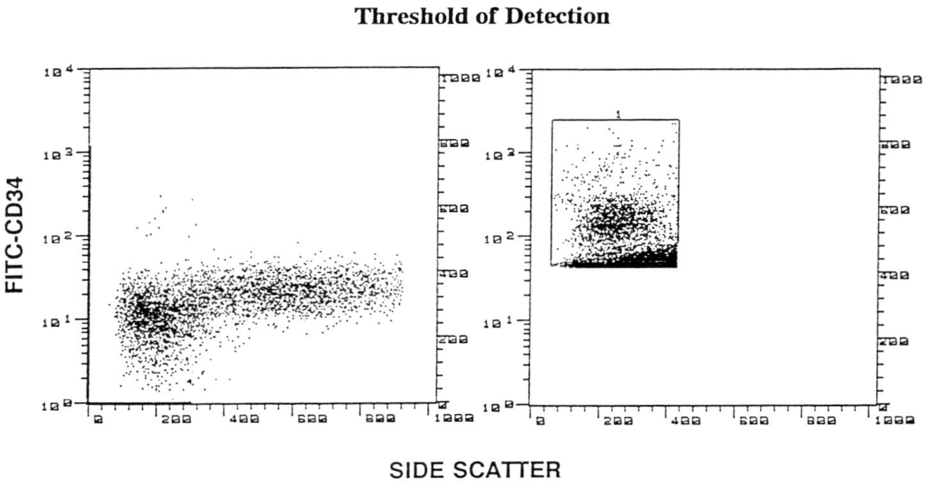

Fig. 4. Threshold of detection of CD34. The limit of detection for CD34 can be determined by the level at which a resolvable cluster of CD34+ cells can be observed within a gated region containing the CD34+ population (right panel).

right panel) and collecting events, allows a "true" and identifiable population or "cluster" to appear. Populations of CD34 greater than 1% create an identifiable cluster of events in this region with little need for gating. At concentrations below 1% it is the definition of this cluster that determines the limits of sensitivity for the measurement of the CD34+ population. At very low percentages (<0.1%), the presence or absence of a defined cluster in this gated region of interest determines the reality or believability of the measurement. Using this type of criteria, populations to almost 0.01% can often be reliably determined. The limit of detection therefore becomes a function of: 1) the development of a cluster when compared to an isotype control sample, 2) the time necessary to acquire enough events in the gated region to see a cluster appear, or 3) the amount of sample, i.e., depletion of sample before a cluster appears. This approach requires the subjective interpretation of the person performing the analysis as to what constitutes a resolved cluster. We await the development of automated multidimensional cluster analysis that would obviate the need for this kind of operator intervention.

A Gallery of Artifacts

In the best of all worlds a perfect measurement can be made every time. In clinical medicine problems are often encountered in the timely delivery and preparation of samples. In addition, the future in the field of transplantation is moving toward more ex vivo manipulation of cells before they are reinfused. Each manipulation can potentially have effects on the measurement of CD34. The separation of mononuclear cells by leukapheresis is a common ex vivo

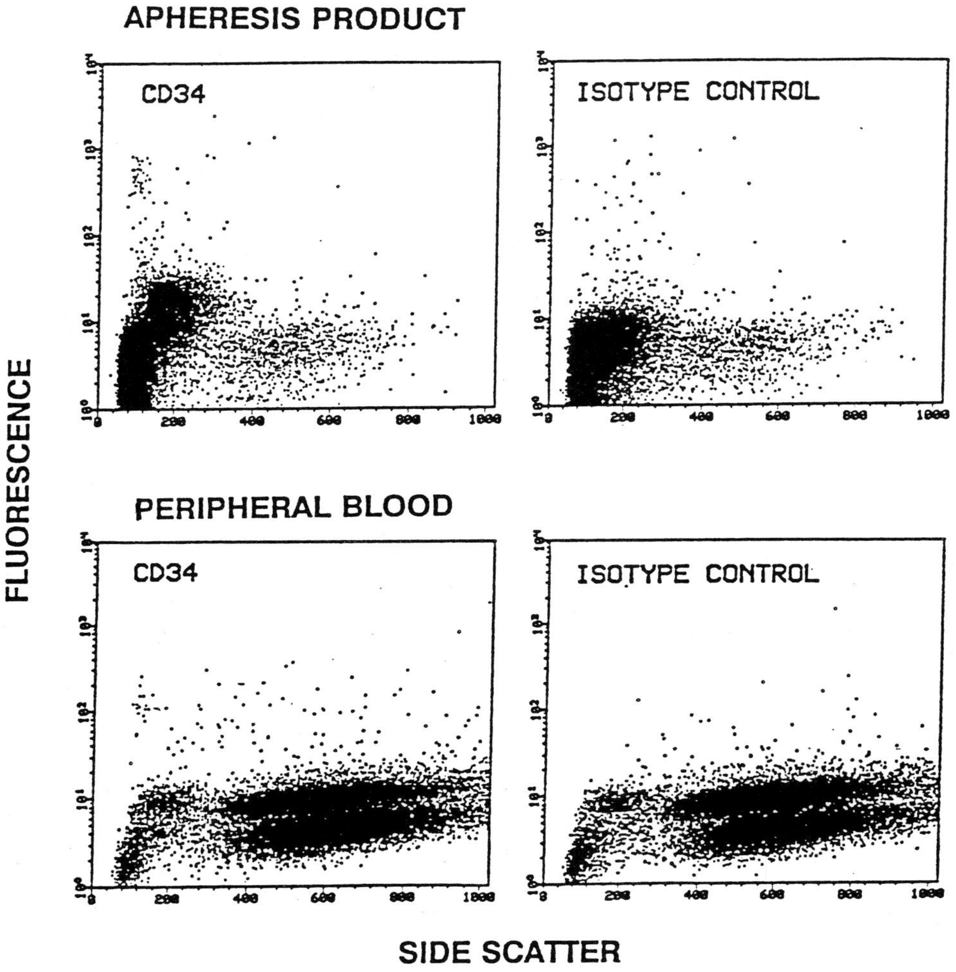

Fig. 5. Artifacts of CD34 analysis. Top panel shows an increase in the fluorescence of the monocyte population in an apheresis product. The bottom panel shows a stain in which an entire subset of cells has stained non-specifically.

manipulation and the effects on the measurement of CD34 can be seen in Figure 5 (top panel) where the monocyte population defined by side scatter has clearly increased its non-specific staining with the PE-HPCA-2 antibody. Other artifacts in which entire subpopulations stain non-specifically such as shown in Figure 5 (bottom panel) are occasionally observed.

References

1 Kessinger A, Armitage JO. Editorial: the evolving role of autologous peripheral stem cell transplantation following high-dose therapy for malignancies. Blood 1991;77:211-213.

2 Zander AR, Lyding J, Bielack S. Transplantation with blood stem cells. Blood Cells 1991;17:301-309.

3 Gianni AM, Siena S, Bregni M, Bonadonna G. The use of GM-CSF and peripheral blood stem cells (PBSC) minimizes hematological toxicity following a myeloablative course of chemo-radiotherapy. Path Biol 1992;39:956.

4 Korbling M, Martin H, Fliedner TM. Autologous blood stem cell transplantation. In: Gale RP, Champlin R, eds. Progress in bone marrow transplantation. UCLA Symposia on Molecular and Cellular Biology, New York: Alan R. Liss, Inc., 1987:877-888.

5 Brown RI. The physics of continuous flow centrifugal cell separation. Artificial Organs 1989;13:4-20.

6 Keilholz U, Klein HG, Korbling M, Brado B, Carter CS, Cullis H, Galm F, Hunstein W. Peripheral blood mononuclear cell collection from patients undergoing adoptive immunotherapy or peripheral blood-derived stem cell transplantation and from healthy donors. J Clin Apheresis 1992;6:131-136.

7 Lasky LC, Ash RC, Kersey JH, Zanjani ED, McCullough J. Collection of pluripotential hematopoietic stem cells by cytapheresis. Blood 1982;59:822-827.

8 Berenson RJ, Bensinger WI, Hill RS, Andrews RG, Garcia-Lopez J, Kalamasz DF, Still BJ, Spitzer G, Buckner CD, Bernstein ID. Engraftment after infusion of CD34+ marrow cells in patients with breast cancer or neuroblastoma. Blood 1991;77:1717-1722.

9 Bensinger WI, Berenson RJ, Andrews RG, Buckner CD, Spitzer G, Garcia-Lopez J, Bernstein ID, Hansen JA. Engraftment after infusion of CD34 enriched marrow cells. Int J Cell Cloning 1992;10(Suppl 1):176-178.

10 Reiffers J, Castaigne S, Tilly H, Lepage E, Leverger G, Hénon P, Douay L. Hematopoietic reconstitution after autologous blood stem cell transplantation: a report of 46 cases. Plasma Ther Transfus Technol 1987;8:360-362.

11 Sheridan WP, Begley CG, Juttner CA, Szer J, To LB, Maher D, McGrath KM, Morstyn G, Fox RM. Effect of peripheral blood progenitor cells mobilized by filgrastim (G-CSF) on platelet recovery after high-dose chemotherapy. Lancet 1992;339:640-644.

12 To LB, Roberts MM, Haylock DN, Dyson PG, Branford AL, Thorp D, Ho JQK, Dart GW, Horvath N, Davy MLJ, Olweny CLM, Abdi E, Juttner CA. Comparison of hematological recovery times and supportive care requirements of autologous recovery phase peripheral blood stem cell transplants, autologous bone marrow transplants and allogeneic bone marrow transplants. Bone Marrow Transplantation 1992;9:277-284.

13 Terstappen LWMM, Johnson D, Mickaels RA, Chen J, Olds G, Hawkins JT, Loken MR, Levin J. Multidimensional flow cytometric blood cell differentiation without erythrocyte lysis. Blood Cells 1991;17:585-602.

14 Harris PE, Ralph P, Litcofsky P, Moore MAS. Distinct activities of lymphokine γ interferon, and cytokine differentiation-inducing factors acting on the human monoblastic leukemia cell line U937. Cancer Res 1985;45:9-13.

15 Weiner RS, Richman CM, Yankee RA. Dilution techniques for optimum recovery of cryopreserved bone marrow cells. Exp Hematol 1979;7:1-6.

16 Visani G, Ricci P, Motta MR, Franchi P, Santucci MA, Bandini G, Tura S. Recovery of CFU-GM after freezing of normal human bone marrow: effect of three dilution techniques after thawing. Cryobiology 1983;20:587-590.

17 Siena S, Bregni M, Brando B, Belli N, Lansdorp PM, Bonadonna G, Gianni AM. Flow cytometry to estimate circulating hematopoietic progenitors for autologous transplantation: comparative analysis of different CD34 monoclonal antibodies. Haematologica 1991;76:330-333.

18 Siena S, Bregni M, Brando B, Belli N, Ravagnani F, Gandola L, Stern AC, Lansdorp PM, Bonadonna G, Gianni AM. Flow cytometry for clinical estimation of circulating hematopoietic progenitors for autologous transplantation in cancer patients. Blood 1991;77:400-409.

19 Bender JG, Williams SF, Myers S, Nottleman D, Lee WJ, Unverzagt KL, Walker D, To LB, Van Epps DE. Characterization of chemotherapy mobilized peripheral blood progenitor cells for use in autologous stem cell transplantation. Bone Marrow Transplantation 1992;10:281-285.

20 Serke S, Sauberlich S, Huhn D. Multiparameter flow-cytometrical quantitation of circulating CD34(+)-cells: correlation to the quantitation of circulating hemopoietic progenitor cells by in vitro colony-assay. Br J Haematol 1991;77:453-459.

21 Fritsch G, Emminger W, Buchinger P, Printz D, Gadner H. CD34-positive cell proportions in peripheral blood correlate with colony-forming capacity. Exp Hematol 1991;19:1079-1083.

22 Ravagnani F, Siena S, Bregni M, Sciorelli G, Gianni AM, Pellegris G. Large-scale collection of circulating hematopoietic progenitors in cancer patients treated with high-dose cyclophosphamide and recombinant human GM-CSF. Eur J Can 1990;26:562-564.

23 Brugger W, Bross K, Frisch J, Dern P, Weber B, Mertelsmann R, Kanz L. Mobilization of peripheral blood progenitor cells by sequential administration of interleukin-3 and granulocyte-macrophage colony-stimulating factor following polychemotherapy with etoposide, ifosfamide, and cisplatin. Blood 1992;79:1193-1200.

Determination of CD34⁺ Hemopoietic Cells by Multiparameter Flow Cytometry: Technical Remarks

Sabine Säuberlich, Andreas Kirsch, Stefan Serke
Abteilung Innere Medizin und Poliklinik, Hämatologie-Onkologie, Hämatologisches Zentrallabor, Universitätsklinikum Rudolf Virchow, Freie Universität Berlin, Berlin, Germany

Key Words. Multiparameter flow cytometry • CD34 antibodies • Whole blood lyse • Mononuclear cells • Statistics • Coefficient of variation (CV)

Introduction

Hemopoietic cells, identified as $CD34^+$ cells, generally are a minor population among all cells of any given sample such as whole blood, whole bone marrow cell suspension, whole leukapheresis sample, or density gradient-separated mononuclear cells from any of the three samples listed above. In the analytical setting, we are heading for two major goals: a) identification and characterization of $CD34^+$ cells, and b) quantitation of $CD34^+$ cells.

The choice of the sample to be studied by flow cytometry will never be a random decision. For exact and biologically true quantitation, one will have to perform analyses on whole blood samples, i.e., applying a red blood cell lyse reagent (also on bone marrow or leukapheresis samples). Density-gradient separated mononuclear cells, however, will be the sample of choice when investigating numbers and/or expression of differentiation antigens of $CD34^+$ cells, correlating these parameters to colonies as grown from these samples by means of in vitro cultures.

The remarks to follow are tentative recommendations for reproducible analyses of $CD34^+$ cells by multiparameter flow cytometry.

Whole Blood versus Mononuclear Cells

When correlating numbers and/or expression of differentiation antigens of $CD34^+$ cells to colonies as grown in tissue culture, using aliquots from the identical samples for both determinations, it is highly recommendable to have the flow cytometrical determinations on the mononuclear cells as used for in vitro cultures. If only quantitation and/or immunophenotyping of $CD34^+$ cells is the subject of the determination, it is highly recommendable to have the determinations on a sample which has passed through a minimum number

Correspondence: Dr. Stefan Serke, Abteilung Innere Medizin und Poliklinik, Hämatologie-Onkologie, Hämatologisches Zentrallabor, Universitätsklinikum Rudolf Virchow, Freie Universität Berlin, Spandauer Damm 130, 14050 Berlin, Germany.

©AlphaMed Press ISBN 1-880854 17-1

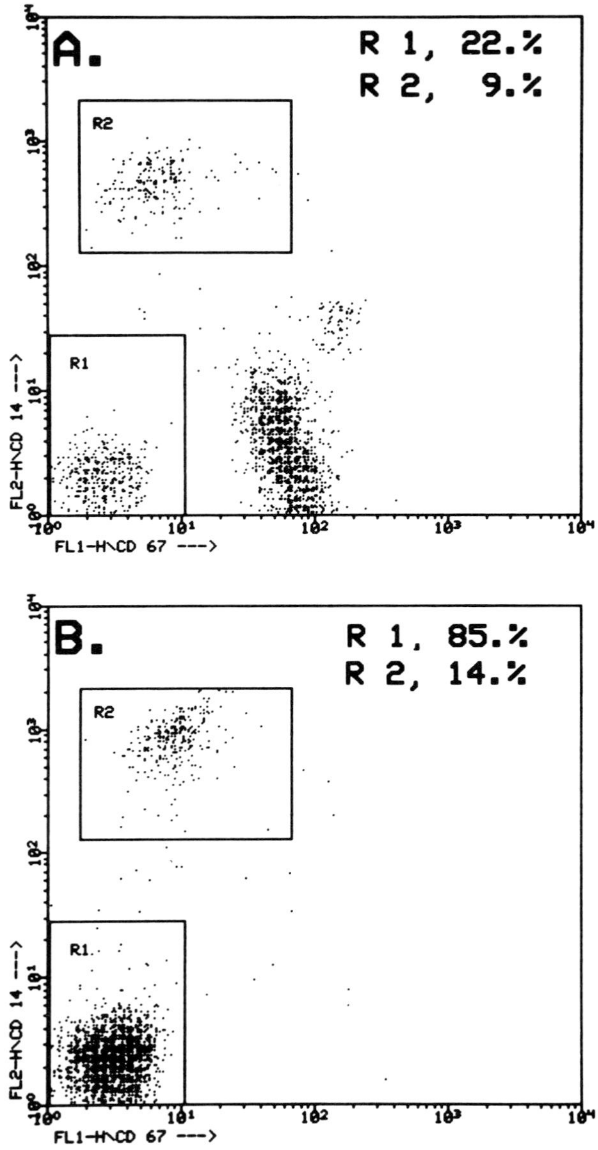

Fig. 1. A) EDTA-anticoagulated blood from healthy adult was stained with CD67-FITC and CD14-PE monoclonal antibodies; samples were processed with FACS lysing reagent; shown is the dot-plot of CD67 to CD14 expression; in R1, lymphocytes, in R2, monocytes; ratio of lymphocytes to monocytes = 2.44:1. B) From the same subject, EDTA-anticoagulated blood was subjected to separation of mononuclear cells by density gradient separation; mononuclear cells were processed as indicated in (A); shown is the dot-plot of CD67 to CD14 expression; in R1, lymphocytes; in R2, monocytes; ratio of lymphocytes to monocytes = 6.1:1.

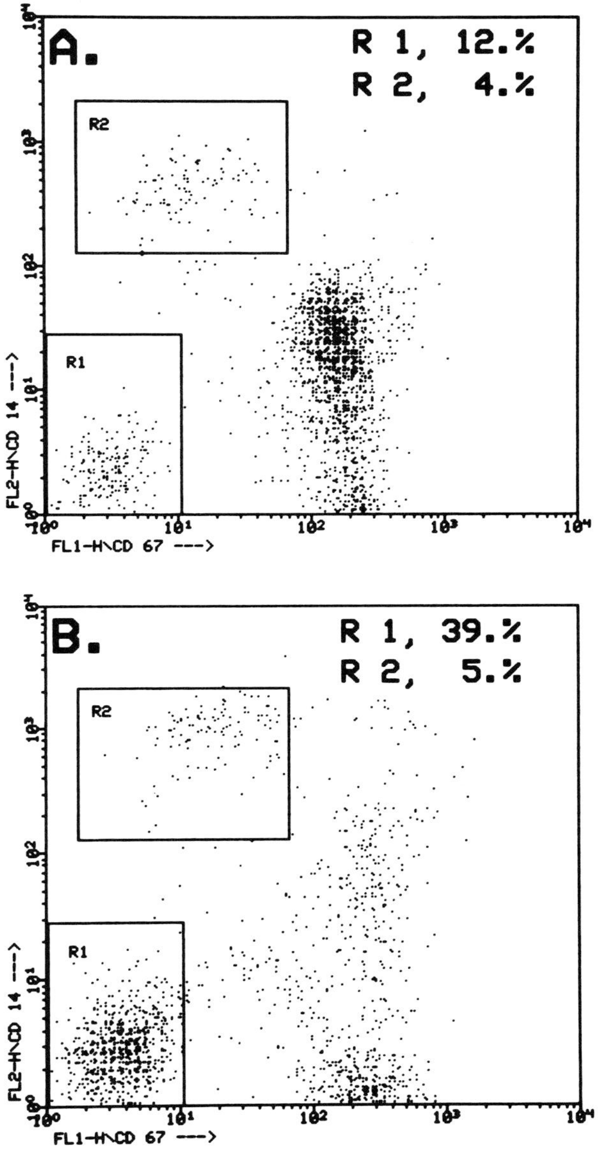

Fig. 2. A) EDTA-anticoagulated blood from a patient on G-CSF therapy was stained with CD67-FITC and with CD14-PE monoclonal antibodies; samples were processed with FACS lysing reagent; shown is the dot-plot of CD67 to CD14 expression; in R1, lymphocytes; in R2, monocytes; ratio of lymphocytes to monocytes = 3.0:1. B) From the same subject, EDTA-anticoagulated blood was subjected to separation of mononuclear cells by density gradient separation; mononuclear cells were processed as indicated in (A); shown is the dot-plot of CD67 to CD14 expression; in R1, lymphocytes; in R2, monocytes; ratio of lymphocytes to monocytes = 7.8:1.

of processing steps. For this reason it is recommended for this purpose to apply a red blood cell lyse reagent and to study the samples without any further processing. Figures 1 and 2 show that the ratios of lymphocytes to monocytes differ substantially from whole blood to mononuclear cells as separated by density gradient. Therefore, while calculating back from the numbers of "mononuclear cells" as determined in whole blood and the percentage of CD34$^+$ cells, as determined studying mononuclear cells as separated by density gradient, one is at major risk to have erroneous determinations. For materials and methodology, see details in section below.

Choice of the Red Blood Cell Lyse Reagent

Although determinations of CD34$^+$ cells on samples processed as little as possible are desirable, currently available flow cytometry devices do not allow for proper determinations of blood, leukapheresis, or bone marrow samples without previous lysis of red blood cells. Although gating on DNA [1] allows for inclusion of nucleated cells only, eliminating red blood cells during data acquisition, this approach leads to extremely large acquisition times. Gating on CD45$^+$ events, however, is not feasible for exact quantitation when nonleukocytes, i.e., CD45$^+$ cells, are present in the sample. This should be taken into account when analyzing bone marrow samples (Figs. 3, 4). In those samples, CD45$^-$ cells, namely erythroblasts, can account for sometimes more than 50% of all cells.

Recently, we have compared two commercially available red blood cell lyse reagents for multiparameter flow cytometry [2]. Whereas with one of these reagents a substantial cell loss occurred with processing, this cell loss was not observed with the other one. Surprisingly, this cell loss was not a random one affecting all leukocyte subsets to the same extent, but it rather was a selective loss, affecting lymphocytes to a much bigger extent than all other leukocyte subsets. Figures 5 and 6 illustrate these different performance characteristics of both those lyse reagents. A further advantage of the lysed reagent we are opting for is that the light scatter patterns of lymphocytes are almost unchanged compared with unprocessed "whole blood" samples. This allows for better characterization of subsets of CD34$^+$ cells according to light scatter patterns.

Materials and Methodology

Sample:

Anticoagulated blood, bone marrow, or leukapheresis sample; adjust cell count to about 5,000 nuclear cells/μl by diluting with Dulbecco's phosphate buffered saline.

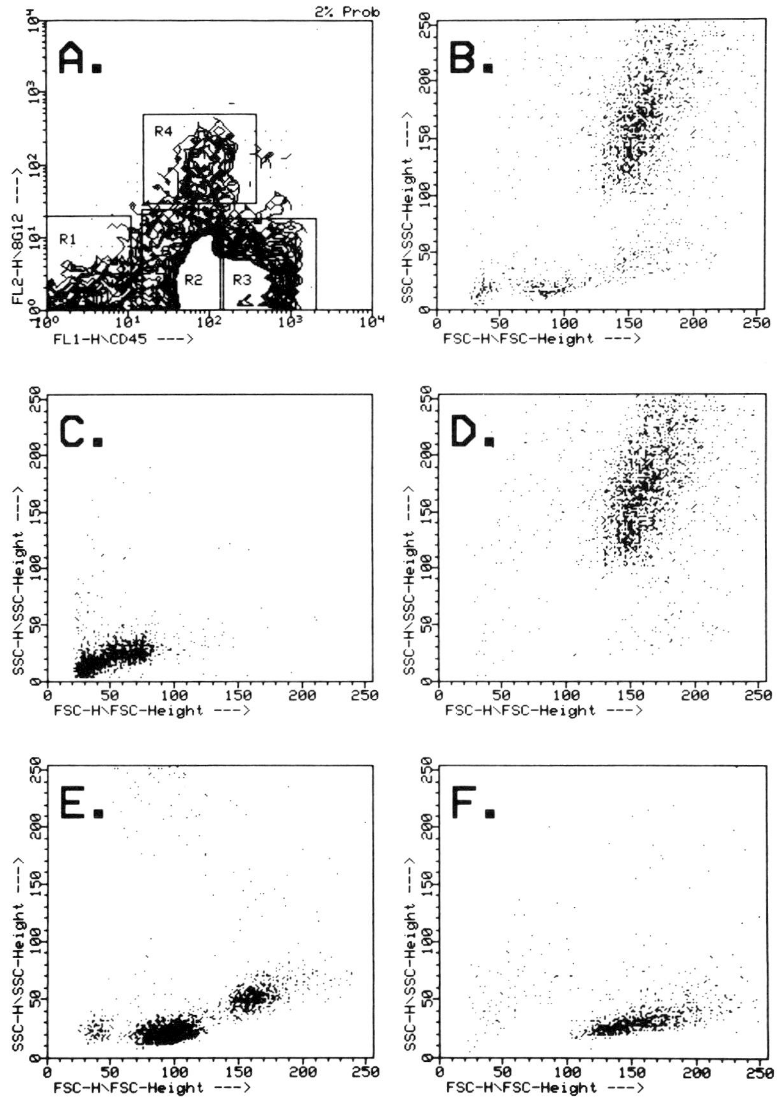

Fig. 3. Native bone marrow sample was stained with CD34 monoclonal antibody (8G12-PE) and with CD45-FITC monoclonal antibody; sample was processed with Opti-Lyse reagent; 5 × 10^4 cells in analysis. A) Correlation contour plot (2% probability) of CD34 expression (y axis) and CD45 expression (x axis); arbitrarily defined analysis regions; R1, erythroblasts (and debris) R2, mature myeloid cells; R3, lymphocytes and immature myeloid cells; R4, $CD34^+$ cells. B) Dot-plot correlating light scatter parameters; all cells of analysis (2,000 dots shown). C) Dot-plot correlating light scatter parameters; cells from R1, erythroblasts and debris (3.6%). D) Dot-plot correlating light scatter parameters; cells from R2, mature myeloid cells (68%). E) Dot-plot correlating light scatter parameters; cells from R3, lymphocytes and immature myeloid cells (25%). F) Dot-plot correlating light scatter parameters; cells from R4, $CD34^+$ cells (1.8%).

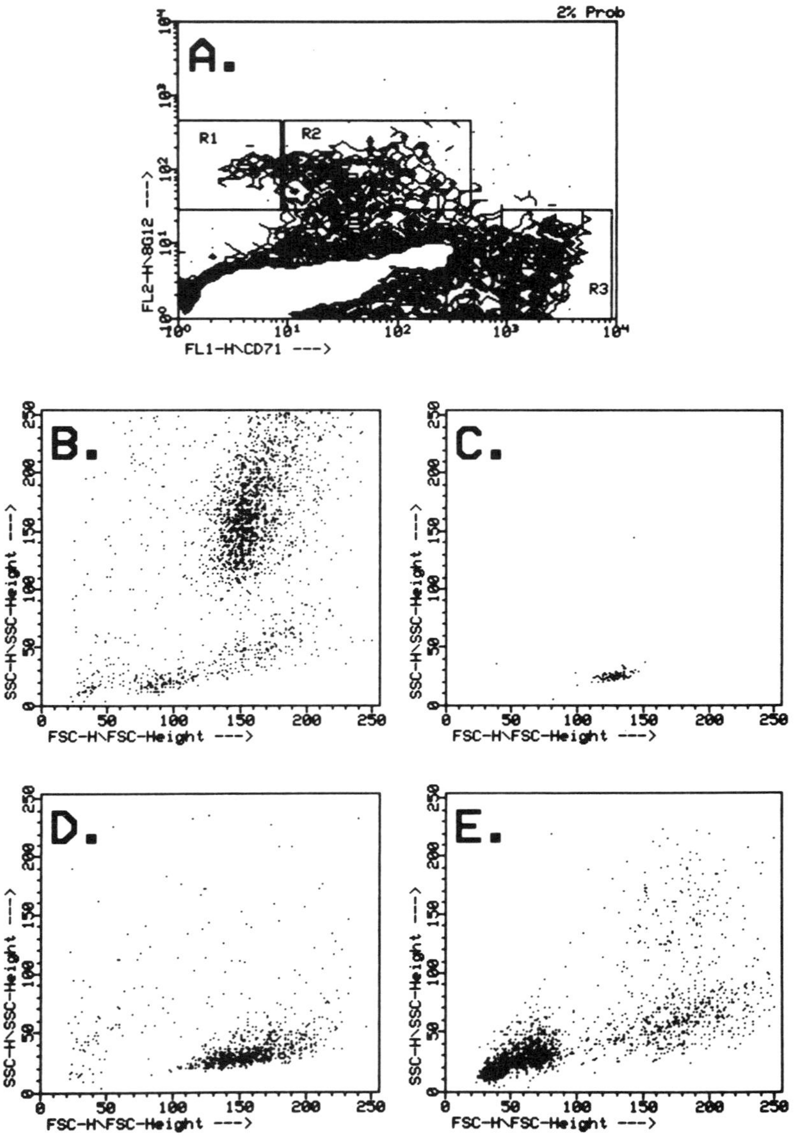

Fig. 4. Native bone marrow sample was stained with 8G12-PE and with CD71-FITC monoclonal antibody; sample was processed with Opti-Lyse reagent; 5×10^4 cells in analysis. A) Correlation contour plot (2% probability) of CD34 expression (y axis) and CD71 expression (x axis); arbitrarily defined analysis regions: R1, resting $CD34^+$ cells; R2, nonresting $CD34^+$ cells; R3, erythroblasts, monocytes and immature myeloid cells. B) Dot-plot correlating light scatter parameters; all cells of analysis (2,000 dots shown). C) Dot-plot correlating light scatter parameters; all cells from R1, resting $CD34^+$ cells (0.16%). D) Dot-plot correlating light scatter parameters; all cells from R2, nonresting $CD34^+$ cells (1.6%). E) Dot-plot correlating light scatter parameters; all cells from R3, erythroblasts, monocytes and immature myeloid cells (3.4%).

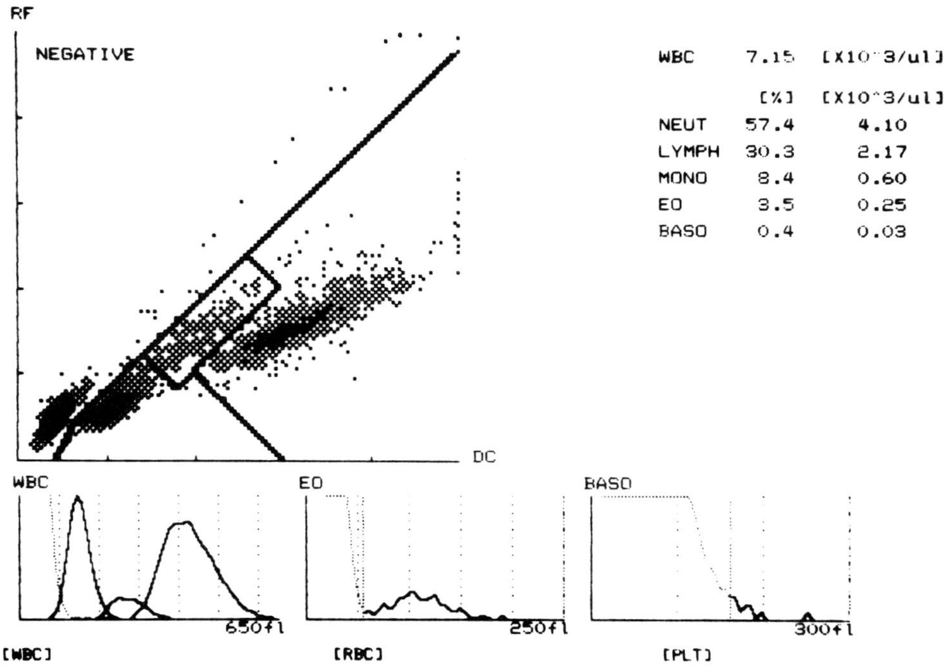

Fig. 5. Five-part differential of leukocytes as determined by a routine CBC device (NE-7000; TOA Medical Electronics, Kobe, Japan). According to differential impedance patterns and according to differential resistance to selective lyse buffers, the five major leukocyte populations are discriminated; EDTA-anticoagulated blood sample from a healthy adult. Note: lymphocytes account for about 30% of all leukocytes.

Antibodies:

QBEND-10, a CD34 monoclonal antibody, PE-conjugate;

8G12, a CD34 monoclonal antibody, PE-conjugate;

CD67-monoclonal antibody, FITC-conjugate;

CD14-monoclonal antibody, PE-conjugate;

CD71-monoclonal antibody, FITC-conjugate;

CD45 monoclonal antibody, FITC-conjugate.

All antibodies, except for 8G12, were purchased from Immunotech/AMAC; 8G12 was purchased from Becton Dickinson.

Lyse Reagents:

a) FACS lysing reagent, Becton Dickinson
b) Opti-Lyse, Immunotech/AMAC

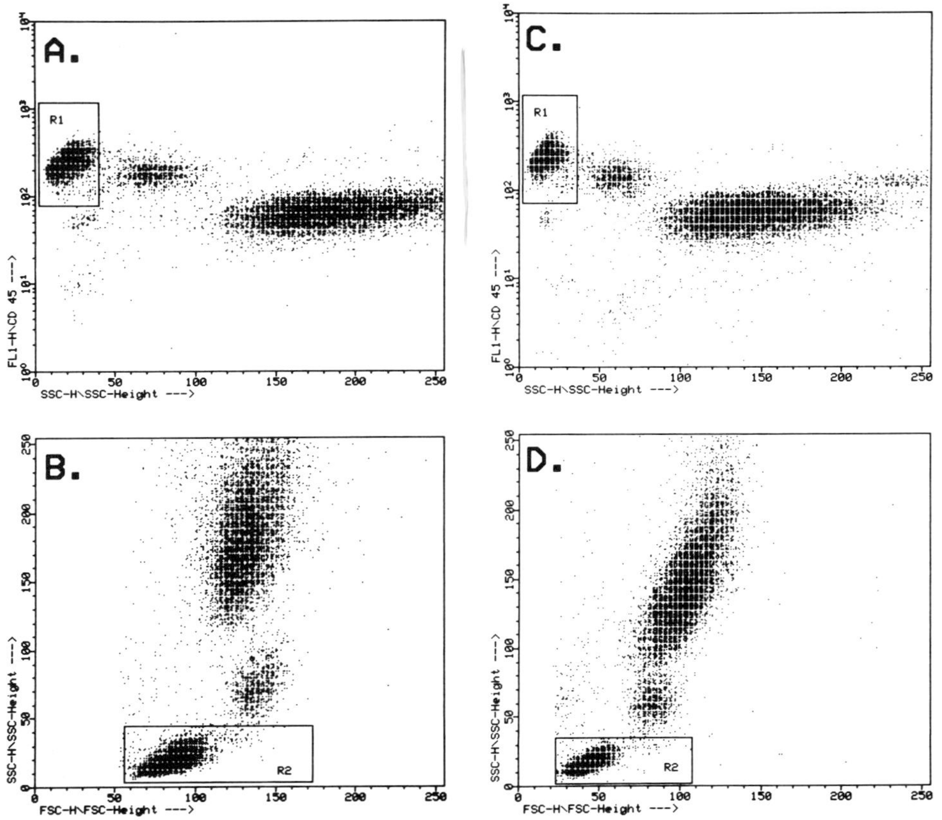

Fig. 6. The blood sample as described in Figure 5 was subjected to staining with CD45 monoclonal antibody and aliquots were processed with Opti-Lyse reagent or with FACS lyse reagent; arbitrary rectangular live-gate on acquisition set on light scatter parameters; 1×10^4 events per analysis. A) Sample processed with Opti-Lyse reagent; dot-plot correlating CD45 expression (y axis) to sideward light scatter (x axis); in R1, lymphocytes (30%). B) Sample processed with Opti-Lyse reagent; dot-plot correlating both light scatter parameters; in R2, lymphocytes (31%). C) Sample processed with Opti-Lyse reagent; dot-plot correlating CD45 expression to sideward light scatter; in R1, lymphocytes (24%). D) Sample processed with FACS lyse reagent; dot-plot correlating both light scatter parameters; in R2, lymphocytes (24%).

Sample processing:

Samples were first stained with monoclonal antibodies, with a sample volume of 100 μl and with 15 μl of the respective monoclonal antibody. After 20 min at room temperature, samples were subjected to a lyse of red blood cells by:

a) applying Becton Dickinson lyse reagent, with further processing performed according to the instructions of the manufacturer (data sheet)

b) applying Opti-Lyse (100 μl) reagent to the sample, followed by immediate vortexing; the sample then was left at room temperature for about 12 min; then 1 ml of distilled water was added, followed again by immediate vortexing; samples were left at room temperature for at least 30 min until performance of flow cytometry.

Flow cytometry:
A FACScan (Becton Dickinson) was used. An arbitrary rectangular live-gate was set on forward to sideward light scatter plot to exclude cell debris. Different numbers of cells were acquired, according to the experimental needs (see legends to figures). Data were analyzed on an LYSY II (Becton Dickinson).

Cell Numbers for Proper Determinations

The complex quantitative determination of blood cells performed by far the most frequently is the leukocyte differential, grouping leukocytes into granulocytes (basophils, eosinophils, neutrophils), monocytes and lymphocytes. Traditionally, 100 whole blood cells are counted by microscopy, and according to the morphological appearance of cells, as present on stained smears, the white blood cell differential is determined. This approach, however, is highly erroneous when intending to quantitate cell subsets accounting for only a few percent or even less. *Rümke* [3] has clearly shown that one has to consider seriously the total numbers of cells necessary per each single determination to have reliable determinations of minor cell subsets. Recently, we have emphasized this fact with special reference to quantitative determinations of $CD34^+$ cells [4]. Generally, one should keep in mind first that the expected standard deviation is about the square root of the mean number ($\bar{x}$) of the cell subset of interest. Second, the coefficient of variation (CV) is the standard deviation (SD) expressed as percent of the mean, according to the equation as follows:

$$\text{CV}(\%) = \frac{\text{SD}}{\bar{x}} \times 100\%$$

Currently available devices for determination of complete blood count (CBC) generally allow for quantitation of leukocytes with a CV of less than 2% while quantitations of a small cell subset such as basophils will not be feasible with a CV of less than 15% [2]. Determinations with a CV greater than 15%, however, are anything else but exact. As devices for CBC are usually working at relatively low numbers of cells per determination, usually on the numbers of leukocytes present in 1 μl blood, there is no way to improve the quality of quantitation of any such minor cell subset with these devices. In contrast, performing determinations by means of multiparameter flow cytometry, we are able to choose freely the total numbers of cells per determination. This allows for exact determination of any cell subset, almost independent from its size among all cells present in the sample. Generally, $CD34^+$ cells are a minor population among all cells in any given sample. For example, we have reported that numbers of $CD34^+$ cells in steady-state healthy adults are about 1,500/ml_{blood}, corresponding to a percentage of about 0.03 [5]. So it is our recommendation to perform determinations of $CD34^+$ cells with a total number of cells large enough to have about 50 $CD34^+$ cells per determination. This number necessary for exact quantitative determinations can be deduced from the equation given above, which reads with 50 $CD34^+$ cells (as the mean number).

$$\text{CV (\%)} = \frac{7}{50} \times 100\% = 14$$

Given a minimum number of 50 $CD34^+$ cells per determination, seen with 5×10^4 cells per determination, the threshold for exact quantitative determinations of $CD34^+$ cells is only about 0.1% of all leukocytes.

Figures 7 to 12 illustrate the impact of total cell numbers on the CV of determinations of $CD34^+$ cells.

The need for sometimes really large numbers of total cells per determination urges one to stain and to process sometimes multiple aliquots of samples. So with a sample from a leukopenic patient, WBC = 1,000/μl, one needs at least a total volume of 300 μl of blood for performing the complete determination, due to cell loss on processing and the need to have cells to pass the cytometer for gating.

Conclusions

Multiparameter flow cytometry is the only method to have exact quantitative determinations and to have detailed studies of coexpression of differentiation

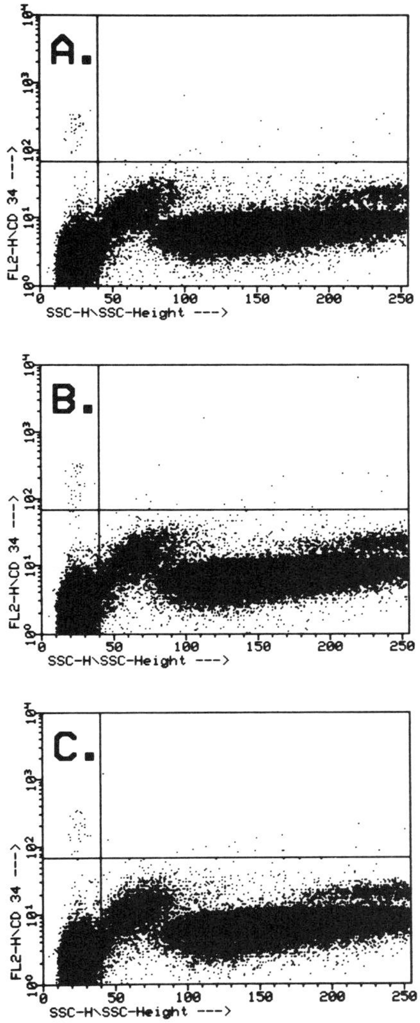

Fig. 7. EDTA-anticoagulated blood from a healthy adult subject was stained with QBEND-10-PE and processed with Opti-Lyse reagent; arbitrary rectangular live-gate on scatter parameters during data acquisition; 5×10^4 cells per determination; dot-plot correlating CD34 expression (y axis) to sideward light scatter (x axis); all dots shown; quadrant statistics; in the upper left quadrant cells considered as CD34⁺ cells. A) Numbers of CD34⁺ cells = 35 = 0.07%. B) Numbers of CD34⁺ cells = 34 = 0.07%. C) Numbers of CD34⁺ cells = 26 = 0.05%. Calculated CV = 15%. Expected CV = 18%

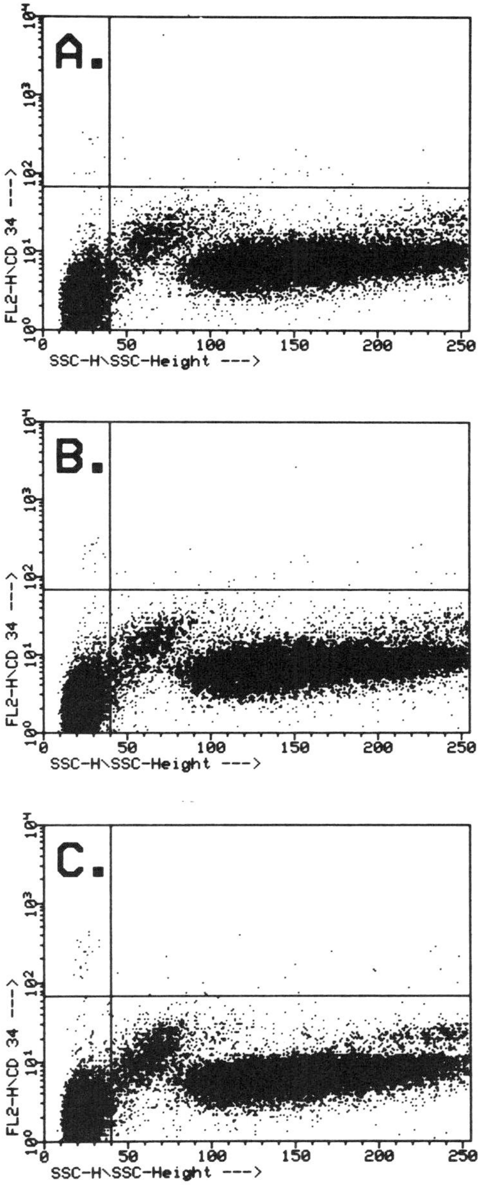

Fig. 8. EDTA-anticoagulated blood from the same subject as described in Figure 7; identical processing and identical data presentation as described in Figure 7; 25×10^3 cells per determination. A) Numbers of CD34⁺ cells = 11 = 0.4%. B) Numbers of CD34+ cells = 13 = 0.05%. C) Numbers of CD34⁺ cells = 20 = 0.08%. Calculated CV = 32%. Expected CV = 26%.

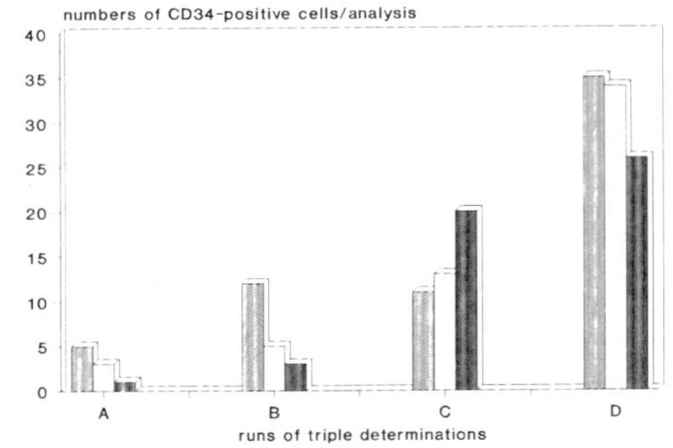

FIGURE 9 A

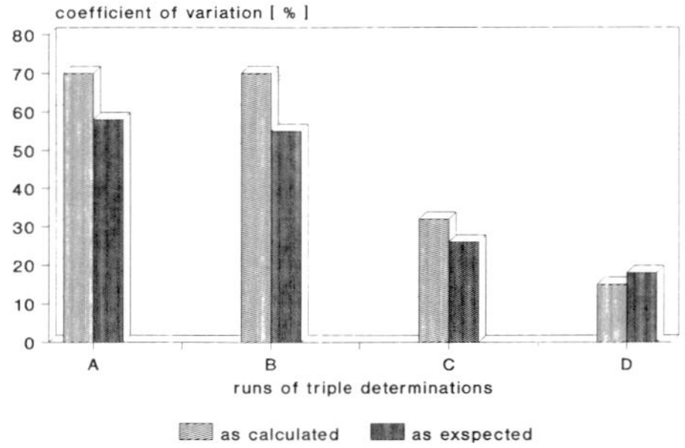

FIGURE 9 B

Fig. 9. Impact of the sample size on the CV of determinations of $CD34^+$ cells in the blood of a healthy adult subject; data were determined performing determination on samples as described in Figures 7 and 8; included are data from triple determinations on 6,250 (A), 12,500 (B), 25,000 (C), and 50,000 (D) cells, respectively. A) Numbers of $CD34^+$ cells per determination. B) CV as calculated from the triple determinations shown in Figure 9A, and CV as expected according to the mean number of $CD34^+$ cells determined.

antigens of $CD34^+$ cells. This method allows for major insights into the biology of hemopoietic cells. Conventionally, most of us working on multiparameter flow cytometry, however, are much more familiar with cells expressed as percentages rather than with cells in terms of absolute numbers. Therefore, a common statement is that $CD34^+$ cells as present in blood of patients on cytokine (for example granulocyte colony stimulating factor or G-CSF) therapy will show an expression of differentiation antigens suggesting that the majority of blood $CD34^+$ cells have entered myeloid differentiation, as evidenced by coexpression of CD33 antigen. A major fear, therefore, seems to be that undifferentiated, $CD33^-$, $CD34^+$ cells might "get lost" with cytokine therapy. Obviously, extreme differences are observed concerning $CD33^+$ or $CD33^-$ subsets of $CD34^+$ cells, when studying steady-state or G-CSF treated adult subjects. But one should keep in mind that accompanying this change in subsets of $CD34^+$ cells in blood there occurs simultaneously an even more drastic change in the absolute numbers of $CD34^+$ cells in blood. This should be illustrated by Figure 13. Figure 13A shows quantitative determination of blood $CD34^+$ cells from a healthy adult subject, with about 0.07% $CD34^+$ cells among all blood leukocytes. Leukocytes in this subject were $6{,}000/\mu l_{blood}$ and therefore a number of about 4,200 $CD34^+$ cells per 1 ml_{blood} can be calculated. Figure 13B shows coexpression of CD33 on gated $CD34^+$ cells. Whereas 65% of all $CD34^+$ cells are lacking CD33 expression, 35% do coexpress CD33. In absolute numbers, about 1,500 $CD34^+$ cells per 1 ml_{blood} are $CD33^+$, whereas about 2,700 are $CD33^-$.

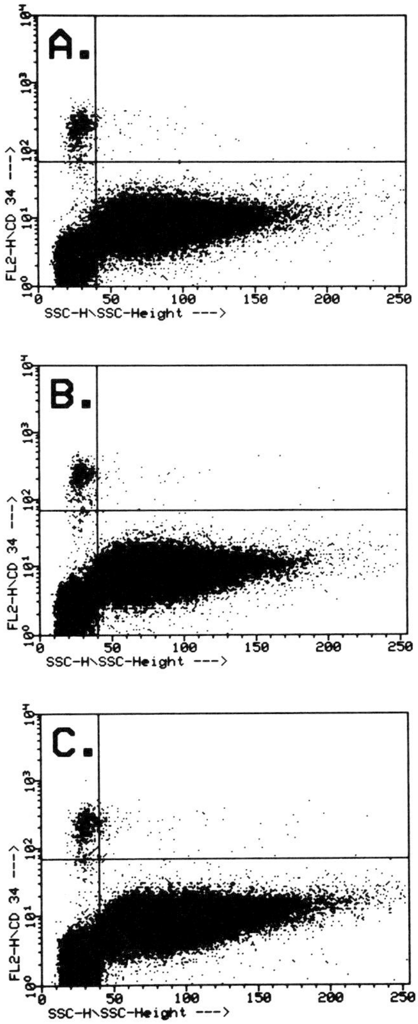

Fig. 10. EDTA-anticoagulated blood from a patient on G-CSF therapy was stained with QBEND-10-PE and processed with Opti-Lyse reagent; arbitrary rectangular live-gate on scatter parameters during data-acquisition; 5×10^4 cells per determination; dot-plot correlating CD34 expression (y axis) to sideward light scatter (x axis); all dots shown; quadrant statistics; in the upper left quadrant, cells considered as $CD34^+$ cells. A) Numbers of $CD34^+$ cells = 508 = 1.02%. B) Numbers of $CD34^+$ cells = 476 = 0.95%. C) Numbers of $CD34^+$ cells = 504 = 1.01%. Calculated CV = 3.5%. Expected CV = 4.5%.

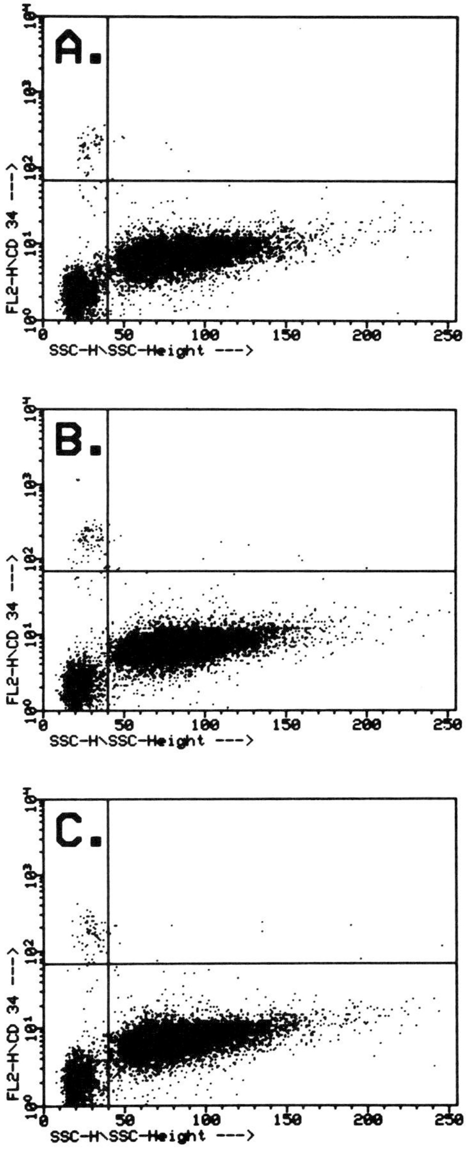

Fig. 11. EDTA-anticoagulated blood from the same subject as described in Figure 10; identical processing and identical data presentation as described in Figure 10; 6,250 cells per determination. A) Numbers of $CD34^+$ cells = 53 = 0.85%. B) Numbers of $CD34^+$ cells = 77 = 1.23%. C) Numbers of $CD34^+$ cells = 68 = 1.09%. Calculated CV = 18%. Expected CV = 12%.

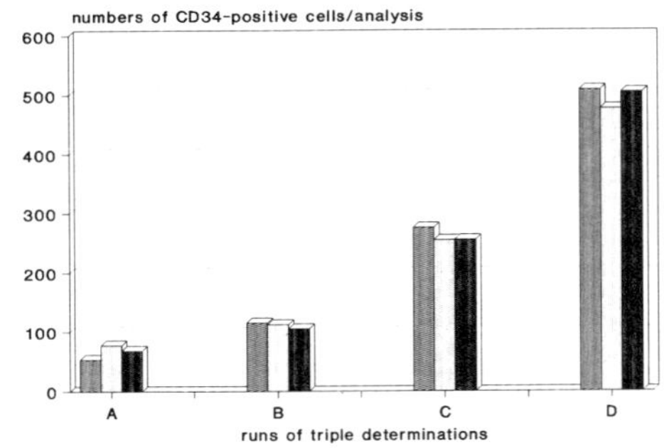

FIGURE 12 A

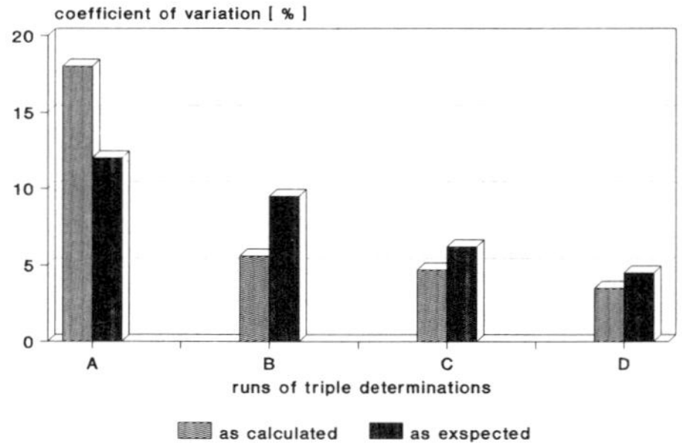

FIGURE 12 B

Fig. 12. Impact of the sample size on the CV of determinations of $CD34^+$ cells in the blood of a patient on G-CSF therapy; data were determined performing determinations on samples as described in Figures 10 and 11; included are data from triple determinations on 6,250 (A), 12,500 (B), 25,000 (C), and 50,000 (D) cells, respectively. A) Numbers of $CD34^+$ cells per determination. B) CV as calculated from the triple determinations shown in (A), and CV as expected according to the mean number of $CD34^+$ cells determined.

Figure 13C shows the quantitation of blood $CD34^+$ cells from a patient on G-CSF therapy, and the WBC of this patient is 9,000/μl. Although only about 3.45% of all $CD34^+$ cells are lacking CD33 expression (Fig. 13C), in absolute numbers, with about 91,000 $CD34^+$ cells per one ml_{blood}, in fact there are about 3,100 $CD34^+$ cells without coexpression of CD33 in the circulation of this patient.

Following the guidelines proposed by us, determinations of $CD34^+$ cells can be performed in the routine diagnostic setting with (at least) the identical reliability as characteristic of the flow cytometric determinations of any other cell subset.

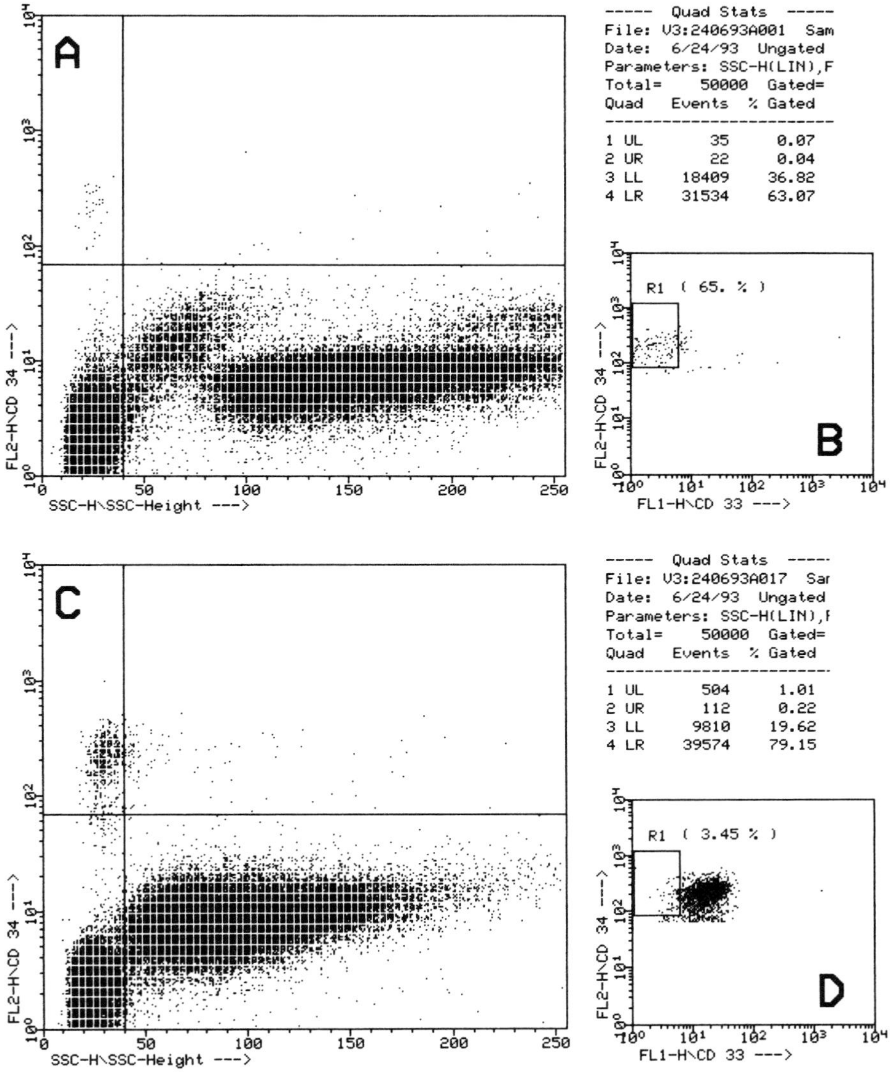

Fig. 13. EDTA-anticoagulated blood from a healthy adult subject and from a patient on G-CSF therapy was stained with QBEND-10-PE and with CD33-FITC, and red blood cells were lysed; an arbitrary rectangular live-gate was set on both scatter parameters during data-acquisition. A) Healthy subject; 5×10^4 cells; dot-plot correlating CD34 expression to sideward light scatter; upper left quadrant, $CD34^+$ cells (35 cells; 0.07%). B) Healthy subject; 200 cells; gated $CD34^+$ cells shown by dot-plot correlating CD34 expression to CD33 expression; cells in R1 are considered to be $CD33^-$ (130 cells; 65%). C) Patient on G-CSF therapy; 5×10^4 cells; dot-plot correlating CD34 expression to sideward light scatter; upper left quadrant, $CD34^+$ cells (504 cells; 1.01%). D) Patient on G-CSF therapy; 2×10^3 cells; gated $CD34^+$ cells shown by dot-plot correlating CD34 expression to CD33 expression; cells in R1 are considered to be $CD33^-$ (69 cells; 3.45%).

References

1 Terstappen LWMM, Johnson D, Mickaels RA, Chen J, Olds G, Hawkins JT, Loken MR, Levin J. Multidimensional flow cytometric blood cell differentiation without erythrocyte lysis. Blood Cells 1991;17:585-602.

2 Serke S, Huhn D. An all leukocyte whole blood lyse method for multiparameter flow cytometry. Clin Lab Haematol (in press).

3 Rümke CL. The statistically expected variability in differential leukocyte counting. In: Differential Leukocyte Counting. Koepke J, ed. College of American Pathologists: Skokie, Illinois, 1978:39-45.

4 Serke S, Huhn D. Quantification of CD34-positive cells. Blood 1992;80:1628-1629. (letter to the editor).

5 Serke S, Säuberlich S, Huhn D. Multiparameter flow cytometrical quantitation of circulating CD34-positive cells: correlation to the quantification of circulating haemopoietic progenitor cells by in vitro colony assay. Br J Haematol 1991;77:453-459.

Multicentric Determination of $CD34^+$ Cells

Hanna Sovalat,[b] *Eckart Wunder,*[b] *Robert Zimmermann,*[a] *Stefan Serke*[a]

[a]Universitätsklinikum Rudolf Virchow-Charlottenburg, Abteilung Innere Medizin und Poliklinik, Hämatologie-Onkologie, Freie Universität Berlin, Berlin, Germany; [b]Institut de Recherche en Hématologie, Hôpital du Hasenrain, Mulhouse, France

Key Words. Multiparameter flow cytometry • CD34 antibodies • Multicentric trial • FITC conjugates • PE conjugates

Introduction

Standardized determination of hemopoietic cells by means of multiparameter flow cytometry promises to be more feasible than by means of in vitro culture. Whereas the potential variables with regard to in vitro cultures are numerous, including choice of the assay method, choice of the growth factors, and finally reading of the culture dishes, in multiparameter flow cytometry they are rather limited. Major effects on the multiparameter flow cytometric determinations can be expected from the sample processing and the antibodies used.

On occasion of the second workshop on determinations of hemopoietic stem and progenitor cells held in Mulhouse, France, in May 1993, we have performed a first multicentric European trial determination of $CD34^+$ cells by multiparameter flow cytometry.

Materials and Methodology

A leukapheresis sample was prepared from a steady-state healthy adult volunteer at the Klinikum Rudolf Virchow, Freie Universität Berlin. Performing a 3 h leukapheresis on an AS104 device (Fresenius, Oberursel, Germany), a product of 400 ml with a cell count of $25 \times 10^3/\mu l$ was prepared. The sample was anticoagulated with ACD/A. Mononuclear cells were then collected by means of density gradient separation at the Mulhouse laboratory. Cells at a count of $1 \times 10^4/\mu l$ were resuspended finally in culture medium (RPMI-1640) supplemented with 10% (v/v) fetal calf serum. Aliquots of about 2 ml were distributed to any participant of the workshop asking for a sample.

Monoclonal antibodies, distributed along with the samples, were generous gifts from Becton Dickinson (France and Europe), and of Immunotech, (France). From Becton Dickinson, both the FITC and the PE conjugates of the CD34 monoclonal antibody 8G12 ("HPCA-2"), and from Immunotech, both the FITC and the PE conjugates of the CD34 monoclonal antibody QBEND10 ("IOM34")

Correspondence: Dr. Stefan Serke, Abteilung Innere Medizin und Poliklinik, Hämatologie-Onkologie, Hämatologisches Zentrallabor, Universitätsklinikum Rudolf Virchow, Freie Universität Berlin, Spandauer Damm 130, 14050 Berlin, Germany.

were provided. Both monoclonal antibodies are mouse IgG1 isotypes. Irrelevant mouse IgG1 isotypic control monoclonal antibodies (PE and FITC conjugates) were provided by Becton Dickinson.

Colleagues were kindly requested to perform determinations (staining as well as flow cytometric analysis) on the samples on the first working day after distribution of the samples. Therefore, all determinations were performed on May 10, 1993, according to the Mulhouse workshop standard protocol. (*See* footnote, p. 66).

A questionnaire was handed out along with the materials, asking for the hard copies of the determinations and asking for the data stored on floppy disks.

Results

Data were sent back to us from 22 laboratories. Viability of the cells was rather heterogeneous, and different methods of viability testing were employed. Figure 1 shows the respective data on viability.

Uniformly, arbitrary acquisition gates were set on the light scatter parameters, according to the respective instruments used. Flow cytometers from five different companies were used. Except for four determinations on less than 2×10^4 cells, all were done on $4\text{-}5 \times 10^4$ cells.

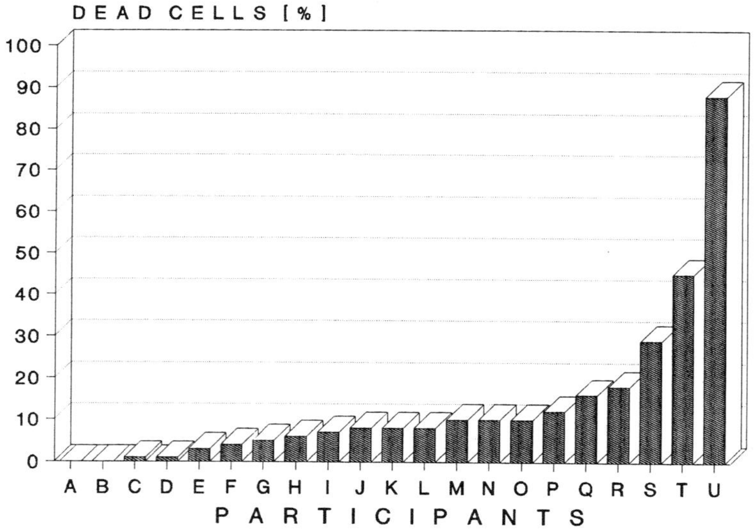

Fig. 1. Percentages of dead cells, as determined by dye-exclusion applying either microscopic or flow cytometric methods; shown are the individual percentages of dead cells as determined by each participant (A to U, participants). The last column (U) is in error. In reality 15.5% dead cells were found.

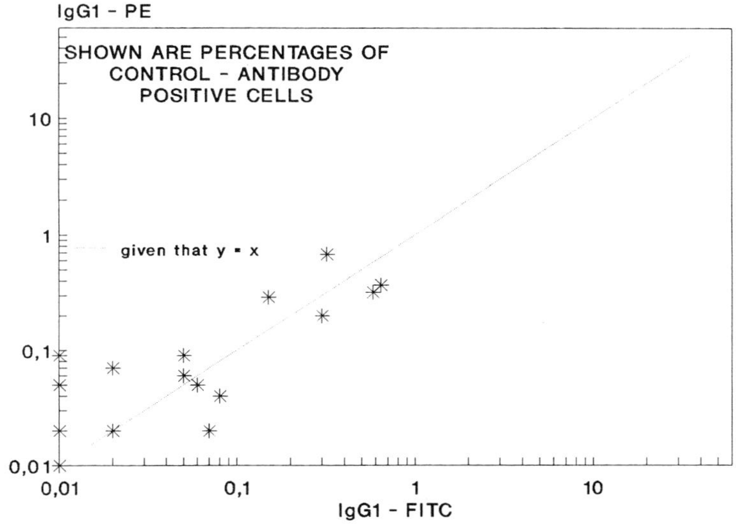

Fig. 2. Percentages of cells staining positive with FITC or with PE conjugated control monoclonal antibody; the respective percentages as determined by each single participant are plotted; x axis, percentages of control FITC positive cells, y axis, percentages of control PE positive cells.

Upon staining samples with the isotypic control antibodies, rather homogeneous results were obtained, with a small range of cells considered to be stain-positive with either the PE or the FITC conjugated control monoclonal antibody, respectively. These data are shown in Figure 2.

Results obtained with the FITC conjugates of the CD34 monoclonal antibodies disclosed major differences between the two epitope-different antibodies. While percentages of $CD34^+$ cells, as determined with 8G12-FITC, ranged from 0.00 to 1.29, this range was 0.17% to 17.8% with QBEND10-FITC. Whereas one colleague found the determination with 8G12-FITC difficult, five colleagues could not get results with QBEND10-FITC. The correlations of the percentages, as determined with the respective antibody, are shown in Figure 3A.

In contrast, determinations with the PE conjugated monoclonal antibodies were much more homogeneous. Whereas all colleagues performed determinations with 8G12-PE, only one colleague did not feel able to make the determination with QBEND10-PE. In spite of the fairly good correlation, however, percentages of $CD34^+$ cells as determined with 8G12-PE tended to be somewhat higher than those stained with QBEND10-PE (Fig. 3B). A representative determination is shown in Figure 4.

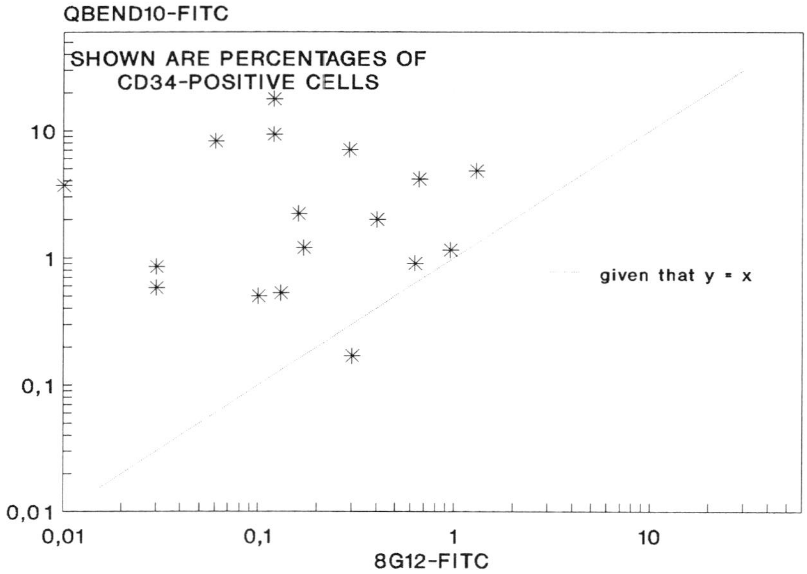

FIGURE 3 A

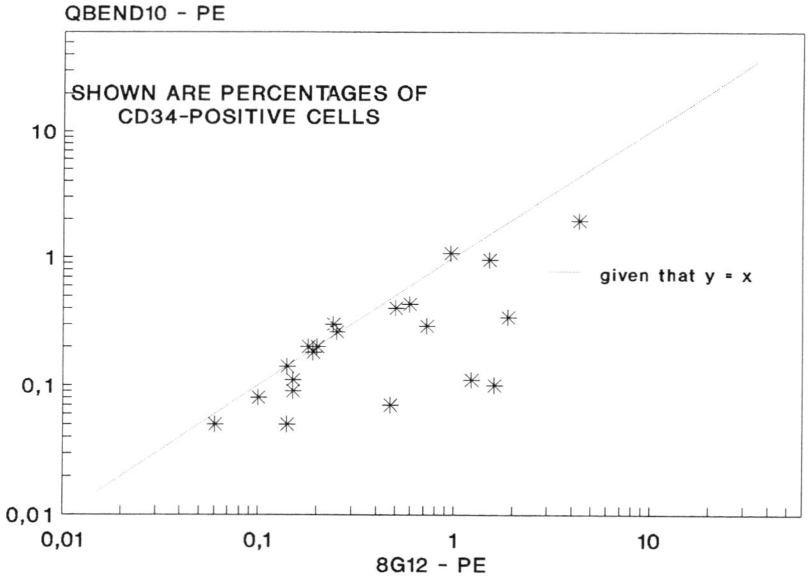

FIGURE 3 B

Fig. 3. Percentages of $CD34^+$ cells as determined with fluorochrome conjugated CD34 monoclonal antibodies; the respective percentages as determined by each single participant are plotted. A) x axis, percentages of 8G12-FITC positive cells, y axis, percentages of QBEND10-FITC positive cells; B) x axis, percentages of 8G12-PE positive cells, y axis, percentages of QBEND10-PE positive cells.

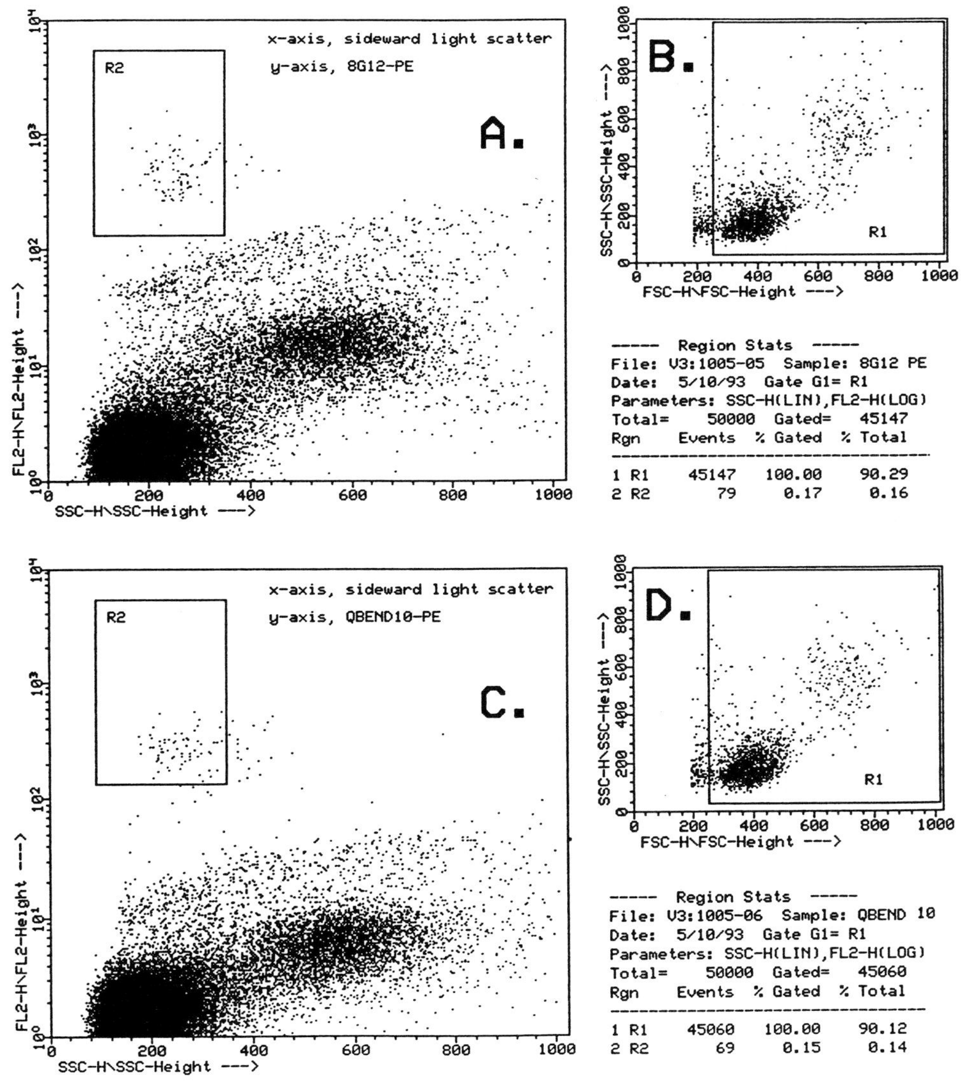

Fig. 4. Representative dot-plot depiction of the leukapheresis sample sent out; graphs were generated from list-mode data files submitted by *Dr. Eli Lien* from Dynal, Norway. A) correlation of 8G12-PE staining (y axis) and sideward light scatter (x axis), cells in R2 are considered as $CD34^+$ cells; B) correlation of sideward light scatter (y axis) and forward light scatter (x axis), events clustering into R1 are considered to be cells, and events outside R1 are considered as debris and platelets; analysis shown in (A) is performed on cells clustering into R1 only; C) correlation of QBEND10-PE staining (y axis) and sideward light scatter (x axis), cells in R2 are considered as $CD34^+$ cells; D) correlation of sideward light scatter (y axis) and forward light scatter (x axis), events clustering into R1 are considered to be cells, and events outside R1 are considered as debris and platelets; analysis shown in (C) is performed on cells clustering into R1 only.

Notably, determinations performed on the sample immediately after harvest (Berlin laboratory) had revealed the percentages of 0.24 (8G12-PE) and 0.21 (QBEND10-PE, quadruplicate determinations on 5×10^4 cells).

Discussion

Our data suggest the feasibility of multicentric determinations of $CD34^+$ cells by multiparameter flow cytometry. We had opted for a leukapheresis sample from a steady-state healthy adult to be distributed to participants for a number of reasons: a) ethical considerations do not permit harvesting the numbers of cells mandatory for this purpose from a patient; b) timing for providing the sample was highly critical; c) an unmodified, i.e., unfixed cell sample was believed to reflect the routine diagnostic setting best.

Furthermore, we have experienced extreme loss of viability in leukapheresis samples from cytokine treated patients within 24 hours, independent from the storage temperature and the count of nucleated cells; so limited viability in the distributed cell samples imitates well the condition of diagnostic cell samples at the time of measurement in clinical settings.

Clearly, the PE conjugates of both 8G12 and QBEND10 are the CD34 monoclonal antibodies of choice. Of both FITC conjugates, only the 8G12 antibody provided relatively reliable staining, while the lot of QBEND10 used at this study produced unusual amounts of nonspecific staining of monocytes.

In conclusion, we feel that consensus determinations of $CD34^+$ cells, with a percentage inferior to 0.5, are feasible. We are strongly recommending, however, the use of PE conjugated CD34 monoclonal antibodies; the efforts to further improve discrimination capacity by applying mixtures of antibodies against different CD34 epitopes promise to yield more reliable results in the future.

Note added in proof: Sovalat H, Serke S. Identification of CD 34+ Cells by Multiparameter Flow Cytometry. In: Wunder EW, Hénon PR, eds. Peripheral Blood Stem Cell Autografts. Springer Verlag Heidelberg, 1993.

Preparation of Samples for Flow Cytometric Analysis: Recommendations from the ISHAGE Course in San José

Adrian P. Gee, Lawrence S. Lamb, Jr.

Division of Transplantation Medicine, Center for Cancer Treatment and Research, Richland Memorial Hospital, University of South Carolina, Columbia, South Carolina, USA

Key Words. Flow cytometry • Progenitor cells • CD34 • Stem cells

Introduction

Quantitation of CD34+ cells in mobilized peripheral blood and bone marrow grafts is now a widely used measure of the engraftment potential of these preparations [1]. In parallel, the search for the true pluripotent hematopoietic progenitor cell has led to the subfractionation of CD34+ populations using additional antigenic markers [2]. The relative scarcity of CD34+ cells in both marrow and blood has, however, resulted in a considerable degree of uncertainty as to how samples should be prepared for flow cytometric analysis, how data analysis should be performed and the best method for reporting the results. The following is a condensed summary of recommended procedures, developed as a result of a workshop on Multidimensional Flow Cytometric Analysis of Bone Marrow and Peripheral Blood Stem Cells held in San José, California, under the direction of *Dr. Leon Terstappen,* and sponsored by the International Society for Hematotherapy and Graft Engineering [3].

General Equipment

Routine staining procedures are most easily performed in 12 × 75 mm disposable polypropylene tubes (Baxter Scientific Products; catalog # T-1280). For simplicity, these can be color coded to distinguish between controls and tests, or between various antibody staining combinations. If glass tubes are substituted, the samples will have to be transferred to plastic tubes for reading on the flow cytometer. Microtiter plates can be used in combination with automated staining and aspiration devices. Incubation of the samples is usually performed in an ice bath or refrigerator, although use of a refrigerated water bath is recommended when large numbers of samples are being processed. Centrifugation of the samples during processing can be performed using any routine laboratory centrifuge. Small (12 tube) centrifuges (e.g., Clay Adams Serofuges or the IEC Centra B centrifuges) with rotors specifically designed for 12 × 75 mm tubes and with rapid up and down times are available, but generally do not come with either sealed carriers or lid lock interfaces. Fully-automated cell washing centrifuges (e.g., the Baxter Scientific Products Dade

Correspondence: Dr. Adrian Gee, Division of Transplantation Medicine, CCTR, 7 Richland Medical Park, Columbia, SC 29203, USA.

©AlphaMed Press ISBN 1-880854 17-1

Automatic Centrifuge III or the IEC Centra-W Centrifuge), which will perform a series of programmed buffer additions, spins and supernatant decantings are ideal, however, these have limited tube capacities (12 places) and their performance should be validated to ensure good cell recovery. Manual washing is facilitated by the use of repeating dispensers (e.g., Labindustries low silhouette Repipet), and by vacuum aspiration of the supernatants. Decanting of fluid from non-fixed cell preparations should be avoided.

Sample Collection

Bone marrow consists of an extremely heterogeneous mixture of cells of all hematopoietic lineages and at all stages of maturity. This variability is compounded by the likelihood of contamination by peripheral blood during sample collection. Marrow cells obtained from cadaveric vertebral bodies or as carefully drawn aspirates represent the "purest" samples, whereas those obtained from large volume harvests may contain anywhere from 30-97% of albumin and cellular mass derived from peripheral blood [4]. In general, the larger the volume of the marrow sample, the greater the risk of contamination by blood. The level of contamination may be determined from the proportion of non-nucleated erythrocytes (which are only found in the vascular channels). These cells may be detected directly by flow cytometry [5], or indirectly by hemoglobin measurements [4]. The source of the sample, together with the methods used for collection, handling and storage may have a major influence on the quality of the data obtained. In addition, many samples are obtained from patients who have had extensive prior therapy which is reflected in the quality of their marrow, and presents an additional source of variability during immunophenotyping.

Samples should be collected into tubes containing sodium heparin (15-20 IU/ml), ACD-A tripotassium ethylenediaminetetraacetate (EDTA), or dipotassium EDTA (1.5 ± 0.25 mg/ml sample—in some applications the chelating properties of EDTA cause difficulties). Lithium heparin has been reported to distort light scatter profiles. For optimal results the sample should be processed immediately, although unfractionated samples may be kept overnight at 4°C. Storage of fractionated samples before staining is not advised.

Sample Preparation

The choice of sample preparation method should reflect the purpose for which the information is required. If $CD34^+$ cells are being enumerated to quantify engraftment potential of a marrow or peripheral stem cell preparation, then the sample preparation should parallel that of the graft, either by taking a sample of the graft itself, or by using the same fractionation procedure on a sample obtained at the time of harvest. In contrast, where patients are being monitored, it is preferable to use a method which perturbs the proportions of nucleated cells within the sample as little as possible.

This approach has resulted in two major forms of sample preparation, namely, erythrocyte lysis and "mononuclear" cell enrichment. These are summarized in the following sections.

Erythrocyte Lysis

This technique is used with the aim of debulking the sample of red cells without affecting the proportions of nucleated cells. As such, it is thought to reflect more accurately the true cellular composition of the sample. It is not suitable for studies in which $CD34^+$ cell content is to be correlated with proportions of colony-forming cells, since colony forming units (CFU) are usually measured by plating enriched mononuclear cells. Two approaches have been used based upon the sequence of lysis and staining.

Post-Lysis Staining

1 Prepare × 10 stock lysing solution

89.9 g NH_4Cl

10.0 g $KHCO_3$

370.0 mg tetrasodium EDTA

Dissolve in distilled water and bring volume to 1 liter. Adjust to pH 7.3 with 1M hydrochloric acid or sodium hydroxide. Filter through a 0.2 μm filter and dilute 1/10 with distilled water before use.

2 The sample is collected as described above.

3 A nucleated cell count is obtained, either manually by a hemacytometer count of a sample diluted in 1% aqueous acetic acid containing 0.01% aqueous gentian violet, or using an automated cell counter with appropriate precautions for analysis of bone marrow samples [6].

4 To 1 volume of the sample add 14 volumes of × 1 lysing solution and mix gently. Incubate the mixture for 3-5 minutes at ambient temperature, or until it develops a transparent red color.

5 Pellet the cells by centrifugation at 300 *g* for 5 minutes at ambient temperature. Aspirate and discard the supernatant. Resuspend the pellet in an equivalent volume of culture medium without *l*-glutamine. Centrifuge at 300 *g* for 5 minutes at 4°C.

6 Repeat Step 5 twice more. Resuspend the final pellet in the staining buffer (usually phosphate buffered saline containing 1% protein and 0.1% sodium azide).

7 Perform a manual or automated cell count (Step 3) and proceed with staining.

Pre-Lysis Staining

1 Perform Steps 2 and 3 of the Post-Lysis Staining procedure.

2 Estimate the potential number of "target" cells (cells to be positively stained) in the sample, allowing for cell losses during sample preparation.

3 Add antibody to cell sample—the exact conditions used must be determined experimentally in each laboratory to ensure that sufficient antibody is provided to saturate all of the antigenic sites. Staining is routinely performed at ambient temperature for 20-30 minutes, with occasional gentle mixing.

4 Add the lysing reagent as in Step 4 of the Post-Lysis Staining procedure.

5 Pellet and wash the cells as described in Steps 5 and 6 above. Resuspend the final pellet in buffer and analyze immediately, or resuspend in paraformaldehyde fixative (see below) and store in the dark at 4°C until analysis.

Evaluation of Erythrocyte Lysis Methods

Whole blood/marrow lysis methods are relatively fast (30-45 minutes) allowing multiple samples to be collected and analyzed during the course of a stem cell apheresis procedure. They produce minimal disruption of the proportions of nucleated cells within the sample, although minor changes have been reported [7], including losses of both granulocytes and lymphocytes, and changes in light scatter properties [8]. The pre-lysis staining method also requires estimation of target cell numbers to ensure that adequate amounts of antibody are used. This usually necessitates optimization of staining conditions by each laboratory, if a standardized procedure is to be used. The procedure can be simplified by the use of commercially available lysing solutions (available from Becton Dickinson; catalog # 30173 and Ortho Diagnostics; catalog # 770520), however some of these preparations contain fixatives, which cannot be used if the cells are also required for CFU assays, or if routine viability measurements are to be made. The efficacy of lysis also varies, in that identical treatment conditions may not always result in complete removal of erythrocytes. This can often be overcome by performing the lysis step at 37°C, or by a second treatment.

Enriched Nucleated Cell Preparations

In these procedures erythrocytes and polymorphonuclear cells are removed by centrifugation of the sample that has been layered onto a solution of defined density (usually $p = 1.077$ g/ml). This results in an interface band of highly enriched mononuclear cells, which can be aspirated, washed and stained. When larger volumes are processed for clinical applications, a two step procedure is often used, in which a buffy coat is first prepared and then separated further by density cushion centrifugation. The most commonly used separation medium is Ficoll-Hypaque [9], which is available commercially from a variety of manufacturers as a solution with a density of 1.077 g/ml (Histopaque [Sigma Chemical Co.; catalog # H8889]; Lymphopaque and Lymphoprep [Nyegaard Diagnostics]; Lymphocyte Separation Medium [Organon Teknika; catalog # 3642], etc.). Cell preparations separated using this material will generally be enriched 2-5 fold for $CD34^+$ cells, with yields in excess of 90%. Use of a density of 1.068 g/ml generally increases the recoveries of progenitor cells, with a total cell recovery of about 10% [10]. A separation procedure using Percoll [11] has also been described [12]. This technique is also useful for removing dead cells from previously frozen marrow samples, in which viabilities may be <40%—see below.

Most laboratories are familiar with these methods, and detailed instructions are also available from the manufacturers. For use with bone marrow, particular attention should be paid to not overloading the gradient and to removal of any cellular debris or spicules prior to layering the sample. Nucleated cell enrichment techniques are slower (45-60+ minutes) than erythrocyte lysis methods, but they produce excellent yields and improved purity of progenitor cells. The cell subpopulations within the preparation are not, however, representative of those in the starting sample, due to the enrichment of mononuclear cells and depletion of large granular cells and erythrocytes. If the preparation is used for CFU assays in addition to flow cytometric analysis, direct comparison between the two assays becomes possible. It is, however, difficult to then back-calculate accurately the original numbers of $CD34^+$ cells or CFU in the starting sample.

Assessment of Cell Viability

A number of methods are available for measuring the viability of cell preparations. In many immunophenotyping laboratories it is now common practice to work with fixed cell preparations, and this necessitates developing a different approach to viability measurements. LDS-751 is a nucleic acid stain which can be added to paraformaldehyde-fixed cells and incubated overnight. The stain is excited by 488 nm light and emits at 670 nm, which allows it to be used in combination with fluorescein isothiocyanate (FITC) and phycoerythrin (PE) conjugated monoclonals. The staining pattern distinguishes three classes of cells a) intensively stained—cells damaged at the time of fixation; b) intermediate stained—intact cells; and c) unstained—platelets and red cells [13]. Staining is performed as follows:

1 Stock stain solution: dissolve 0.2 mg LDS 751 stain (Exciton, Dayton, OH; catalog #07510) in 1 ml methanol.

2 Prepare the working solution by adding 500 μl stock solution to 49.5 ml phosphate-buffered saline containing 0.1% sodium azide.

3 Add 10 μl of the working stock to 1 ml paraformaldehyde fixed stained cell suspension. Store in the dark at 4°C and analyze within 1 week.

Where unfixed preparations are used, viability may be determined using vital stains such as trypan blue or eosin. These may either be purchased in solution or prepared by mixing 4 parts of 0.2% w/v aqueous trypan blue solution with 1 part 4.25% w/v aqueous sodium chloride. An aliquot of the stain solution is mixed with a sample of the cells, incubated at ambient temperature for about 5 minutes and examined in a hemacytometer. The stain is excluded by viable cells, whereas dead cells stain blue.

An alternative technique is to use propidium iodide (PI) to stain dead and dying cells [13]. PI is excited at 488 or 605 nm and emits light at >603 nm which is detectable in the PE/Texas Red range. This method can therefore be used in combination with FITC-stained cells, but not with PE or Texas Red conjugates.

1 Stock stain solution: dissolve 50 μg propidium iodide in 1 ml phosphate-buffered saline. Note that PI is a potent carcinogen and should be handled with care.

2 Immediately before analysis, add 10 μl of the stain to unstained cells and the positive staining control for FITC.

3 Set gates to ensure clear discrimination between brightly stained dead cells (FL2), while capturing all FITC-stained cells (FL1).

4 Dying cells may exclude the stain, but can generally be gated out based on a combination of their light scatter properties and their non-specific binding of the test monoclonal antibodies and controls.

Recovery of Viable Cells from Cryopreserved Marrow

In some cases it is necessary to work with samples of frozen bone marrow. This often results in technical problems since the material will tend to gel upon handling, due to release of DNA from lysed cells. Rapid thawing and slow dilution of the sample often help, as does inclusion of 0.1-0.2 U/ml Staph. Micrococcal Nuclease (Sigma) in the medium. *Dr. Terry Thomas* of the Terry Fox Laboratories in Vancouver, Canada, has also developed a procedure for removing dead cells by centrifugation on Percoll [11].

1 Prepare stock Percoll by adding 1 part of × 10 buffered saline to 10 parts Percoll (Pharmacia, Upsala, Sweden). Adjust the pH to 7.4 ± 0.05 with 1M hydrochloric acid. Measure the density of the stock and store at ambient temperature.

2 Thaw the cells quickly, and dilute the sample slowly with medium.

3 Wash once, and then incubate the cells for 4 hours at 37°C or overnight at 4°C. Allow the cells to reach ambient temperature.

4 Add the stock Percoll to cells to obtain a final density of 1.045 g/ml – see sample calculation:

$$\text{Volume of stock} = \frac{1.045 - \text{density of medium } (1.010)}{\text{Density of stock} - 1.045} \times \text{Volume of Medium}$$

For 5 ml of cells and a Percoll stock of 1.0677 g/ml

$$\text{Volume of stock} = \frac{1.045 - 1.010 \times 5 \text{ ml}}{1.0677 - 1.045} = 7.71 \text{ ml}$$

5 Mix and overlay with 0.5 ml medium.

6 Centrifuge at 1400 *g* for 30 minutes at ambient temperature.

7 Recover cells in pellet and resuspend in medium.

In a summary of eight separations the percent recovery of $CD34^+$ cells was 105 ± 8.6% and the proportion of dead cells removed was 96 ± 1.4% (*Thomas*, personal communication).

Staining Methods

For enumeration of progenitor cell populations a direct staining method, in which fluorescently tagged monoclonal antibodies are used, should always be chosen in preference to an indirect method. This technique is faster and the background is substantially lower, since a secondary antibody is not required. Each laboratory should optimize staining conditions; the following is a standardized procedure.

1 Adjust the cell concentration to 1×10^7/ml in phosphate-buffered saline containing 1% bovine serum albumin (or 2% heat inactivated fetal bovine serum) and 0.1% sodium azide. The cell viability should be at least 90%.

2 Remove any aggregates from the fluorescently tagged antibody by centrifugation at 10,000 *g* for 5-10 minutes immediately before use.

3 Add 100 μl cell suspension to the optimal volume of test monoclonal antibody (this should be specified by the supplier, or may be determined experimentally by titration). Mix and incubate for 20-30 minutes at 4°C (or on ice) in the dark.

4 Wash the cells by addition of 2 ml cold buffer, followed by centrifugation at ~300 *g* for 5 minutes at 4°C and aspiration of the supernatant.

5 Resuspend the cell pellet by gentle vortexing, and add buffer if the sample is to be analyzed immediately, otherwise add fixative and store at 4°C in the dark.

Indirect Staining

1 Stain with unconjugated primary antibody as described above (Steps 1-3 for Direct Staining).

2 Remove any aggregates from the fluorescently tagged secondary antibody by centrifugation at 10,000 *g* for 5-10 minutes immediately before use.

3 Dilute the secondary antibody to the optimal concentration (as determined by the manufacturer or by prior titration).

4 Add the required volume of the secondary antibody to the resuspended cell pellet. Mix gently and incubate for 20-30 minutes at 4°C (or on ice) in the dark.

5 Follow Steps 4 and 5 of the Direct Staining procedure.

Controls

Appropriate controls must always be included to allow correct interpretation of staining patterns. These should include monoclonals to aid in identifying cell subpopulations within the sample e.g., anti-CD45 and anti-CD14, etc., in addition to isotype controls (available in conjugated and unconjugated forms from most monoclonal antibody suppliers), secondary antibodies alone (and in combination with isotype controls), viability controls and unstained cells. Other controls that must be considered pertain to the set-up and performance of the flow cytometer [14]. Daily calibrations and service records should be documented, and performance may be validated using commercially available pre-stained fixed blood cells e.g., CD Chex—Immunology Control for Cluster Determination—Human Source Fixed Nucleated Cells (Streck Laboratories; catalog # 213205). Where data is provided for clinical applications, both hard copies and electronic storage systems should be available.

Non-Specific Staining

Use of a direct staining procedure minimizes the problem of non-specific staining. If difficulties persist $F(ab')_2$ conjugates can be used to avoid binding via the Fc receptor. If the monoclonal is not available in this form, non-specific binding may be reduced by pre-incubating the cells in 1/5 to 1/10 dilution of normal rabbit serum.

Fixation of Samples

To reduce the risk of infection from samples it is advisable to work with fixed preparations whenever possible. Some erythrocyte lysing solutions contain fixative. Stained mononuclear cells may be fixed using the following procedure [15], and stored at 4°C in the dark for at least three days prior to analysis.

1 Prepare stock 2% w/v paraformaldehyde solution by adding 2 g paraformaldehyde (Mallinckrodt or Eastman Kodak) to 100 ml phosphate-buffered saline containing 0.1% sodium azide. Dissolve by heating in a 56°C water bath for up to an hour.

2 Cool solution to ambient temperature and bring pH to 7.4 using 0.1M sodium hydroxide or hydrochloric acid. Store at 4°C.

3 Prepare working solution by adding 10 ml 2% stock solution to 30 ml phosphate-buffered saline. Store at 4°C and use within a week.

4 Add 0.3-1.0 ml cold fixative solution to resuspended stained cell pellet and vortex immediately. The suspension can be stored at 4°C for at least 3 days before analysis.

Analysis of $CD34^+$ Cells

Methods for the detailed analysis of $CD34^+$ cells are discussed elsewhere in this volume. In spite of remaining controversies, a general consensus seems to be emerging both in the United States and Europe [3, 8, 16].

1 Erythrocyte lysis techniques should be used for cell preparation. These methods are rapid and produce minimal distortions in the proportions of nucleated cells. A single treatment may not, however, result in lysis of all red cells in the sample. Results obtained using erythrocyte lysed marrow, machine-prepared buffy coat cells, machine-prepared Ficoll-Hypaque cells and manually-prepared Ficoll-Hypaque cells are shown in Figure 1.

2 Direct staining is preferred over indirect techniques, and many FITC and PE conjugated anti-CD34 monoclonal antibodies are now commercially available [17]. In general, PE conjugates provide optimal discrimination of the stained populations. Figure 1 shows anti-CD34 staining using different antibody conjugates on the same bone marrow preparations.

3 The choice of controls is critical to ensure correct interpretation of the data, particularly when the aim is analysis of $CD34^+$ cell subsets.

Cytometer calibration and performance should be documented [14].

4 For simple $CD34^+$ cell analysis, fluorescence should be plotted on the ordinate versus orthogonal light scatter on the abscissa. $CD34^+$ progenitors are discriminated as a discrete population with low side scatter and with positive fluorescence. In some cases, the staining intensity may be such that the population "smears" into the non-stained area, making it difficult to set a region. Under these circumstances, improved definition may be achieved by the use of several anti-CD34 monoclonals conjugated to different fluorochromes, and directed toward different epitopes on the CD34 antigen.

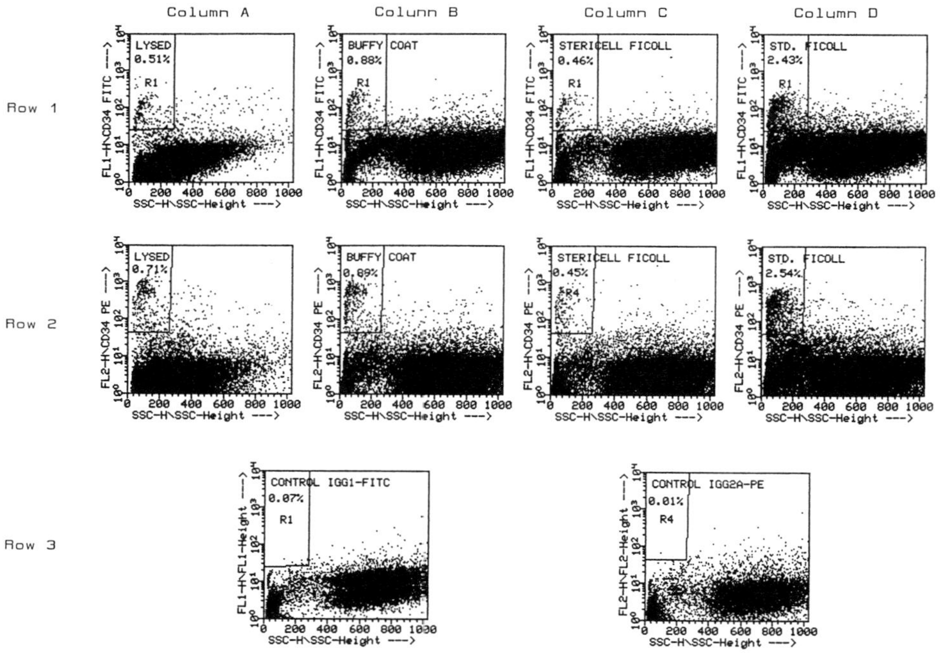

Fig. 1 Staining of nucleated bone marrow cell preparations using anti-CD34 conjugates. Enriched nucleated cells were prepared from the same bone marrow by erythrocyte lysis using the Becton Dickinson (B-D) lysing solution (Column A); by buffy coat preparation on a Terumo Stericell cell processor (Column B); by automated Ficoll-Hypaque density cushion centrifugation of the buffy coat preparation (Column C); and by manual Ficoll-Hypaque separation of whole marrow (Column D). Each sample was stained with anti CD34-FITC (Row 1) or anti-CD34-PE (Row 2) obtained from B-D. Fifty thousand ungated events were collected on a calibrated FACSort flow cytometer (B-D) and analyzed using Lysys II software (B-D). Cells were gated for positive expression of CD45 prior to analysis for CD34 expression. Values shown are the percentage of positively stained cells in the region drawn. Controls are shown (Row 3) for only the Ficoll-Hypaque separated cells.

5 $CD34^+$ cells may be quantitated as a percentage of a) total events; b) nucleated cells—as determined by light scatter properties; or c) leukocytes—as determined by anti-CD45 staining. In our hands, the last format provides more reliable, reproducible, comparative data.

6 $CD34^+$ subset analysis is most reliably undertaken by multidimensional analysis, as described previously [2]. It is in this area that the greatest variability between investigators is usually seen.

7 Automated CD34 analysis software is likely to be available in the near future. This will facilitate direct comparison of data generated at different centers by providing a standardized procedure for analysis.

Acknowledgments

This paper is based in part on a course run by The International Society for Hematotherapy & Graft Engineering.

References

1 Bender JG, To LB, Williams S, Schwartzberg LS. Defining a therapeutic dose of peripheral blood stem cells. J Hematotherapy 1992;1:329-342.

2 Terstappen LWMM. Assessment of hematopoietic cell differentiation by multidimensional flow cytometry. J Hematotherapy 1993;2 (in press).

3 Multidimensional flow cytometric analysis of bone marrow and peripheral blood stem cells. J Hematotherapy 1993;2(in press).

4 Holdrinet RS, von Egmond J, Wessels JM, Haanen C. A method for quantification of peripheral blood admixture in bone marrow aspirates. Exp Hematol 1980;8:103-111.

5 Terstappen LWMM, Levin J. Bone marrow cell differential counts obtained by multidimensional flow cytometry. Blood Cells 1992;18:311-330.

6 Read EJ, Carter CS. Enumeration of cells in bone marrow and peripheral blood stem cell collections: technical issues and prospects for standardization. J Hematotherapy 1992;1:175-182.

7 Fritsch G, Emminger W, Buchinger P, Printz D, Gadner H. CD-34 positive cell proportions in peripheral blood correlate with colony forming capacity. Exp Hematol 1991;19:1079-1083.

8 Wunder E, Sovalat H, Fritsch G, Silvestri F, Hénon P, Serke S. Report on the European workshop on peripheral blood stem cell determination and standardization. J Hematotherapy 1992;1;131-142.

9 Böyum A. Isolation of mononuclear cells and granulocytes from human blood. Scand J Clin Lab Invest 1968;21:77-89.

10 Sutherland HJ, Eaves CJ, Eaves AC, Dragowska W, Lansdorp PM. Characterization and partial purification of human marrow cells capable of initiating long term hemopoiesis in vitro. Blood 1989;74:1563-1570.

11 Thomas TE, Abraham SJR, Phillips GL, Lansdorp PM. A simple procedure for large scale density gradient separation of bone marrow cells for transplantation. Transplantation 1992;53:1163-1165.

12 Terstappen LWMM, Loken MR. Five dimensional flow cytometry as a new approach for blood and bone marrow differentials. Cytometry 1988;9:548-556.

13 Current protocols in immunology—Cytometry analysis using FACScan. In: Coligan J, Kruisbeer A, Margulies D, Shevach E, eds. New York, New York: John Wiley and Sons, 1992.

14 Recktenwald D. Introduction to flow cytometry, principles, fluorochromes, instrument setup and calibration. J Hematotherapy 1993;2 (in press).

15 Lanier LL, Warner NL. Paraformaldehyde fixation of hematopoietic cells for quantitative flow cytometry (FACS) analysis. J Immunol Methods 1981;47:25-30.

16 Bender J. Flow cytometric analysis of peripheral blood stem cells. J Hematotherapy 1993;2 (in press).

17 Linscott's directory of immunological and biological reagents. 7th ed. Linscott's Directory, Santa Rosa, California. 1992.

Quantitative Expression of P-Glycoprotein Encoded by a Multidrug-Resistant Gene (MDR1) on Human CD34+ Cells

Hanna Sovalat

Institut de Recherche en Hématologie et Transfusion, Hôpital du Hasenrain, Mulhouse, France

Key Words. $CD34^+$ cells and subsets • P-gp 170 expression • Quantitative immunofluorescence • Bone marrow • Umbilical cord blood • Mobilized and steady state peripheral blood

Introduction

Isolation and characterization of pluripotent stem cells is a major goal of research in hematopoiesis. Human hematopoietic cells have been characterized by expression of several surface antigens. The surface marker associated with human immature blood cells is the CD34 antigen [1]. CD34 expression is found in stem cells, precursor cells and in progenitor cells proliferating in short- and long-term cultures. The latter, long-term culture-initiating cells (LTC-IC), express CD34 at high level and have been shown to be $CD33^-HLA\text{-}DR^{low}$ [2, 3] or $CD34^{++}CD38^-lin^-$ [4]. A further characteristic property of earlier immature hematopoietic cells being frequently used for their identification is their low staining with the fluorescent dye rhodamine-123 (Rh 123). In the mouse model, the Rh 123^{dull} cell population is enriched for marrow repopulating cells [5] and for LTC-IC [6].

Rh 123 is a substrate of a membrane pump consisting of the so-called P-glycoprotein (P-gp, molecular weight 170 kD), which is the product of the multidrug resistance gene 1 (MDR1). This gene has originally been identified in leukemia cells having acquired resistance against several cytostatic drugs [7]. *Chaudhary* and *Roninson* [8] showed that P-gp is expressed in all progenitors found in normal human bone marrow and most intensely in LTC-IC. *Drach et al.* [9] have studied levels of MDR1-mRNA by the polymerase chain reaction (PCR) in human marrow cells. They detect them in total $CD34^+$ cells as well as in myeloid progenitors ($CD34^+CD33^+$), while there is insignificant expression in $CD34^-CD33^+$ cells and no detectable expression in monocytes ($CD34^-CD33^{++}$).

In view of analyzing and comparing $CD34^+$ cells of different origin, enumeration of the frequency of $CD34^+$P-gp^+ cells and average numbers of P-gp antigenic sites on the cell surface of the respective cell populations appears worthwhile. To this end, cells are specifically marked with an anti-P-gp monoclonal antibody (MAb) stemming from mice, followed by binding of a

---

Correspondence: Hanna Sovalat, Institut de Recherche en Hématologie et Transfusion, Hôpital du Hasenrain, 87 Avenue d'Altkirch, 68051 Mulhouse, France.

 ISBN 1-880854 17-1

second anti-mouse antibody which is carrying the fluorescent dye. For distinguishing $CD34^+$ cells from mature cells being present in natural cell populations, these cells are identified by an anti-CD34 MAb stained with a different fluorescent dye, and an evaluation of their degree of maturation should be possible by measuring the degree of P-gp expression.

Materials and Methods

P-gp expression can be tested on $CD34^+$ cells by cytofluorimetry in any kind of hematopoietic cell population: in bone marrow in steady state or regeneration after transplantation, in cytapheresis products after mobilizing treatments and even in the rare immature cells circulating in peripheral blood of adults or in the more frequent ones in umbilical cord blood from newborns.

For testing the anti-P-gp MAb and the quantitative evaluation, it is useful to apply test cell lines. The well-growing human multiple myeloma cell line 8226/S does not express P-gp and is sensitive to doxorubicin, while two available sublines are resistant to different concentrations of this cytostatic drug: 8226/DOX6 and 8226/DOX 40 support 6 mg/ml and 40 mg/ml doxorubicin and carry low or high amounts of P-gp 170 [10].

Cell Preparation

MNC fractions are prepared from bone marrow aspirates or cytapheresis products in the usual way by density gradient centrifugation over Lymphoprep (density 1.077 g/ml; Flobio, France) at 20°C, 800 *g*, 20 min washed twice in RPMI 1640 (Eurobio, France), resuspended at 1×10^7 cells/ml in RPMI 1640 containing 2% fetal calf serum (FCS) and kept on melting ice until labeling with MAb.

The test cell lines—which are cultured in RPMI 1640 containing 10% FCS, 1% penicillin, 1% streptomycin, and 1% L-glutamine at 37° in humidified 5% CO_2—are washed twice in RPMI 1640, adjusted to 10^7 cells/ml in RPMI 1640 containing 2% of FCS and kept on melting ice until labeling with MAb in the same way.

Labeling with Anti-P-gp and Anti-CD34 MAbs

MI66 (IgG2a isotype) MAb against P-gp was developed by *Dr. Cianfriglia* (Istituto di Sanita, Roma), and kindly provided by *Dr. Lohri* (Kantonsspital, Basel).

The cells are stained at three steps: two steps for indirect immunofluorescence and one for direct staining. First, 100 μl of cell suspension containing 10^6 cells are pipetted in a round bottom plastic tube (5 ml, f.expl. Falcon) and put on an ice bath. 50 μl of M166 MAb at saturating concentration (at beginning of plateau of saturation, as tested before by titration) are added and mixed briefly on a Vortex, placed on the ice bath and covered for protection against light. After incubation for 45 min, two washes with phosphate-buffered saline (PBS) containing 2% v/v FSC are made. Second, cells are incubated for 45 min with 100 μl of fluorescein isothiocyanate (FITC)-conjugated $F(ab')_2$ fragment of sheep anti-mouse IgG (Silenus, Eurobio, France) diluted 1:100 in PBS with 2% FSC, washed twice in PBS with 2% FSC and then mouse IgG (40 μg) is added to block any free reactive sites on the secondary antibody. Third, 20 μl of phycoerythrin (PE)-conjugated anti-CD34 MAb (IgG1 isotype, HPCA-2, Becton Dickinson, France) are added for 45 min. Appropriate isotype control antibodies are prepared in parallel. Cells labeled with individual antibodies: HPCA-2 PE and M166 plus FITC-$F(ab')_2$ anti-mouse IgG are used to set the optimal voltage and electrical compensation of the spectral overlap between green and red fluorescence on the flow cytometer. Cells are maintained at 4°C during all steps of antibody labeling, including centrifugation. All MAbs are used at saturating dose.

Technique of Quantitative Indirect Immunofluorescence (QIIF)

Poncelet et al. [11, 12] have demonstrated a linear correlation between mean fluorescence intensity and average number of MAb molecules being bound. A series of beads carrying a precisely defined amount of anti-CD5 MAb (ST1, IgG2a isotype) serve to construct a standard-curve relating the net mean fluorescence intensity measured by flow cytometer to the mean number of anti-CD5 MAb molecules per bead.

Working Protocol

The series of beads carries anti-CD5 MAb at eight different densities (QIFIKIT, Biocytex, France). In the lot used here, the number of anti-CD5 MAb molecules bound to the surface of beads varies between zero for tube A and 6.6×10^5 for tube H. 100 μl of each bead suspension are incubated for 45 min with 100 μl of FITC-conjugated $F(ab')_2$ fragment of sheep anti-mouse IgG diluted (1:100) with 2% of FSC in PBS. The beads are maintained on ice water and protected from light. After two washes in PBS with 2% FSC, the beads are resuspended with 500 μl of PBS with 2% FSC. The experimental conditions (incubation-time, second-step reagent) are the same for all cells including the test lines and the beads.

Flow Cytometric Analysis

The analysis can be done with any common cytofluorimeter and does not depend on a specific software. The details are given here for the FACStar (Becton Dickinson, Mountain View, CA) equipped with an argon laser (Coherent, France) operated at 488 nm and 250 mW, and green (FITC) and red (PE) fluorescence is detected by 530/30 nm and 585/40 nm bandpass filters. Spectral

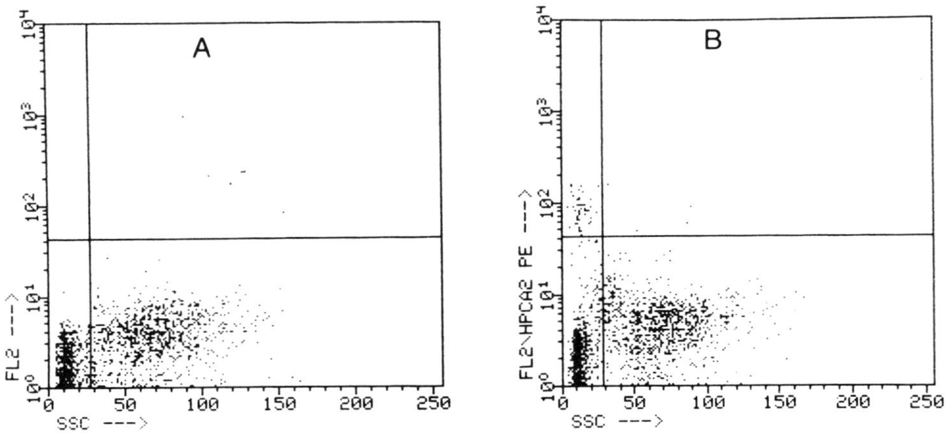

Fig. 1. Cytograms displaying the side scatter (x-axis) versus red fluorescence intensity (y-axis) of normal human bone marrow MNC. A) Staining with IgG1-control antibody coupled to PE, 50×10^3 MNC per determination. 5×10^3 cells are shown. No cells in the lymphocyte region show staining with this control antibody (upper left quadrant); B) Direct staining with PE-conjugated HPCA-2 MAb. 50×10^3 MNC per determination; 5×10^3 cells are shown. The cells in the upper left quadrant are considered $CD34^+$ cells.

overlap between green and red fluorescence is electronically compensated (see below). Data acquisition and analysis are performed with Consort 30 software (B-D). Forward scatter (FSC) and side scatter (SSC) are collected using linear scale, and fluorescence signals are collected on logarithmic scale. The cells, test cell lines and immunostained calibration beads are analyzed during the same experiment and with the same tension of PMT of fluorescence. Average fluorescence intensity per cell is calculated automatically after relinearization of the data by the program. Data acquisition is made on 5×10^4 mononuclear cells (MNC) after elimination of dead cells and debris by an FSC/SSC gate.

Fluorescence analysis of beads is guided by a gate set according to their FSC and SSC. The $CD34^+$ cells are defined by gating according to SSC and red fluorescence intensity: cells with SSC like lymphocytes and red fluorescence above isotype control are considered $CD34^+$ cells (Fig. 1) and acquisition narrows down on $CD34^+$ cells (Fig. 2). The acquisition of the cells incubated with only the second FITC-conjugated MAb and/or anti CD34 MAb is done the same way.

Evaluation of QIIF

Fluorescent beads

Corrected mean intensity is calculated from flow cytometer histograms for each sample of beads (100% of population) (Fig. 3a) according to the following formulas:

$$\overline{m} = \left[\sum_{i=a}^{i=b} i \times n_i \Big/ \sum_{i=a}^{i=b} n_i \right] \quad \text{and} \quad m_c \equiv \overline{m} - \overline{m}_0$$

where i = channel number; b = number of channel of histogram; n_i= number of events in channel i; m_c = corrected mean fluorescence; m_0 = mean fluorescence of the negative control [12]. As negative control, beads A (without anti-CD5 MAb) are incubated with a second fluorescent antibody. The values obtained are plotted against the number of anti-CD5 MAb molecules bound per bead. (QIIF standard-curve Fig. 3b). The linear regression is calculated with Cricket Graph (Computer Associates) software.

Cells

The mean fluorescence intensity as assessed from 10^4 acquired $CD34^+$ cells indicates the average amount of P-gp expression on $CD34^+$ cells and is calculated from the histogram according to the formula indicated above. Control histograms are obtained by fluorescent second antibody and/or anti-CD34 MAb. The mean intensity of the controls is subtracted. The equation of the linear regression curve as determined on the beads is used to calculate, from the mean fluorescence intensity value, the mean number of anti P-gp MAb molecules bound per CD34 positive cell (Fig. 4).

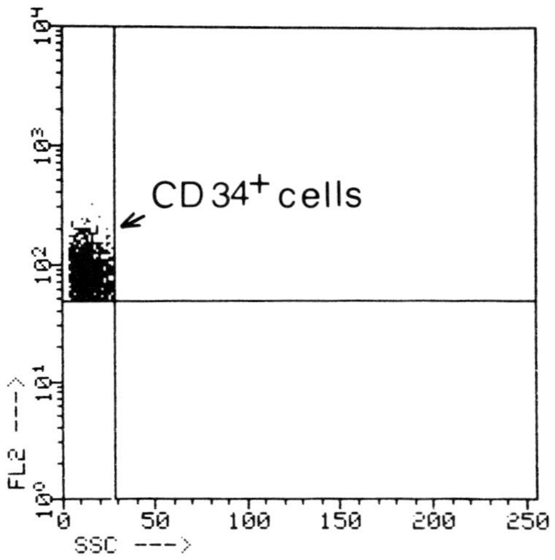

Fig. 2. Cytogram displaying side scatter (x-axis) versus red fluorescence intensity (y-axis) of human bone marrow $CD34^+$ cells; 10^4 gated $CD34^+$ cells per determination; all cells are shown.

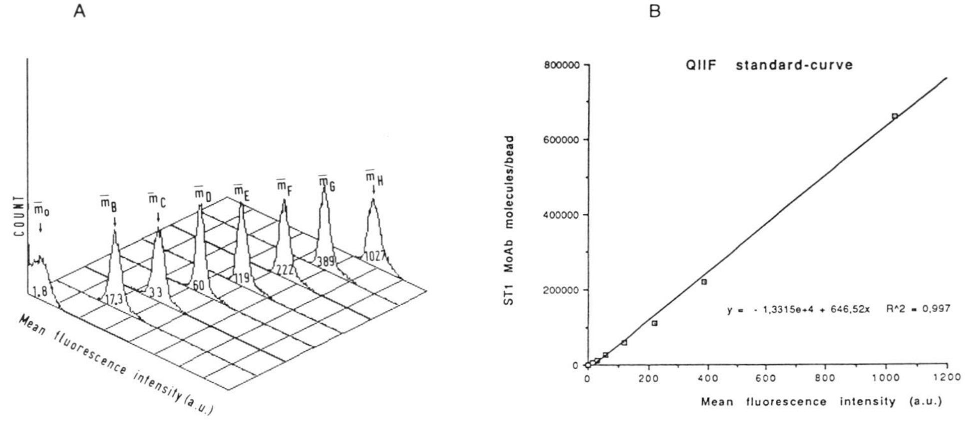

Fig. 3. Data processing for quantification by indirect immunofluorescence. Eight preparations of beads with a stable and precisely defined amount of MAb ST1 (from zero to 6.6 × 10^5) were used to construct the standard curve. A) Histograms of mean fluorescence intensities (arbitrary units) from eight preparations of beads (A-H) incubated with FITC conjugated F $(ab')_2$ fragment of sheep anti-mouse IgG. B) QIIF standard-curve for correlation between the mean number of anti-CD5 MAb molecules and the corrected mean intensity of fluorescence.

Results

By means of double staining and QIIF methods at the same time, the frequency of CD34⁺P-gp⁺ cells as well as the degree of their expression of P-gp can

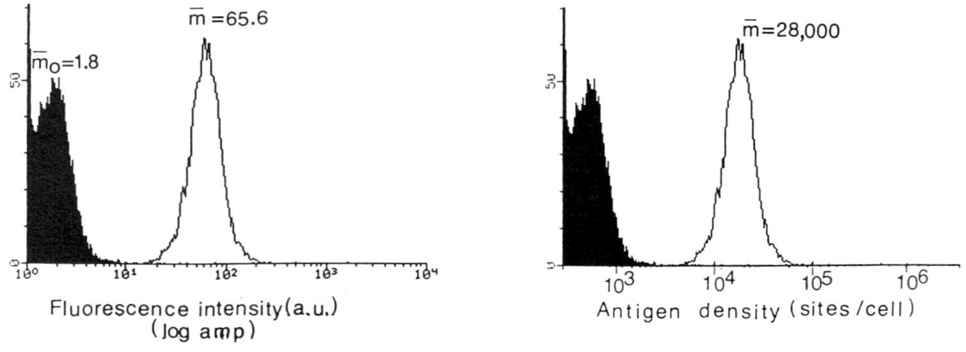

Fig. 4. Analysis of antigen density of P-gp on $CD34^+$ cells in normal bone marrow. The mean fluorescence intensity of negative control cells (incubated with HPCA-2-PE and FITC-F $(ab')_2$ fragment of sheep anti-mouse IgG), and of the $CD34^+P\text{-}gp^+$ cells (incubated with M166 anti-P-gp MAb plus FITC-F $(ab')_2$ anti-mouse IgG and HPCA-2-PE) is positioned. By use of linear regression as determined on the beads, the fluorescence intensity expressed in arbitrary units can be replaced by the antigen density expressed as number of M166 MAb molecules being bound per cell.

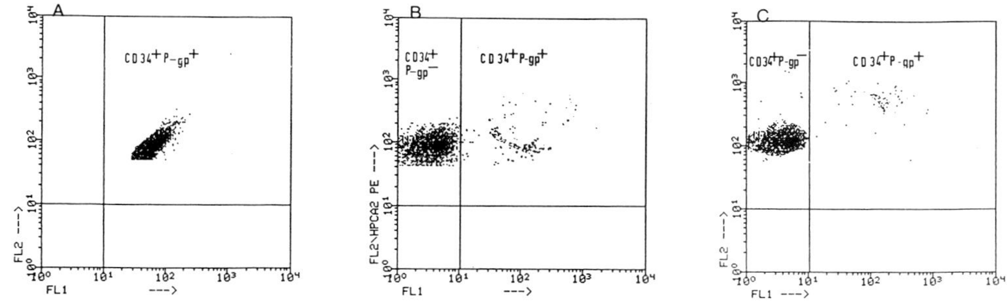

Fig. 5. Determination of P-gp positive subset cells among CD34⁺ cells in different cellular materials. A) bone marrow, B) cytapheresis product and C) peripheral blood in steady state.

be determined in different cellular materials (Fig. 5). Examples are given in Table I.

Discussion

By application of this technique the primary results—given as a histogram of frequency of events with arbitrary intensities of fluorescence on channel zero to 255 of the display—can be processed for obtaining the absolute number of bound antigenic sites per cell. Accordingly, antigen density can be determined for defined subsets of the $CD34^+$ cell population. In the given examples with small frequencies of $CD34^+$ cells (0.10 – 2.08% of MNC), there are in fact P-gp expressing subsets, and the average intensity of expression can be quantified. For obtaining these results on a complete MNC fraction, certain strategic points must be underlined:

1. Acquisition narrows down on $CD34^+$ cells, which are defined by electronic gating. In order to get statistical significance, independent from $CD34^+$ cell frequency in individual samples, sufficient numbers of MNC should be processed for allowing acquisition of a standard number of 10^4 $CD34^+$ cells.
2. The number of beads acquired should be on the same order as the number of $CD34^+$ cells analyzed.
3. In the negative controls, appropriate cell numbers should be measured for safely determining the background, including calculation of the numbers of molecules bound corresponding to this fluorescence.
4. The same batch of FITC-conjugated second antibody should be used throughout a study.
5. All experimental conditions should be identical for the beads and cells being tested.
6. All MAbs need to be used at saturation concentration (see above), since in such condition binding of MAbs is mainly monovalent.

Table I. Frequency of $CD34^+$P-gp^+ cells and degree of their expression of P-gp in different cellular materials

material	$CD34^+$ cells % of MNC	P-gp^+ cells % of $CD34^+$ cells (determined in 10^4 $CD34^+$ cells)	P-gp antigen density on $CD34^+$ cells[a] [× 10^3]
Cytapheresis product (samples taken from two patients)	1) 1.65 2) 0.37	1 5	133 89
Peripheral blood in steady state	0.10	2	85
Bone marrow in steady state	2.08	100	28
Bone marrow seven months after PBSCT	0.51	21.7	600
Umbilical Cord blood at birth	0.70	0	0
Test cell lines			
8226/S			1
8226/ DOX6			26
8226/ DOX40			110

[a]Expressed as mean number of antibody molecule bound/cell

Provided these points are considered, results produced in consecutive analyses and in different laboratories should be comparable. The results given here result from unselected volunteers. For determining ranges of variation, an extension of the data base is necessary. It is of note, however, that large differences are encountered in cells from different origins: while in normal bone marrow the majority of $CD34^+$ cells are P-gp positive, their antigen density is on average three times lower than in the mobilized $CD34^+$P-gp^+ cells, which constitute only 5% of all hematopoietic cells in cytapheresis products. The cut-off corresponds to 10^3 molecules/cell, which is equivalent in negative controls and in the parental cytostatic sensitive line 8226/S. Furthermore it should be pointed out, that there is no gradual transition from P-gp positive expression to non-expression. Cells may express P-gp strongly or moderately, but in any case this is well distinguished from non-expressing cells.

References

1 Civin CI, Strauss LC, Brovall C, Fackler MJ, Schwartz JF, Shaper JH. Antigenic analysis of hematopoiesis. III. A hematopoietic progenitor cell surface antigen defined by a monoclonal antibody raised against KG-1a cells. J Immunol 1984;133:157-165.

2 Sutherland HJ, Eaves CJ, Eaves AC, Dragowska W, Lansdorp PM. Characterization and partial purification of human marrow cells capable of initiating long-term hemopoiesis in vitro. Blood 1989;74:1563-1570.

3 Andrews RG, Singer JW, Bernstein ID. Precursors of colony-forming cells in humans can be distinguished from colony-forming cells by expression of the CD33 and CD34 antigens and their light scatter properties. J Exp Med 1989;169:1721-1731.

4 Terstappen LWMM, Huang S, Safford M, Lansdorp PM, Locken MR. Sequential generations of hematopoietic colonies derived from single nonlineage-committed $CD34^+CD38^-$ progenitor cells. Blood 1991;77:1218-1227.

5 Ploemacher RE, Brons NHC. Cells with marrow and spleen repopulating ability and forming spleen colonies on day 16, 12 and 8 are sequentially ordered on the basis of increasing rhodamine-123 retention. J Cell Physiol 1988;136:531-536.

6 Van der Sluijs JP, De Jong JP, Brons NHC, Ploemacher RE. Marrow repopulating cells, but not CFU-S, establish long-term in vitro hemopoiesis on a marrow-derived stromal layer. Exp Hematol 1990;18:893-896.

7 Michieli M, Giacca M, Fanin R, Damiani D, Geromin A, Baccarani M. MDR-1 gene amplification in acute lymphoblastic leukaemia prior to antileukaemic treatment. Br J Haematol 1991;78:288-289.

8 Chaudhary PM, Roninson IB. Expression and activity of P-glycoprotein, a multidrug efflux pump, in human hematopoietic stem cells. Cell 1991;66:85-94.

9 Drach D, Zhao S, Drach J, Mahadevia R, Gattringer C, Huber H, Andreef M. Subpopulations of normal peripheral blood and bone marrow cells express a functional multidrug resistant phenotype. Blood 1992;80:2729-2734.

10 Dalton WS, Grogan TM, Rybski JA, Scheper RJ, Richter L, Kailey J, Broxterman HJ, Pinedo HM, Salmon SE. Immunohistochemical detection and quantitation of P-glycoprotein in multiple drug resistant human myeloma cells: association with level of drug resistance and drug accumulation. Blood 1989;73:747-752.

11 Poncelet P, Carayon P. Cytofluorometric quantification of cell surface antigens by indirect immunofluorescence using monoclonal antibodies. J Immunol Methods 1985;85:65-74.

12 Poncelet P, Lavabre-Bertrand T, Carayon P. Quantitative phenotypes of B chronic lymphocytic leukemia B cells established with monoclonal antibodies from the B cell protocol. In: Reinherz EL, Haynes BF, Nadler LM, Bernstein ID, eds. Leukocyte Typing II. New York: Springer-Verlag, 1986:329-343.

Subsets of Early CD34+ Cells in Cord Blood, Bone Marrow, and Peripheral Blood

Hans-Jörg Bühring,[a] *Wolfgang Brehm,*[b] *Michaela Burkhardt,*[a] *Claudia A. Müller,*[a] *Rupert Handgretinger*[b]

[a]Section for Transplantation Immunology and Immunohematology, Second Department of Internal Medicine, University of Tübingen, Tübingen, Germany; [b]Children's Hospital, University of Tübingen, Tübingen, Germany

Key Words. Antibody • c-*kit* • CD38 • HLA-DR • Purified CD34+ cells • Three-color fluorescence • Cytofluorimetric analysis

Introduction

Hematopoietic stem cells have the capacity for both self renewal and differentiation into a variety of hematopoietic lineages [1, 2]. Recently, a common precursor of hematopoietic and stromal cells expressing the phenotype $CD34^+CD38^-HLA\text{-}DR^-$ was identified in fetal bone marrow [3]. Furthermore, it was reported that the most primitive hematopoietic cells, assayable in long-term bone marrow cultures (LTBMC), express the phenotype $CD34^+HLA\text{-}DR^-p145c\text{-}kit^+$, while cells with the phenotype $CD34^+HLA\text{-}DR^-p145c\text{-}kit^-$ did not respond to a combination of steel factor (SLF) and IL-3 [4] in LTBMC. However, the maintenance of primitive, long-term culture-initiating cells (LTC-IC), which most likely express the phenotype $CD34^+CD38^-HLA\text{-}DR^-$ [5, 6], is alternatively supported by SLF or by a combination of interleukin (IL)-3 and granulocyte-macrophage-colony stimulating factor (GM-CSF) [7], suggesting the presence of a second, $CD34^+p145c\text{-}kit^-$ totipotent hematopoietic stem cell population. In conclusion, the most primitive hematopoietic stem cells most likely express the phenotype $CD34^+p145c\text{-}kit^+CD38^-HLA\text{-}DR^-$, although the existence of an alternative, equally primitive stem cell bearing the phenotype $CD34^+p145c\text{-}kit^-CD38^-HLA\text{-}DR^-$ cannot be excluded.

In the present studies the stem cell pools from cord blood, bone marrow, and peripheral blood were phenotypically characterized, using monoclonal antibodies (MAb) with specificities for CD34, p145c-*kit*, CD38, and HLA-DR. In order to accurately identify CD34+ subpopulations, cells labeled with a biotinylated CD34 MAb were separated on streptavidin-loaded affinity columns [8]. The enriched cells were triple-stained with MAb specific for CD34 (PerCP conjugate) and MAb combinations with specificities for p145c-*kit* (phycoerythrin (PE)) and CD38 (fluorescein isothiocyanate (FITC)), p145c-*kit* (PE) and HLA-DR (FITC), or CD38 (PE) and HLA-DR-(FITC), respectively, and analyzed on a flow cytometer.

Correspondence: Dr. Hans-Jörg Bühring, Medical University Clinic II, FACS-Laboratory, Otfried-Müller-Str.10, 72076 Tübingen, Germany.

Materials and Methodology

Antibody Conjugates

HLA-DR-FITC, HPCA-2-FITC (CD34) and Leu17-PE (CD38) were purchased from Becton Dickinson, Mountain View, CA, and IOM-38-FITC (CD38) was obtained from Dianova GmbH, Hamburg, Germany. HPCA-2-PerCP (CD34) was a kind gift from *Dr. Ken Davis* (Becton Dickinson, San José, CA) and 95C3-PE (p145c-*kit*) was generously supplied by *Drs. André van Agthoven* and *Caroline Zuber* (Immunotech S.A., Marseille, France).

Cells

Buffy coat peripheral blood (PB) leukocytes were obtained from the Blood Center of the University Hospital, Tübingen. Heparinized cord blood (CB) cells collected immediately after delivery were obtained from the Women's Hospital of the University Hospital, Tübingen, and bone marrow (BM) cells, extracted from femoral bones of patients undergoing artificial hip joint replacements, were obtained from the Berufsgenossenschaftliche Unfallklinik, Tübingen.

Collected cells were separated by centrifugation on Ficoll-Hypaque (density 1.077 g/ml) (Pharmacia, Freiburg, Germany) and the interphase fraction (mononuclear cells) was used for further experiments.

Affinity Column Purification of CD34+ Cells

$CD34^+$ cells were purified on Ceprate™LC CD34 affinity columns (CellPro, Bothell, WA). Gravity flow separations of $1\text{-}5 \times 10^8$ mononuclear cells were performed according to the manufacturer's instructions ($1\text{-}2 \times 10^9$ cells were used for separation of peripheral blood cells). To determine the yield of separated cells, the following formula was used:

$$\text{yield} = \frac{\#\text{adsorbed cells} \times \%\text{CD34}^+ \text{ cells adsorbed}}{\#\text{start cells} \times \%\text{CD34}^+ \text{ cells start}} \times 100\%$$

Cell numbers before and after separation were estimated microscopically using trypan dye exclusion. The percentage of $CD34^+$ cells obtained from unseparated, HPCA-2-FITC labeled specimens was determined on a flow cytometer (FACScan, Becton Dickinson; software: Lysis 2) by plotting the side scatter (SSC) versus the HPCA-2-FITC fluorescence (FL1) signals and calculating the percentage of HPCA-2-positive cells within the population with low SSC intensity. The percentage of $CD34^+$ cells obtained after separation was calculated by setting a primary gate in a forward scatter (FSC) versus SSC plot (left lanes) to exclude debris and aggregates, and a secondary gate in a SSC versus FL3 (HPCA-2-PerCP) plot (Fig. 1) (right lanes).

Immunofluorescence Staining

1 Unseparated cells: for blocking of binding to Fc receptors cells were incubated with 10% human AB serum (Behringwerke, Marburg, Germany) for 10 min on ice. In the next step, cells were incubated with 10μl HPCA-2-FITC for 30 min and washed prior to analysis on a FACScan flow cytometer.

2 Separated cells: after blocking of Fc receptors, cells were triple-stained with 10μl of both, HPCA-2-PerCP, and combinations of 95C3-PE and HLA-DR-FITC, 95C3-PE and IOM-38-FITC, or Leu17-PE and HLA-DR-FITC, respectively. Additionally, aliquots were labeled either with HPCA-2-PerCP, HLA-DR-FITC, or Leu17-PE. For further control experiments, cells were double-labeled with HLA-DR-FITC and Leu17-PE and triple-stained with HPCA-2-PerCP, control-IgG1-FITC and control IgG1-PE.

Flow Cytometric Analysis

To properly set compensations for acquisition of triple-stained cells on the FACScan flow cytometer, the following procedures were sequentially conducted:

1 In the first step, a live gate around the cells with low SSC signals in the dual scatter plot was set (Fig. 1, left lanes).

2 In the next step, cells labeled with only one conjugate were analyzed. The FL2-%FL1 compensation of HLA-DR-FITC labeled cells was set so that the FITC-positive cells were negative on the PE detector while the FL1-%FL2 compensation was set so that the Leu17-PE-positive cells were negative on the FITC detector. In the final step, HPCA-2-PerCP-positive cells were corrected by FL2-%FL3 and Leu17-PE labeled cells by FL3-%FL2 compensation. Subsequently, the three single-stained controls were re-analyzed in order to definitively confirm that compensations were properly set: the resulting dual fluorescence plots showed a single, double-negative population in the "irrelevant" dual fluorescence plot (example: analysis of HLA-DR-FITC labeled cells resulted in a double-negative population in the FL2/FL3 plot). In "relevant" plots, negative and positive populations were orthogonally located (example: cells labeled with HLA-DR-FITC resulted in a negative and single-positive population in the FL1/FL2 and FL1/FL3 displays).

3 In an additional control, the FL1/FL2 display of cells triple-stained with HPCA-2-PerCP, HLA-DR-FITC and Leu17-PE was compared with the FL1/FL2 display of cells double-stained with HLA-DR-FITC and Leu17-PE. The resulting plots were essentially the same, confirming again that compensations were properly set.

4 Prior to acquisition of cells and list mode storage of the resulting data, the live gates were inactivated.

5 Analysis: in the first step a gate in the dual scatter display was set as described in 1), in the next step a second gate was set on the $CD34^+$ population in the SSC/FL3 plot (Fig. 1,

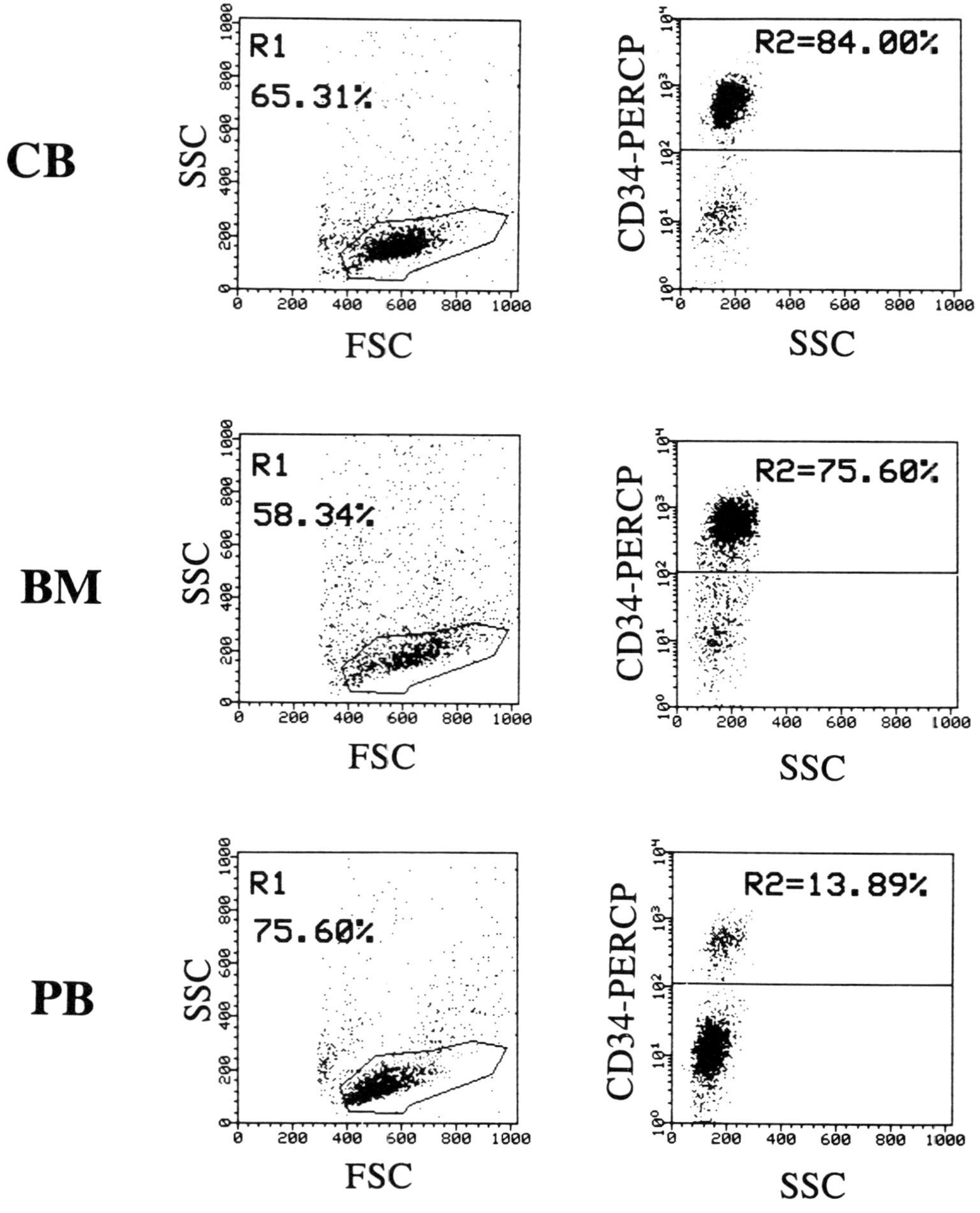

Fig. 1 *Left lane:* Dual scatter dot plot displays of affinity column selected cells (Ceprate™LC CD34; CellPro, Bothell) from cord blood (CB), bone marrow (BM), and peripheral blood (PB). To exclude debris and cell aggregates only gated cells were considered for further analysis.

Right lane: SSC versus FL3 plot displays of gated CD34-selected cells triple-stained with HPCA-2-PerCP and antibody combinations described in Materials and Methodology and in Figure 2. Only the CD34$^+$ population was considered for analysis described in Figure 2.

right lanes), and finally, by logically combining the two gates, the resulting FL1/FL2 plots were displayed (Fig. 2). To discriminate between negative and positive populations, the cut-off lines of a probe triple-stained with HPCA-2-PerCP, control IgG1-FITC and control IgG1-PE were set so that 98% in the FL1/FL2 display were double-negative.

Results

Prior to purification of the CD34⁺ population, the cells were counted and the percentage of CD34⁺ cells determined. Table I shows that cord blood contained 0.5-1.0% of CD34⁺ cells while in BM the percentage ranged between 1.3% and 2.5%. The low frequency of CD34⁺ cells in PB prevented us from estimating the percentage of this population. Because of the low frequency of CD34⁺ cells in unseparated cells the precise phenotype of CD34⁺ subpopulations is difficult to determine. Therefore, enrichment of CD34⁺ cells with Ceprate™LC affinity columns was performed prior to further analysis. Since the yields of the purified cells were not 100% and ranged between 43% and 65% (Table I), information about the lost CD34⁺ cells will be of interest. Have the lost CD34⁺ cells been statistically removed or did the separation result in a selective enrichment of CD34 high-positive cells because of insufficient affinity of CD34 low-positive cells to the streptavidin column? In the latter case the percentage of CD34⁺ B cells and the progenitors of advanced maturational stages should be decreased.

Table I. Selection of CD34⁺ cells from CB, BM, and PB[1]

	% CD34⁺ (starting pop.)[2]	% CD34⁺ (purified pop.)[3]	Yield (%)[4]
CB (1)	0.8%	76.5%	56%
CB (2)	1.0%	80.0%	65%
CB (3)	0.7%	63.2%	49%
CB (4)	0.5%	82.7%	44%
BM (1)	1.8%	89.6%	63%
BM (2)	1.3%	75.6%	43%
BM (3)	2.5%	84.8%	51%
PB (1)	–	11.2%	–
PB (2)	–	13.9%	–
PB (3)	–	56.3%	–

[1]See Materials and Methodology section for description of cell collection and density gradient enrichment of CB, BM, and PB.
[2]Calculation of %positive cells is based on ungated cells.
[3]Calculation of %positive cells is based on the gated populations shown in Figure 1. Cell aggregates with high SSC signals and debris (low FSC signals) were excluded from further analysis.
[4]Yield of cells was calculated as described in the Materials and Methodology section.

Alternatively, separation may result in the selective removal of the most immature CD34 high-positive cells because of increased difficulty in detaching this population from the column. However, the latter possibility seems unlikely because affinity column purified $CD34^+$ cells were successfully used for stem cell transplantations [9].

After column separation, the purity and the yield of the cells were estimated as described in the Materials and Methodology section. CD34-enriched CB cells were 63-83%, BM cells 76-90% and PB cells 11-56% pure (Table I). The yields ranged between 43% and 65%. Exclusion of debris and aggregates (and a few remaining granulocytes) by gating on cells with low SSC intensity in the dual scatter plot (Fig. 1, left lanes) and subsequent gating on the CD34 high-positive population (Fig. 1, right lanes) was performed as described in Materials and Methodology. Cells with low and intermediate fluorescence intensities had to be excluded from further analysis to ensure that rare populations like $CD34^+HLA\text{-}DR^-$ cells could be appropriately assessed. Consequently, the further analysis of surface markers excludes many of the CD34 low-positive B cells, myeloblasts and the more mature progenitor cells. However, the aim of these studies was the characterization of the more immature progenitors and stem cells which are exclusively found in the CD34 high-positive population.

Figure 2 shows the dual-fluorescence displays of HPCA-2-PerCP-positive (CD34-positive) CB, BM, and PB cells labeled with combinations of MAb directed against p145c-*kit* (SCFR), HLA-DR, and CD38, respectively.

Comparison of CB, BM, and PB cells labeled with MAb specific for SCFR and HLA-DR revealed that cells from CB express the highest SCFR levels, BM cells intermediate levels, and PB the lowest levels; 88-92% of CB, 60-70% of BM and 9-18% of PB cells coexpress SCFR and HLA-DR (Table II). These findings may well explain the fact that CB progenitors grow faster than their BM and PB counterparts (colonies derived from CB are enumerated on day 12, while colonies derived from BM are evaluated on day 14). Furthermore, $CD34^+HLA\text{-}DR^-$p145c-kit^+ cells, which comprise the potentially most immature stem cell population, are preferentially found in CB cells. Table II shows that 2.9% of CB, 1.1-1.2% of BM and 0.5-1.8% of PB cells express this phenotype.

$CD34^+$ cells labeled with MAb specific for SCFR and CD38 are shown in the second lane of Figure 2 and in Table II. In contrast to PB cells, a smooth transition of CD38-positive to CD38-negative/low-positive cells is observed in $CD34^+$ CB and BM cells. The highest percentage of $CD34^+CD38^-$p145c-kit^+ cells was found in CB while cells expressing this phenotype were not found in

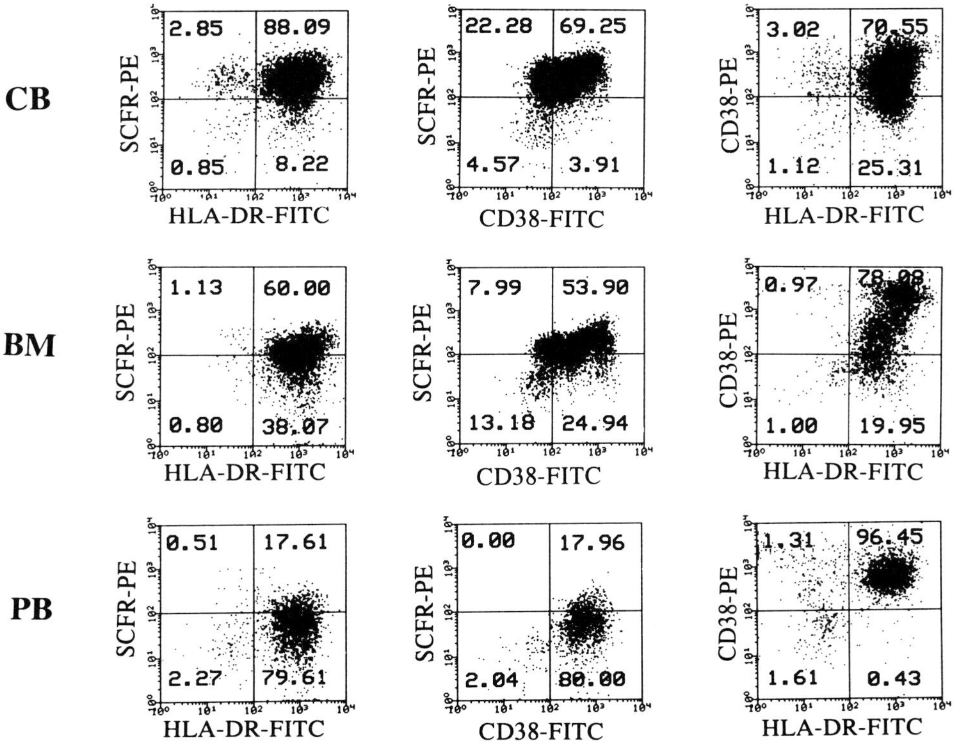

Fig. 2 Double fluorescence dot plot displays of triple-stained CB, BM, and PB cells preselected as described in Figure 1. Cells were labeled with HPCA-2-PerCP (CD34) and combinations of either 95C3-PE (p145c-*kit*) and HLA-DR-FITC (left lane), 95C3-PE and IOM38-FITC (CD38) (center lane), or Leu17-PE (CD38) and HLA-DR-FITC (right lane), respectively.

PB. The high percentages of CD38-negative cells in CB and BM should be carefully interpreted because definite discrimination between positive and negative populations is only precise if distinct, clearly separated subpopulations can be distinguished.

Coexpression analysis of CD38 and HLA-DR on $CD34^+$ cells of different sources (Fig. 2, right lanes) revealed that there are no significant differences in the population size of $CD34^+CD38^-HLA\text{-}DR^-$ cells; 1.1-2.4% were found in CB, 1.0-2.5% in BM and 1.6-2.2% in PB cells (Table II). Therefore, it can be concluded that the majority of the $CD34^+HLA\text{-}DR^-p145c\text{-}kit^+$ cells (Fig. 2, top left) coexpress CD38 (Fig. 2, top right). In order to investigate the functional properties of the phenotypically characterized cells, distinct populations may be separated for studying the growth behavior of sorted cells in LTBMC, LTC-IC, or CFUs, respectively.

Table II. Coexpression of HLA-DR, p145c-*kit*, and CD38 on CD34-positive CB, BM, and PB cells[1]

	CB 1	CB 2	BM 1	BM 2	PB 1	PB 2
HLADR+SCFR+:	92.0%	88.1%	70.2%	60.0%	17.6%	9.4%
HLADR+SCFR−:	3.9%	8.2%	26.1%	38.1%	79.6%	85.8%
HLADR−SCFR+:	2.9%	2.9%	1.2%	1.1%	0.5%	1.8%
HLADR−SCFR−:	1.1%	0.8%	2.5%	0.8%	2.3%	3.0%
CD38+SCFR+:	78.9%	69.2%	57.8%	53.9%	18.0%	9.8%
CD38+SCFR−:	2.4%	3.9%	20.3%	24.9%	80.0%	86.9%
CD38−SCFR+:	16.8%	22.3%	9.6%	8.0%	0.0%	0.0%
CD38−SCFR−:	1.9%	4.6%	12.3%	13.2%	2.0%	3.7%
HLADR+CD38+:	71.4%	70.6%	78.1%	75.9%	96.5%	94.2%
HLADR+CD38−:	24.7%	25.3%	19.9%	20.1%	0.4%	0.8%
HLADR−CD38+:	1.5%	3.0%	1.0%	1.5%	1.3%	2.8%
HLADR−CD38−:	2.4%	1.1%	1.0%	2.5%	1.6%	2.2%

[1]Fluorescence conjugates of antibodies are described in Materials and Methodology. Threshold settings for determination of positive populations are shown in Figure 2.

Discussion

If triple-stained, purified CD34+ cells are to be analyzed, the initial instrument setting should be established preferably with peripheral blood cells, because high cell numbers are easily available. 5×10^6 unseparated mononuclear cells for each probe and control allow proper compensation without the necessity for quick (and perhaps imprecise) decisions caused by the low CD34+ cell numbers which are generally available after enrichment. A good conjugate combination for this purpose is Leu8-PE, CD3-FITC and CD4-PerCP, because both triple-negative and triple-positive populations can be detected. Since the autofluorescence signal of gated lymphocytes is comparable to CD34+ cells, storage of these instrument settings is very helpful for analysis of CD34+ cells requiring only minor modifications.

Accurate three-color analysis of CD34+ subpopulations requires a precise gating on the CD34+ population. This is of particular importance if the percentage of CD34+HLA-DR− or CD34+CD38− is to be determined, in view of the risk to include false-CD34+HLA-DR/CD38− cells if setting the cutoff line too close to the CD34− population.

The use of biotinylated antibodies for further analysis of Ceprate™LC purified cells should be avoided, because many biotinylated CD34 antibodies used for separation remain bound after separation, and therefore compete for the binding of streptavidin conjugates. In addition, it is important to use CD34 conjugates which recognize an epitope distinct from the determinant occupied by the antibody used for the separation.

Acknowledgments

We are indebted to *Dr. Ken Davis* (Becton Dickinson, San José) for providing us with HPCA-2-PerCP (CD34), to *Drs. Caroline Zuber* and *André van Agthoven* (Immunotech, Marseille) for their generous supply with 95C3-PE (c-*kit*), and to *Dr. Graham Pawelec* (Tübingen), and *Dr. Eckart Wunder* (Mulhouse) for helpful discussions.

References

1 Suda T, Suda J, Ogawa M. Single-cell origin of mouse hematopoietic colonies expressing multiple lineages in variable combinations. Proc Natl Acad Sci USA 1983;80:6689-6693.

2 Spangrude GJ, Heimfeld S, Weissman IL. Purification and characterization of mouse hematopoietic stem cells. Science 1988;241:58-62.

3 Huang S, Terstappen LWMM. Formation of hematopoietic microenvironment and hematopoietic stem cells from single human bone marrow stem cells. Nature 1992;360:745-749.

4 Briddell RA, Broudy VC, Bruno E, Brandt JE, Srour F, Hoffman R. Further phenotypic characterization and isolation of human hematopoietic progenitor cells using a monoclonal antibody to the c-*kit* receptor. Blood 1992;79:3159-3167.

5 Terstappen LWMM, Huang S, Safford M, Lansdorp PM, Loken MR. Sequential generations of hematopoietic colonies derived from single nonlineage-committed $CD34^+CD38^-$ progenitor cells. Blood 1991;77:1218-1227.

6 Brandt JE, Srour EF, van Besien K, Briddell RA, Hoffman R. Cytokine-dependent long-term culture of highly enriched precursors of hematopoietic progenitor cells from human bone marrow. J Clin Invest 1990;86:932-941.

7 Sutherland HJ, Hogge DE, Cook D, Eaves JC. Alternative mechanisms with and without steel factor support primitive human hematopoiesis. Blood 1993;81:1465-1470.

8 Berenson RJ, Bensinger WI, Kalamasz D. Positive selection of viable cell populations using avidin-biotin immunoadsorption. J Immunol Meth 1986;91:11-19.

9 Berenson RJ. Transplantation of $CD34^+$ hematopoietic precursors: clinical rationale. Transpl Proc 1992;24:3032.

Stem Cell Mobilization: Role of Blood Cell Growth Factors

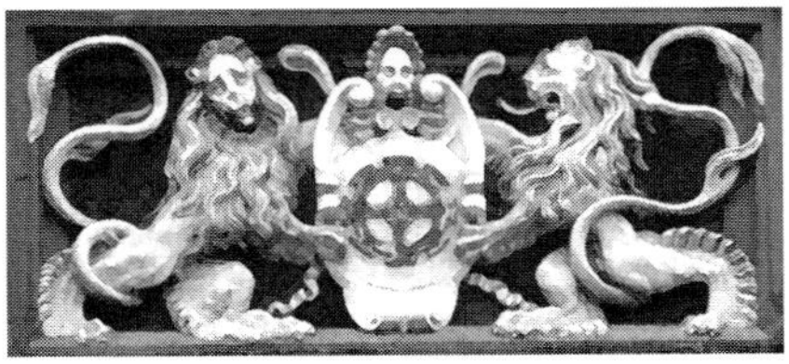

Peripheral Blood Stem Cell Mobilization: A Critical Review

Philippe R. Hénon
Institut de Recherche en Hématologie et Transfusion, Hôpital du Hasenrain, Mulhouse, France

Key Words. Peripheral blood stem cells • Mobilization • Chemotherapy • Cytokines • CFU-GM • $CD34^+$ cells

Introduction

So called "peripheral blood stem cells" (PBSC) are increasingly used worldwide for autotransplantations in malignancies [1] and even are now proposed for allografts [2]. One of the critical issues to ensure their further successful engraftment is to collect sufficient amounts of both already committed cells (recognized as $CD34^+$, 33^+, 38^+ cells) and very immature cells ($CD34^+$, 33^-, 38^-), responsible for accelerated short term and sustained long term hematopoietic reconstitution, respectively [3]. Although likely capable of long-term hematopoietic reconstitution, PBSC collected in steady-state without any mobilization method do not result in hastened engraftment [4], and it is now admitted that only mobilized PBSC can achieve such a result.

Richman et al. were the first to demonstrate in 1976 in solid tumors that the rebound of peripheral blood cell counts generally observed after myeloablative chemotherapy was most of the time preceded or accompanied by the transient appearance into the blood of high amounts of colony forming units granulocyte-macrophage (CFU-GM) [5]. A similar observation was reported later after high-dose chemotherapy in acute myeloid leukemia (AML) by *To et al.* [6], and in fact was the actual starting point of clinical experiments using PBSC for autotransplants. More recently, cytokine(s), singly or combined with chemotherapy, have been recommended to improve PBSC enhancement and are still currently being explored.

Mobilization of PBSC Induced by Chemotherapy

Not all chemotherapies are capable of PBSC mobilization which is also relevant to various factors such as the type of disease, eventual prior treatments or individual factors. PBSC mobilization is generally observed at the "rebound phase" following the transient aplastic period, provided that the myelosuppression was deep enough. Indeed, the amplitude of the rebound phase and, consequently, of mobilization of hematopoietic stem cells from bone marrow into peripheral blood, strongly correlates to the intensity of the preceding myelosuppression but also to its briefness [6, 7].

Correspondence: Dr. Philippe R. Hénon, Institut de Recherche en Hématologie et Transfusion, Hôpital du Hasenrain, 87 Avenue d'Altkirch, 68051 Mulhouse, France.

Both different combination chemotherapy and single high-dose chemotherapy have been used, also depending on the type of disease. For example, using the daunorubicin, cytosine arabinoside (Ara-C), and 6-thioguanine (DAT) chemotherapy regimen in AML patients, *To et al.* observed in 1984 a mean 25-fold increase from baseline values in circulating CFU-GM [6]. High-dose Ara-C, singly or combined with daunorubicin and/or etoposide, was demonstrated to similarly increase circulating CFU-GM levels in AML patients [8]. Studying the incidence of various chemotherapy regimens on CFU-GM yields in acute lymphoblastic leukemias (ALL), we have ourselves demonstrated a little later that, at least in this category of disease, the more intensive the chemotherapy regimen in previously untreated patients, the higher the peak of CFU-GM and the better their collection, except in patients with a t(9;22) or t(4;11) chromosome translocation, who failed to mobilize PBSC satisfactorily [9]. Chemotherapy regimens associating cyclophosphamide (CTX) with either Ara-C, carmustine and etoposide, or adriamycin, vincristine and prednisone (C_2H_2OP) have been successfully proven to be a mobilizing regimen in non-Hodgkin's lymphomas (NHL) and in multiple myeloma [10, 11]. Other miscellaneous chemotherapy protocols have also been reported in the literature.

Single high doses of alkylating agents (HD-CTX, or melphalan HDM) have been recommended by many groups as mobilizing chemotherapy in NHL, solid tumors and multiple myeloma [12-15]. HD-CTX (4 to 7 g/m^2) is generally preferred in the first two types of diseases, both because it is usually active against their tumor loads and because it is seldom associated with prolonged cytopenia, and the following rebound-phase PBSC peak will be consequently highly increased (up to 100-fold from the baseline values) [12]. For this second reason, the use of HD-CTX is also proposed by several groups instead of HDM in multiple myeloma, while the latter is generally much more active against the tumor plasma cells [15].

Even using one of these chemotherapy regimens, however, mobilization attempts are sometimes unsuccessful, due either to disease-related impaired hematopoiesis or to chemotherapy-related exhaustion of the bone marrow stem cell pool. For example, an inhibition of total hematopoiesis, both by decreased absolute levels of $CD34^+$ cells contained in bone marrow and by their impaired stimulation by accessory cells, has been demonstrated in about one third of high-risk myeloma patients prior to any therapy [16]. In chronic myeloid leukemia as well, "mobilizing" chemotherapies applied in chronic phase often seem to enhance the expansion of the Philadelphia-positive (Ph^+) clone instead of the proliferation of the residual normal stem cells [17]. In Hodgkin's disease (HD) or in low-grade NHL, attempts to collect

PBSC are most often performed in second complete remission after the patients have relapsed. This implies that they have previously been heavily treated with six or more chemotherapy courses and additional radiotherapy. Addition of a further "mobilizing" chemotherapy course may fail to enhance the amounts of circulating stem cells. Probably such chemotherapy regimens are capable of inflicting physiologically important damages on the stem cell compartment, such as recently demonstrated in experimental murine studies [18]. Moreover, the mobilizing chemotherapy itself may be directly toxic against the stem cell pool, even without prior treatment. For example, while usually achieving a marked anti-tumor effect, HDM may induce severe marrow aplasia of unpredictable duration without subsequent rebound phase, and consequently cannot be considered as the best PBSC mobilizing agent, at least if used alone [19].

More generally, chemotherapy mobilization, when successful, is also profitable in terms of reduction of the tumor cell load, acting as in vivo purging both on the graft and the recipient, but it may entail infectious complications and even occasional mortality during aplasia.

Cytokine Enhancement of PBSC

At the end of the 1980s, several authors, arguing from preliminary investigations in animals indicating that cytokines were capable of inducing a significant increase in total peripheral blood counts [20], introduced the use of such cytokines in human clinical trials. Dramatic increase of circulating hematopoietic progenitors has been reported after administration of recombinant human granulocyte-macrophage colony stimulating factor (rhGM-CSF), granulocyte CSF (rhG-CSF) and interleukin 3 (rhIL-3) [21-23], which also seems to reduce significantly the length of the chemotherapy-related aplasia and, consequently, the risk of the chemotherapy-related morbidity/mortality. Such risk might even be avoided if cytokines might be used for PBSC mobilization without any prior chemotherapy. Preliminary studies have effectively suggested that using only cytokines, singly or in combination, might allow adequate PBSC collection with a single leukapheresis. Such a chemotherapy-free process may of course be beneficial in nonmalignant situations and especially in view of PBSC collection in healthy donors [2]. But it may likely be detrimental in malignancies by managing a PBSC enhancement lacking an associated reducing effect on the tumor load and also acting as in vivo purging upon leukapheresis products. So presently the goal must be to find both the best PBSC enhancement procedure and the highest tumor load reduction, balanced with the lowest chemotherapy-related morbidity.

rhGM-CSF

Socinski et al. showed in 1988 in a sarcoma patient series that rhGM-CSF used alone expands the circulating pools of CFU-GM and erythroid burst forming units (BFU-E) by a factor of 18, and even more (up to 60-fold) when it was substantially given after high-dose chemotherapy [21]. A few months later, *Dührsen et al.* reported in a phase I/II clinical trial that the administration of rhG-CSF in 30 patients with metastatic cancer treated with a single injection of melphalan (25 mg/m^2) was followed by a pronounced increase in the number of circulating progenitor cells, associated in most patients with a slight reduction in the frequency of bone marrow progenitor cells [22]. All lineage precursor cells were concerned by this mechanism. *Gianni et al.,* combining HD-CTX (7 g/m^2) and rhGM-CSF in a short series of previously untreated (except one) NHL patients, obtained a dramatic increase from baseline values (up to 1,000-fold) in the number of circulating CFU-GM, which were afterwards harvested by two to four leukaphereses [24]. At the same time, *Siena et al.,* from the same Milano group, investigated whether CD34$^+$ cells were detectable in the peripheral blood of cancer patients after treatment with HD-CTX with or without rhGM-CSF [25]. They reported not only that CD34$^+$ cells effectively circulate in blood during the hematopoietic recovery following the aplasia induced by HD-CTX, but also that their circulation was highly enhanced by administration of rhGM-CSF, even allowing a higher yield of CD34$^+$ cells by leukapheresis than can generally be harvested from bone marrow. Last but not the least, such circulating CD34$^+$ cells seemed not to significantly differ from their marrow counterpart in the steady-state, particularly in terms of their trilineage cloning efficiency. In this way, a linear correlation was found between the number of CD34$^+$ cells and day-14 CFU-GM progenitors present in the same samples, which was later confirmed by some other groups.

So these various reports demonstrated that, in blood, rhGM-CSF was really capable of enhancing significantly both committed progenitors responsible for short-term hematopoietic recovery and more immature cells involved in a further trilineage differentiation.

rhGM-CSF has been clinically used for PBSC priming essentially in HD. For example, in a series reported by *Haas et al.* [26], seven patients with sensitive relapsed HD, who had responded well to a salvage therapy consisting of dexamethasone, carmustine (BCNU), etoposide, Ara-C and melphalan (Dexa-BEAM), received a further cycle of Dexa-BEAM followed by i.v. continuous infusion of rhGM-CSF (250 μg/m^2 daily). Blood stem cells were collected in the leukocyte recovery phase with an average of six leukaphereses.

Despite low yields of CFU-GM (median 0.61 × 10^4/kg body weight, ranging from 0.077 to 4.8) as compared with that reported by *Gianni* [24], these patients were autografted with leukapheresis products and hematopoiesis recovered satisfactorily, although a little slower (17 days to reach 0.5 × 10^9/l granulocytes) than that described in the literature with PBSC collected after chemotherapy priming alone [27, 28]. In advanced HD again, *Körbling* compared chemotherapy priming alone (Ara-C + daunorubicin) with chemotherapy plus rhGM-CSF (250 μg/m^2 daily) [29]. He showed that the CFU-GM yield during rhGM-CSF application exceeded the yield after chemotherapy priming by a factor of five (average yield of 25.4 versus 5.4 CFU-GM/kg body weight, respectively). The rhGM-CSF approach was also more efficient in terms of number of apheresis procedures. In our own experience in HD patients heavily pretreated with ABV chemotherapy (unpublished data), we failed to achieve higher yields of either circulating $CD34^+$ cells or circulating CFU-GM after C_2H_2OP chemotherapy regimen + rhGM-CSF priming as the yield observed after chemotherapy priming alone. *Elias et al.* also used a PBSC priming combining chemotherapy (doxorubicin, 5-fluorouracil, methotrexate) and rhGM-CSF (5 μg/kg/d) administered by i.v. continuous infusion on days 6-15, in two groups, of 12 patients each with metastatic breast cancer [30]. Two such priming courses were administered, PBSC being collected each time in two apheresis procedures between days 14-18 of each cycle. One group of patients received PBSC alone, while the other group received both PBSC and bone marrow. Unfortunately, although the authors considered that "mobilization of PBSC by rhGM-CSF appears to facilitate collection of adequate numbers of peripheral blood progenitor cells with fewer leukaphereses," they omitted to support this assertion with any information about the PBSC yields achieved or about the amounts of PBSC reinfused for transplantation. They only reported that all patients engrafted, without any difference between the two groups in terms of rapidity of hematopoietic reconstitution, faster than patients did following autologous bone marrow transplantation (ABMT).

rhG-CSF

Bronchud et al. in 1987 [31] and *Gabrilove et al.* in 1988 [32] first demonstrated, in cancer patients receiving rhG-CSF in addition to cytotoxic chemotherapy, an increase in blood granulocyte count similar to that observed in animal models.

rhG-CSF priming alone has been recently clinically tested. *Sheridan et al.* [33] demonstrated an average 63-fold increase of CFU-GM from baseline in 17 patients with nonmyeloid disorders (ALL, HD, NHL) of poor prognosis, heavily pretreated, after continuous s.c. infusion of rhG-CSF (12 μg/kg daily for 6 days). That allowed the collection of a median of 33×10^4 CFU-GM/kg body weight by three consecutive daily apheresis. PBSC were reinfused together with bone marrow harvests in 14 patients, the cell infusion being immediately followed by further additive treatment with rhGM-CSF. A significantly faster platelet recovery was observed in these patients in comparison with controls transplanted with autologous bone marrow without rhGM-CSF. More recently, the same group also reported that rhG-CSF-mobilized PBSC reinfused without bone marrow cell contribution allowed rapid granulocyte and platelet recovery and was safe in terms of long-term hematopoiesis [34].

The combination of various chemotherapy regimens with subsequent rhG-CSF infusion was also tested for PBSC mobilization in patients with various malignancies by three other groups [35-37]. In two studies, such a mobilization protocol was applied in patients with newly diagnosed malignancies [35, 36], while in the third one, most of the patients had already received prior chemotherapy [37]. rhG-CSF was generally administered at dosages varying from 50 $\mu g/m^2$ [36] to 230 $\mu g/m^2$ daily [34] from the second day after the completion of chemotherapy, and continued until collection of PBSC was completed. Whatever the rhG-CSF dosage, a number of CFU-GM and/or $CD34^+$ cells sufficient for further engraftment was achieved with an average of no more than one to three leukaphereses in most of the patients. In one series, where chemotherapy + rhG-CSF priming was compared with chemotherapy priming alone, analysis of progenitor cells within the apheresis product showed a 3.9-fold increase in daily CFU-GM and a 2.1-fold increase in $CD34^+$ cells for chemotherapy + rhG-CSF compared with chemotherapy alone [37]. In all three studies, the post-transplant platelet recovery was significantly accelerated.

Using again a Dexa-BEAM regimen, but followed by s.c. administration of rhG-CSF instead of rhGM-CSF, as he did before [26], the *Haas* group has observed in an additional series of eight HD patients a median increase from blood baseline values of 194-fold for CFU-GM and 54-fold for BFU-E [38]. In parallel, a consistent median increase of circulating $CD34^+$ cells was also achieved (median peak: 4,550/ml). All patients transplanted with these mobilized PBSC achieved complete engraftment with a median of 15 days for 0.5×10^9/l neutrophils and 22 days for 20×10^9/l platelets.

rhIL-3

rhIL-3 is an earlier acting cytokine than rhGM-CSF and rhG-CSF, and its impact on PBSC enhancement is also being investigated. *Vose et al.* have evaluated the ability of three different dosages (125 μg, 250 μg and 500 $\mu g/m^2$)

of IL-3 to mobilize PBSC in eight patients with lymphoid malignancies [39]. The CFU-GM values increased in six patients with "peak" values of only 0.25, 0.15 and 0.02 × 10^4/kg body weight, respectively, according to the growing IL-3 dosages. Furthermore, two heavily pretreated patients failed to mobilize PBSC. The median BFU-E and CFU megakaryocyte (CFU-Meg) values did not rise consistently. The six "mobilized" patients were subsequently transplanted with PBSC. Engraftment was extremely slow, needing 41 days and 26 days, corresponding with the 125 μg and 250 μg/m^2 dosages, respectively, to achieve 0.5 × 10^9/l granulocytes. We were not more successful in mobilizing PBSC with a combination priming of HDM and rhIL-3, given daily for 14 days from chemotherapy completion in a very evolutive heavily pretreated myeloma patient. The total yields of CFU-GM and $CD34^+$ cells that we could obtain with five leukaphereses were 3.63 × 10^4/kg and 2.63 × 10^7, respectively, i.e., similar to the values we had obtained in some patients of a previous series of chemotherapy-mobilized myeloma patients [15]. So rhIL-3 priming only seems to lead to minor elevations of circulating progenitor cells.

Combination of an early (IL-3) and a late (rhGM-CSF) acting cytokine after chemotherapy might enhance PBSC more satisfactorily than does rhIL-3 alone. *Brugger et al.* [40] have recently demonstrated that a chemotherapy consisting of etoposide (VP16), ifosfamide and cisplatin (VIP), followed by the combined sequential administration of rhIL-3 and rhGM-CSF allowed the recruitment by a single leukapheresis of amounts of myeloid, erythroid and multipotential progenitors at least comparable to data published with HD-CTX and rhGM-CSF by *Gianni* [24]. Other studies also suggest that sequential treatment with rhIL-3 and rhGM-CSF [41] or rhG-CSF [42] is superior to treatment with single factors with regard to enhancement of circulating progenitor cells. We have personally started a phase I trial to evaluate the ability of a combination of HDM (100 mg/m^2) and of sequential administration of rhIL-3 and rhG-CSF to mobilize PBSC in patients with high risk myeloma. Even if the very preliminary results seem to be encouraging, further patients have to be included in this trial before drawing any conclusion.

Conclusion

Harvesting enough PBSC to constitute adequate grafts is difficult in steady-state, and mobilization regimens are usually required to achieve such a goal. Combining cytokine(s) with chemotherapy mobilization may allow further recruitment of higher amounts of circulating hematopoietic progenitors—provided sufficient numbers of residual stem cells remain in bone marrow to be stimulated—thus avoiding the too poor PBSC yield sometimes collected after mobilization chemotherapy alone in particular diseases. Furthermore, hematopoietic recovery—especially platelet recovery—following reinfusion of cytokine-mobilized hematopoietic progenitor cells often occurs faster than previously described with chemotherapy priming alone. The use of cytokine(s) may also significantly reduce the side effects often associated with chemotherapy-related aplasia, therefore decreasing the morbidity/mortality rate of the procedure.

It is presently too early, however, to actually determine what is the most appropriate single cytokine or cytokine combination to improve PBSC enhancement and recruitment, since new cytokines which are still being investigated in animals, such as stem cell factor, could even further enhance peripheral blood cell harvesting in humans. The clinical tolerance and the effective cost of such processes have also to be taken into account to reach such a conclusion. Finally, it must be remembered that many neoplastic cell lines have receptors for cytokines, which consequently could stimulate tumor cells in various malignant diseases such as AML and adversely affect their clinical course. Perhaps in vitro cytokine enhancement could be more appropriate in such diseases.

References

1 Hénon PR. Peripheral blood stem cell transplantations: past, present and future. Stem Cells 1993;11:154-172.

2 Dreger P, Suttorp M, Haferlach T, Löffler H, Schmitz N, Schroyens W. Allogenic granulocyte colony-stimulating factor-mobilized peripheral blood progenitor cells for treatment of engraftment failure after bone marrow transplantation. Blood 1993;81:1404-1409.

3 Bender JG, Unverzagt KL, Walker DE, Lee W, Van Epps DE, Smith DH, Stewart CC, To LB. Identification and comparison of CD34 positive cells and their subpopulations from normal peripheral blood and bone marrow using multicolor flow cytometry. Blood 1991;77:2591-2596.

4 Kessinger A, Armitage J, Landmark J, Smith D, Weisenburger D. Autologous peripheral hematopoietic stem cell transplantation restores hematopoietic function following marrow ablative therapy. Blood 1988;71:723-727.

5 Richman CM, Weiner RS, Yankee RA. Increase in circulating stem cells following chemotherapy in man. Blood 1976;47:1031-1037.

6 To LB, Haylock DN, Kimber RJ, Juttner CA. High levels of circulating haemopoietic stem cells in very early remission from acute non-lymphoblastic leukaemia and their collection and cryopreservation. Br J Haematol 1984;58:399-410.

7 Reiffers J, Bernard P, Marit G, Sarrat A, Froideval JL, Broustet A, Vezon G. Collection of blood-derived hemopoietic stem cells and applications for autologous transplantation. Bone Marrow Transplant 1986;1(suppl 1):371-372.

8 Reiffers J, Leverger G, Marit G, Castaigne S, Tilly H, Lepage E, Hénon P, Douay L, Troussard X. Haematopoietic reconstitution after autologous blood stem cell transplantation. In: Gale RP, Champlin RE, eds. Bone Marrow Transplantation: Current Controversies. New York: Alan Liss, Inc., 1988:313-320.

9 Hénon PR, Debecker A, Lepers M, Eisenmann JC, Kandel G, Dörr R, Selva J. Collection of circulating stem cells and their use for autograft in adults with acute lymphoblastic leukemia. Nouv Rev Fr Hematol 1988;30:229-235.

10 Kessinger A, Armitage JO. Peripheral stem cell transplantation for patients with non-Hodgkin's lymphoma. Int J Cell Cloning 1992;10(suppl 1):127-128.

11 Fermand JP, Levy Y, Gerota J, Benbunan M, Cosset JM, Castaigne S, Seligmann M, Brouet JC. Treatment of aggressive multiple myeloma by high dose chemotherapy and total body irradiation followed by blood stem cell autologous autografts. Blood 1989;73:20-23.

12 To LB, Haylock DN, Dyson PG, Rawlings TP, Bayly JL, Rawling CM, Canty AN, Wake B, Thorp D, Juttner CA. A comparison between 4 g/m^2 and 7 g/m^2 cyclophosphamide for peripheral blood stem cell mobilization. Int J Cell Cloning 1992;10(suppl 1):33.

13 Boiron JM, Marit G, Fabéres C, Cony-Makhoul P, Foures C, Ferrer AM, Cristol G, Sarrat A, Girault D, Reiffers J. Collection of peripheral blood stem cells in multiple myeloma following single high-dose cyclophosphamide with and without recombinant human granulocyte-macrophage colony-stimulating factor (rhGM-CSF). Bone Marrow Transplant 1993;12:49-55.

14 Tarella C, Boccadoro M, Omedi P, Bondesan P, Caracciolo D, Frieri R, Bregni M, Siena S, Gianni AM, Pileri A. Role of chemotherapy and GM-CSF on hemopoietic progenitor cell mobilization in multiple myeloma. Bone Marrow Transplant 1993;11:271-277.

15 Hénon P, Eisenmann JC, Beck-Wirth G, Liang H. A two phase intensive therapeutic approach in high risk myeloma. Follow up. Int J of Cell Cloning 1992;10(suppl 1):142-144.

16 Wunder E, Sovalat H, Liang H, Eisenmann JC. Mobilization of peripheral stem cells after high dose chemotherapy in multiple myeloma. Int J Cell Cloning 1992;10(suppl 1):38-40.

17 Hénon PR, Eisenmann JC, Becker M, Beck-Wirth G, Wunder E, Sovalat H. Difficulties in collecting peripheral blood stem cells in chronic myeloid leukemia related to persistence of the leukemic cell clone. Stem Cells Jan. 1994 (in press).

18 Hornung RL, Longo DL. Hematopoietic stem cell depletion by restorative growth factor regimens during repeated high-dose cyclophosphamide. Blood 1992;80:77-83.

19 To LB, Juttner CA. Stem cell mobilization by myelosuppressive chemotherapy. In: Wunder E, Hénon P, eds. Peripheral Blood Stem Cell Autografts. Heidelberg: Springer-Verlag, 1993:132-144 (in press).

20 Metcalf D. The colony stimulating factors. Discovery, development, and clinical applications. Cancer 1990;65:2185-2195.

21 Socinski MA, Elias A, Schnipper L, Cannistra SA, Antman KH, Griffin JD. Granulocyte-macrophage colony stimulating factor expands the circulating haemopoietic progenitor cell compartment in man. Lancet 1988;i:1194-1198.

22 Dührsen U, Villeval JL, Boyd J, Kannourakis G, Morstyn G, Metcalf D. Effects of recombinant human granulocyte colony-stimulating factor on hematopoietic progenitor cells in cancer patients. Blood 1988;72:2074-2081.

23 Saeland S, Caux C, Favre C, Aubry JP, Mannoni P, Pebusque MJ, Gentilhomme O, Otsuka T, Yokota T, Arai N, Arai K, Banchereau J, de Vries JE. Effects of recombinant human interleukin-3 on CD34-enriched normal hematopoietic progenitors and on myeloblastic leukemia cells. Blood 1988;72:1580-1588.

24 Gianni AM, Siena S, Bregni M, Tarella C, Stern AC, Pileri A, Bonadonna G. Granulocyte-macrophage colony-stimulating factor to harvest circulating haemopoietic stem cells for autotransplantation. Lancet 1989;ii:580-585.

25 Siena S, Bregni M, Brando B, Ravagnani F, Bonadonna G, Gianni AM. Circulation of CD34$^+$ hematopoietic stem cells in the peripheral blood of high-dose cyclophosphamide-treated patients: enhancement by intravenous recombinant human granulocyte-macrophage colony-stimulating factor. Blood 1989;74:1905-1914.

26 Haas R, Hohaus S, Egerer G, Ogniben E, Witt B, Hunstein W. Autologous blood stem cell transplantation in relapsed Hodgkin's disease. Int J Cell Cloning 1992;10(suppl 1):138-140.

27 Hénon P, Liang H, Beck-Wirth G, Eisenmann JC, Lepers M, Wunder E, Kandel G. Comparison of hematopoietic and immune recovery after autologous bone marrow or blood stem cell transplants. Bone Marrow Transplant 1992;9:285-291.

28 To LB, Roberts MM, Haylock DN, Dyson PG, Branford AL, Thorp D, Ho JQK, Dart GW, Horvath N, Davy MLJ, Olweny CLM, Abdi E, Juttner CA. Comparison of haematological recovery times and supportive care requirements of autologous recovery phase peripheral blood stem cell transplants, autologous bone marrow transplants and allogenic bone marrow transplants. Bone Marrow Transplant 1992;9:277-284.

29 Körbling M. The role of stem cell mobilization in autologous blood stem cell transplantation (ABSCT). In: Dicke KA, Armitage JO, Dicke-Evinger MJ, eds. Autologous Bone Marrow Transplantation, Fifth International Symposium. The University of Nebraska Medical Center, Omaha, Nebraska, 1991:791-799.

30 Elias A, Mazanet R, Wheeler C, Anderson K, Ayash L, Schwartz G, Tepler I, Pap S, Gonin R, Critchlow J, Schnipper L, Griffin J, Frei E, Antman K. Peripheral blood progenitor cells (PBPC): Two protocols using GM-CSF potentiated progenitor cell collection. In: Dicke KA, Armitage JO, Dicke-Evinger MJ, eds. Autologous Bone Marrow Transplantation, Fifth International Symposium. The University of Nebraska Medical Center, Omaha, Nebraska, 1991:875-879.

31 Bronchud MH, Scarffe JW, Thatcher N, Crowther D, Souza LM, Alton NK, Testa NG, Dexter TM. Phase I/II study of recombinant human granulocyte colony-stimulating factor in patients receiving intensive chemotherapy for small cell lung cancer. Br J Cancer 1987;56:809-813.

32 Gabrilove JL, Jakubowski A, Scher H, Sternberg C, Wong G, Grous J, Yagoda A, Fain K, Moore MAS, Clarkson B, Dettgen HF, Alton K, Welte K, Souza L. Effect of granulocyte colony-stimulating factor on neutropenia and associated morbidity due to chemotherapy for transitional-cell carcinoma of the urothelium. N Engl J Med 1988;318:1414-1422.

33 Sheridan WP, Begley CG, Juttner CA, Szer J, To LB, Maher D, McGrath KM, Morstyn G, Fox RM. Effect of peripheral-blood progenitor cells mobilized by filgrastim (G-CSF) on platelet recovery after high-dose chemotherapy. Lancet 1992;339:640-644.

34 Sheridan W, Begley G, Juttner CA, de Luca E, To LB, Szer J, Maher D, Watson D, Grigg A, Cebon J, Morstyn G, McGrath K, Green M, Tomita D, Hoffman E, Fox RM. The impact of R-Methug-CSF (filgrastim) dose on the mobilization of mononuclear and progenitor cells in peripheral blood in patients with malignancy. Blood 1992;80(suppl 1):420a.

35 Pettengel R, Demuynck H, Testa NG, Dexter TM. The engraftment capacity of peripheral blood progenitor cells (PBPC) mobilized with chemotherapy ± G-CSF. Int J Cell Cloning 1992;10(suppl 1):59-61.

36 Shimazaki C, Oku N, Ashihara E, Okawa K, Goto H, Inaba T, Ito K, Fujita N, Tsuji H, Murakami S, Haruyama H, Nishio A, Nakagawa M. Collection of peripheral blood stem cells mobilized by high dose Ara-C plus VP-16 or aclarubicin followed by recombinant human granulocyte-colony stimulating factor. Bone Marrow Transplant 1992;10:341-346.

37 Schwartzberg LS, Birch R, Hazelton B, Tauer KW, Lee P Jr, Altemose R, George C, Blanco R, Wittlin F, Cohen J, Muscato J, West WH. Peripheral blood stem cell mobilization by chemotherapy with and without recombinant human granulocyte colony-stimulating factor. J Hematotherapy 1992;1:317-327.

38 Hohaus S, Goldschmidt H, Ehrhardt R, Haas R. Successful autografting following myeloablative conditioning therapy with blood stem cells mobilized by chemotherapy plus rhG-CSF. Exp Hematol 1993;21:508-514.

39 Vose JM, Kessinger A, Bierman PJ, Sharp G, Garrison L, Armitage JO. The use of rhIL-3 for mobilization of peripheral blood stem cells in previously treated patients with lymphoid malignancies. Int J Cell Cloning 1992;10(suppl 1):62-64.

40 Brugger W, Bross KJ, Meterlsmann R, Kanz L. IL-3 plus GM-CSF induced recruitment of high numbers of peripheral blood progenitor cells following standard dose chemotherapy. In: Wunder E, Hénon PR, eds. Peripheral Blood Stem Cell Autografts. Heidelberg: Springer-Verlag, (in press).

41 Ottmann OG, Brücher J, Geissler G, Martin H, Claude R, Schulz G, Hoelzer D, Ganser A. Effect of sequential treatment with interleukin 3 (rh IL-3) and granulocyte-macrophage colony-stimulating factor (rhGM-CSF) on circulating CFU-GM. Int J Cell Cloning 1992;10(suppl 1):65-67.

42 Guillaume T, D'Hondt V, Symann M. IL-3 and peripheral blood stem cell harvesting. Stem Cells 1993;11:173-181.

Mobilization of Peripheral Blood Stem Cells with Cytotoxic Chemotherapy and Granulocyte Colony-Stimulating Factor (G-CSF) in Malignant Lymphoma

R. Haas, R. Möhle, S. Fruehauf, M. Pförsich, B. Witt, W. Hunstein
Department of Internal Medicine V, University of Heidelberg, Heidelberg, Germany

Key Words. Peripheral blood stem cells (PBSC) • G-CSF • Autologous blood stem cell transplantation

Introduction

For patients with refractory or relapsed malignant lymphoma, high-dose therapy with stem cell support has been proposed [1, 2]. Infections and bleeding complications are related to the duration of severe pancytopenia and therefore directly depend on the quantity of hematopoietic progenitor cells autografted [3]. Treatment with recombinant human granulocyte colony-stimulating factor (G-CSF) during steady-state hematopoiesis or after cytotoxic chemotherapy is associated with an increase of hematopoietic progenitor cells in peripheral blood [4, 5]. Characterization is done by immunofluorescence analysis with monoclonal antibodies against the CD34 antigen which is expressed on virtually all hematopoietic progenitor cells including primitive stem cells with the capacity to generate mesenchymal cells of the bone marrow microenvironment [6-8].

Focusing on the assessment of $CD34^+$ cells, it was the objective of our study to find parameters which may help to improve the collection of blood stem cells in patients with malignant lymphoma.

Materials and Methodology

Patients

Since May 1991, 35 patients (23 males, 12 females) with malignant lymphoma were included into our study. The median age was 35 years (range 21–58). Thirteen patients had Hodgkin's disease, while 22 had non-Hodgkin's lymphoma (NHL; 6 high-grade, 16 low-grade). Patients received conventional chemotherapy such as high-dose ara-C/mitoxantrone and DexaBEAM (dexamethasone, BCNU, etoposide, ara-C, melphalan). Twenty-four hours after chemotherapy had been completed, G-CSF (filgrastim, five μg/kg bodyweight, s.c.) was started. At the time of peripheral blood stem cell (PBSC)

Correspondence: Dr. R. Haas, Medizinische Klinik & Poliklinik V, University of Heidelberg, Hospitalstr. 3, 69115 Heidelberg, Germany.

©AlphaMed Press ISBN 1-880854 17-1

mobilization, nine patients were in complete remission (CR), 20 in partial remission (PR), while four had a relapse and two had progressive disease.

Pretreatment comprised a median number of two different regimens (range zero to seven). Additionally, nineteen patients had irradiation such as mantle-field, inverted "Y" or total-nodal. Histopathological examination prior to cytotoxic chemotherapy followed by G-CSF revealed bone marrow involvement in six patients. The study was conducted under the ethical guidelines of the joint committee on clinical investigation of the University of Heidelberg.

Informed consent was obtained from each patient. The cut-off date of this report is June 10, 1993.

Stem Cell Collection and Cryopreservation Procedure

Stem cell collection was performed with a Fenwal CS 3000 (Baxter Deutschland GmbH, München). PBSC harvesting was started when a white blood count (WBC) > 1×10^9/l was reached, and a total of 10 l blood per apheresis was processed at a flow rate of 50–70 ml/min. The apheresis product of 50 ml cell suspension was mixed with the same volume of minimal essential medium (MEM) containing 20% dimethylsulfoxide (DMSO, Merck, Darmstadt, Germany). The final 100 ml cell suspension was transferred into freezing bags (Delmed Inc., New Brunswick, NJ) and frozen to –100°C with a computer-controlled cryopreservation device (Cryoson BV-6, Cryoson Deutschland GmbH). The frozen cells were transferred into the liquid phase of nitrogen and stored at –196°C.

Clonogenic Assay for Hemopoietic Progenitor Cells

The concentration of hematopoietic progenitor cells in each single leukapheresis product and in the peripheral blood was assessed using a semisolid clonogenic culture assay (Terry Fox Laboratories, Vancouver, British Columbia, Canada). The culture medium consisted of 30% fetal calf serum, 10% medium conditioned by phytohemagglutinin-stimulated leukocytes (PHA-LCM), 1 IU recombinant human erythropoietin, 5×10^{-5} M 2-mercaptoethanol, and 0.9% methylcellulose. 2×10^5/ml mononuclear cells were plated in duplicate and incubated at 37°C and 5% CO_2 in humidified atmosphere.

After 14 days, colonies were scored using an inverted microscope. Hematopoietic progenitor cells in the peripheral blood were assessed on the day of leukapheresis.

Immunofluorescence Staining and Flow Cytometry

For immunofluorescence analysis 20 μl of whole blood or 1×10^6 mononuclear cells were incubated for 30 min at 4°C with the fluorescein isothiocyanate (FITC)-conjugated monoclonal antibody (MAb) HPCA2 (CD34) (Becton Dickinson, Heidelberg).

The cells were analyzed with a Becton Dickinson FACScan with a two watt argon ion laser as a light source. Excitation was allowed at 488 nm and fluorescence was measured at 530 nm.

We used a forward scatter (FSC) versus CD45 fluorescence dot plot to discriminate between the smallest lymphohematopoietic cell population and erythrocytes or debris. The $CD34^+$ cell population was analyzed in a FL-1 versus side scatter (SSC). Only cells with lymphoid or lymphoblastoid characteristics (low SSC) were counted as $CD34^+$ cells and further assessed for their FSC characteristics. The percentage of $CD34^+$ cells was calculated as follows:

$$[\%] = \frac{CD34^+ \text{ cells}}{CD45^+ \text{ cells}} \times 100$$

To evaluate $CD34^+$ cells/ml of peripheral blood, the percentage of $CD34^+$ cells was multiplied by the WBC. We defined a concentration of 1/μl $CD34^+$ cells as the detection limit. As negative control, 0.05% false positive events were considered the upper limit. For the first 12 patients, the individual peak value of $CD34^+$ cells in the peripheral blood was derived from measurements on days of leukaphereses. From then on, daily measurements (except for weekends) were available.

Statistical Analysis

The clinical and laboratory data were retrieved from the transplant data base and analyzed according to standard statistical methods using a commercially available computer program (Statworks, Cricket Software, Philadelphia, PA). The relationship between the different hematological parameters of the peripheral blood and leukapheresis products was estimated by simple linear regression and correlation analysis.

Results

Circulating Hematopoietic Progenitor Cells

Cytotoxic chemotherapy and blood stem cell collection with G-CSF support was associated with non-hematological toxicity not exceeding grade two (World Health Organization toxicity grading). We started PBSC collection when the WBC exceeded 1.0×10^9/l. G-CSF was administered during the entire collection period. The WBC reached a median of $12.2 \times 10^9/l$ (range $1.0–57.1 \times 10^9/l$) on days of leukaphereses. Bands and polymorphonuclear cells predominated (median $9.82 \times 10^9/l$, range $0.04–44.76 \times 10^9/l$), while the mononuclear cells (MNC) comprising the hematopoietic progenitor cells rose to a median of $2.16 \times 10^9/l$ with a range between 0.13 and $12.3 \times 10^9/l$.

Looking for parameters of the peripheral blood count which may be related to the number of circulating $CD34^+$ cells, we found a close correlation between the MNC and the level of $CD34^+$ cells/μl ($r = 0.80$, $p < 0.001$). In contrast, no relationship was found between the $CD34^+$ cells/μl and the WBC.

Individual peak levels of colony forming units (CFU) and $CD34^+$ cells during the collection period are shown in Figure 1. It should be noted that the values were influenced by the repeated leukapheresis procedures. colony-forming units granulocyte-macrophage (CFU-GM) and burst-forming units-erythroid (BFU-E) were spread over a 3-log range. The individual peak concentration

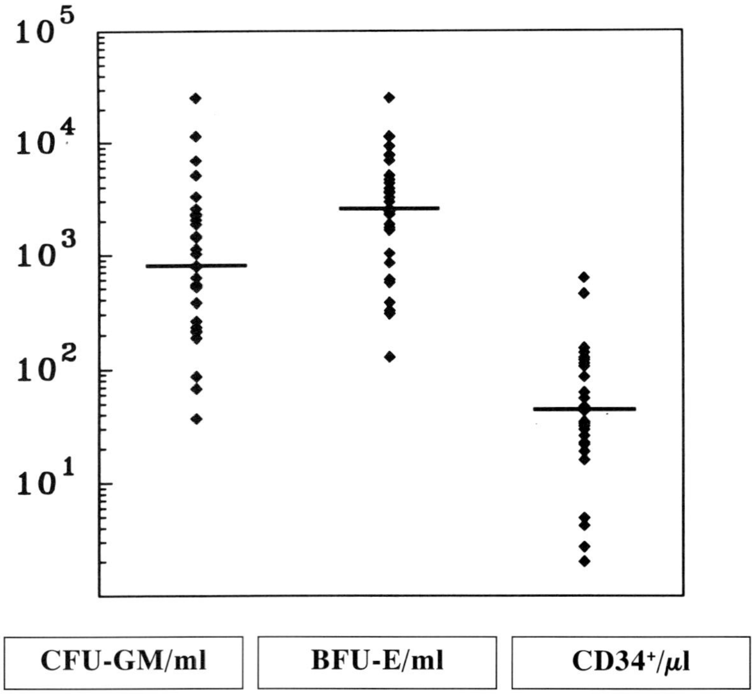

Fig. 1. Number of circulating hematopoietic progenitor cells (CFU-GM/ml and BFU-E/ml) and $CD34^+$ cells/μl in peripheral blood during G-CSF-supported marrow recovery and blood stem cell collection. The individual peak values of the patients are shown and the horizontal lines indicate the median.

of CD34+ cells varied between 0 and 619/μl (median 44.1/μl), while baseline values were below 5/μl. However, one patient with relapsed high-grade NHL was exceptional with 67/μl CD34+ cells during steady-state hematopoiesis.

The close relationship between the peak values of CD34+ cells/μl and CFU-GM/ml or BFU-E/ml is demonstrated by a correlation coefficient of R = 0.87 ($p < 0.001$) (Fig. 2).

Blood Stem Cell Collection

We performed a median of four leukaphereses (range two to ten) starting when a WBC of at least $1.0 \times 10^9/l$ had been reached. In the first 10 patients, blood stem cell collection was stopped when a target quantity of $0.4 \times 10^9/kg$

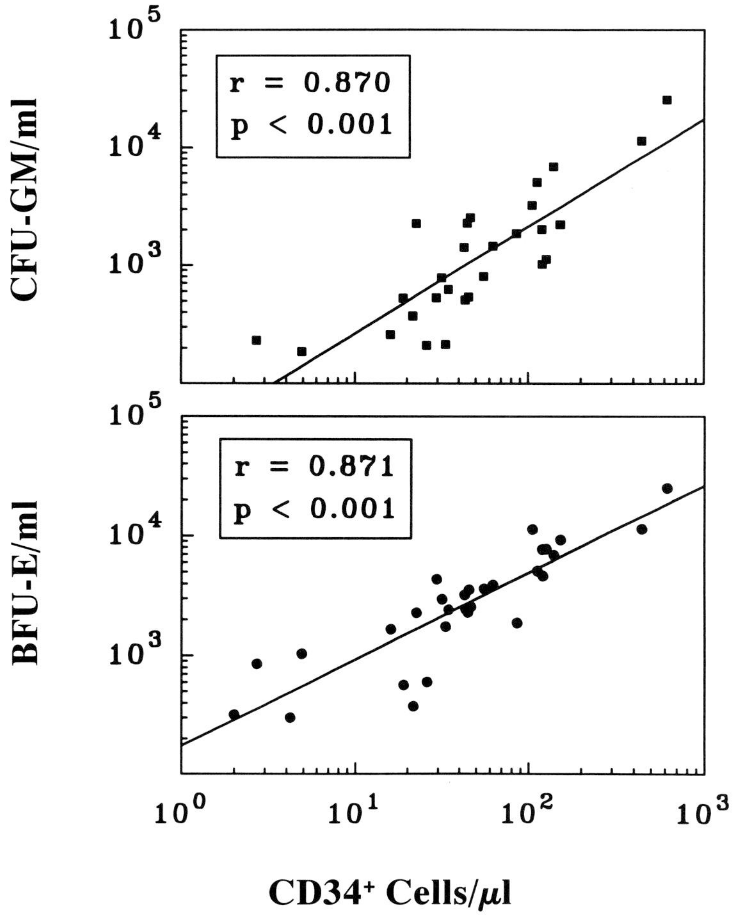

Fig. 2. Correlation analysis by linear regression between the number of CFU-GM/ml or BFU-E/ml and CD34+ cells/μl in peripheral blood. The correlation coefficient was identical for both CFU.

total nucleated cells (TNC) had been obtained. An interim analysis then showed that patients autografted with more than 5 × 10^6 $CD34^+$ cells/kg achieved complete engraftment with a rapid platelet recovery to an unsubstituted count > 20.0 × 10^9/l in less than 14 days. The decision to finish PBSC harvesting was therefore no longer based on the number of TNC collected but on the quantity of $CD34^+$ cells obtained.

The kinetics of hematological reconstitution after high-dose therapy and PBSC autografting in the 35 patients presented here suggest that a number of 2.5 × 10^6 $CD34^+$ cells/kg is sufficient to allow platelet recovery within less than 14 days (Fig. 3). We then looked for characteristic features of patients who reached this target quantity of $CD34^+$ cells.

In 27 of the 35 patients presented here, this number was achieved with a median of three leukaphereses (range two to six). They had a history of six cycles of chemotherapy (median, range zero–15); additionally, 11 had previous irradiation such as mantle-field or inverted Y. Conversely, in eight patients total harvests did not exceed 2.5 × 10^6 $CD34^+$ cells/kg, although a

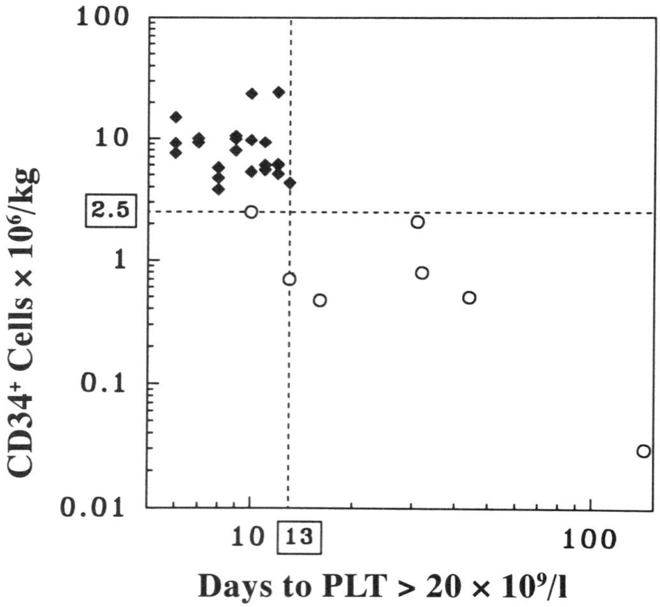

Fig. 3. The number of $CD34^+$ cells transplanted was predictive for platelet recovery. Above a threshold of 2.5 × 10^6/kg $CD34^+$ cells autografted, platelet reconstitution (unsubstituted count > 20 × 10^9/l) was observed within less than 14 days.

median of seven leukaphereses (range four to ten) was performed. These patients had 11 cycles of chemotherapy (median, range four to nineteen), while six of them had irradiation.

The most suitable parameter to discriminate between the two groups was the peak level of $CD34^+$ cells/μl in the peripheral blood. Patients with autografts containing more than 2.5×10^6 $CD34^+$ cells/kg had values above 20/μl $CD34^+$ cells (Fig. 4). Interestingly, 21 patients achieved this harvest with a single leukapheresis.

Discussion

The discussion will address two questions: How many stem cells are needed for hematological reconstitution after high-dose therapy, and how many patients will fulfill this requirement? Answers were given operationally based on the kinetics of hematopoietic recovery. The number of TNC, MNC or clonogenic progenitor cells has been used to describe the cellular composition of the autograft. Suggestions were made for CFU-GM and varied from center to center, mainly

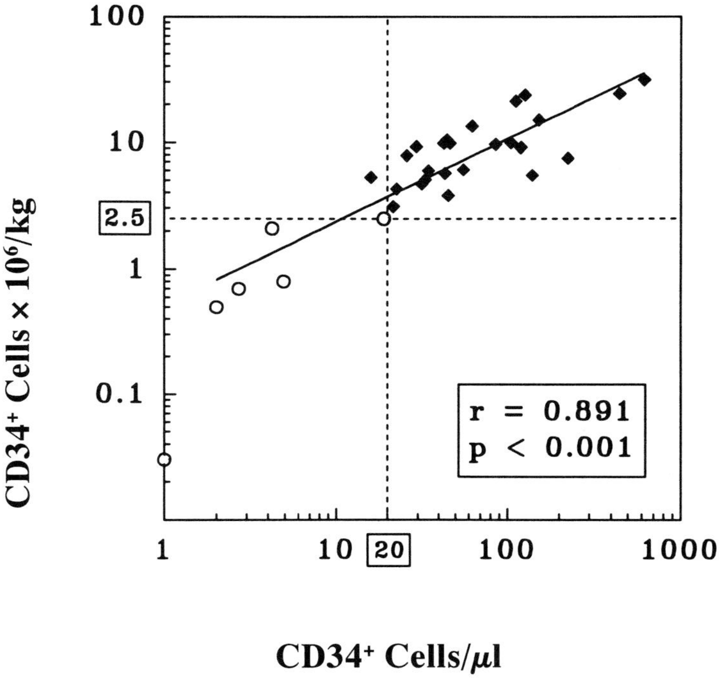

Fig. 4. The peak level of circulating $CD34^+$/μl cells in the peripheral blood is related to the total harvest.

reflecting the inter-laboratory differences in culture techniques [9]. Culture assays are no longer needed to monitor the collection of blood stem cells especially considering the close relationship between CFU and $CD34^+$ cells. With an incubation period of 14 days, the culture methods cannot provide the information necessary to decide when to start and how long to proceed with the leukaphereses to obtain a sufficient autograft. The clonogenic assays, however, may still serve to evaluate the proliferative capacity of the progenitor cells harvested and as quality control of the freezing and thawing procedures. Considering the final endpoint of rapid and complete engraftment, we now rely on the assessment of $CD34^+$ cells which has been first proposed by *Siena et al.* [7]. Autografts containing more than 2.5×10^6 $CD34^+$ cells/kg allowed rapid hematological reconstitution after high-dose therapy.

Yields above this threshold were obtained in patients with a concentration of circulating $CD34^+$ cells greater than 20/μl. Therefore, we consider the peak level of $CD34^+$ cells in the peripheral blood as an indicator for the individual hematopoietic reserve, being highly predictive for the total harvest. As observed by other investigators using different cytokine regimens for PBSC mobilization, the amount of previous chemotherapy appears to have an adverse effect on the yield of PBSC [10].

Summary

PBSC mobilized by G-CSF are capable of restoring hematopoiesis after high-dose conditioning therapy without additional bone marrow or cytokine support. Assessing the number of $CD34^+$ cells in the peripheral blood allows us to monitor blood stem cell collection and avoid unnecessary leukapheresis procedures. Traditionally, the number of TNC harvested per kg bodyweight served to define an adequate blood stem cell graft. This parameter, however, can be misleading. Patients with autografts of more than 2.5×10^6 $CD34^+$ cells/kg achieved platelet recovery in less than 14 days. All patients with circulating $CD34^+$ cells >20/μl obtained this target quantity. These patients had substantially less previous cytotoxic chemotherapy compared to the group of patients who did not exceed the threshold of 2.5×10^6 $CD34^+$ cells/kg in the autografts. For an upfront approach in patients with a high risk of relapse or slow response to first-line therapy, we suggest harvesting PBSC as early as possible during the course of the disease.

References

1 Peterson FB, Appelbaum FR, Hill R, Fisher LD, Bigelow CL, Sanders JE, Sullivan KM, Bensinger WI, Witherspoon RP, Storb R, Clift RA, Fefer A, Press OW, Weiden PL, Singer J, Thomas ED, Buckner CD. Autologous marrow transplantation for malignant lymphoma: a report of 101 cases from Seattle. J Clin Oncol 1990;8:638-647.

2 Kessinger A, Armitage JO, Smith DM, Landmark JD, Bierman PJ, Weisenburger D. High-dose therapy and autologous peripheral blood stem cell transplantation for patients with lymphoma. Blood 1989;74:1260-1265.

3 Saral R. Infectious diseases. In: Armitage JO, Antman KH, eds. High-Dose Cancer Therapy. Baltimore: Williams and Wilkins 1992:456-472.

4 Dührsen U, Villeval JL, Boyd J, Kannourakis G, Morstyn G, Metcalf D. Effects of recombinant human granulocyte colony stimulating factor on hematopoietic progenitor cells in cancer patients. Blood 1988;72:2074-2081.

5 Haas R, Hohaus S, Ehrhardt R, Goldschmidt H, Hunstein W. Autologous blood progenitor cell transplantation in relapsed Hodgkin's disease—the role of hematopoietic growth factors. Bone Marrow Transplant 1993;11(Suppl 2):30-35.

6 Civin CI, Strauss LC, Brovall C, Fackler MJ, Schwartz JF, Shaper JH. Antigenic analysis of hematopoiesis. III. A hematopoietic progenitor cell surface antigen defined by a monoclonal antibody raised against KG-1a cells. J Immunol 1984;133:157-165.

7 Siena S, Bregni M, Brando B, Belli N, Ravagnani F, Gandola L, Stern AC, Lansdorp PM, Bonadonna G, Gianni AM. Flow cytometry for clinical estimation of circulating hematopoietic progenitors for autologous transplantation in cancer patients. Blood 1991;77:400-409.

8 Huang S, Terstappen LW. Formation of hematopoietic microenvironment and hematopoietic stem cells from single human bone marrow stem cells. Nature 1992;360:745-749.

9 To LB, Dyson PG, Juttner CA. Cell-dose effect in circulating stem-cell autografting. Lancet 1986;2:404-405.

10 Brugger W, Bross K, Frisch J, Dern P, Weber B, Mertelsmann R, Kanz L. Mobilization of peripheral blood progenitor cells by sequential administration of interleukin-3 and granulocyte-macrophage colony stimulating factor following polychemotherapy with etoposide, ifosfamide and cisplatin. Blood 1992;79:1193-1200.

Purification of $CD34^+$ Cells

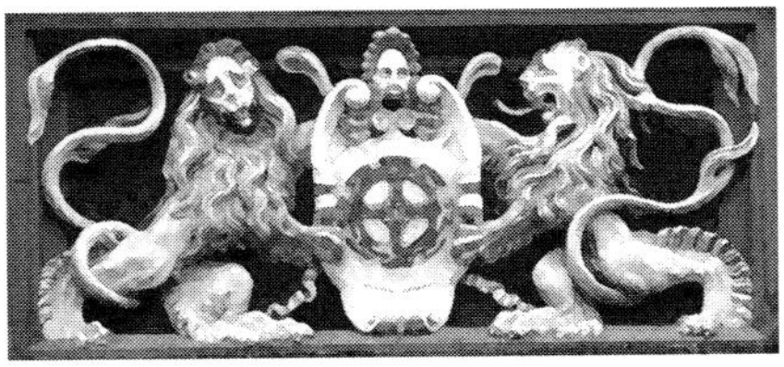

Basics of CD34+ Cell Purification, Evaluation and Use of the Separated Products

Eckart Wunder,[a] *Erika de Wynter*[b]

[a]Institut de Recherche en Hématologie et Transfusion, Hôpital du Hasenrain, Mulhouse, France; [b]Paterson Institute for Cancer Research, CRC Department of Experimental Hematology, University of Manchester, United Kingdom

Key Words. Isolated CD34+ cells • Purity • Yield • Immunoadsorption • Colony growth • Cytofluorimetry • Positive selection • Applications

Introduction

In the rapidly expanding fields of bone marrow transplantation and stem cell research, the demand for purified or enriched populations of immature hematopoietic cells is increasing. In the past, depletion methods were employed to remove the more abundant differentiated cells of various lineages, often utilizing specific "end-cell" functions which the immature cells do not express. These traditional methods were adequate for some purposes (e.g., T cell depletion), though the degree of enrichment obtained was comparatively low.

Recent advances in the characterization of cell surface markers using specific monoclonal antibodies (MAb) have led to new purification strategies. In the analysis of cell surface markers, a fundamental difference was observed between mature and immature hematopoietic cells in both blood and bone marrow, that is, the expression of the CD34 surface marker. This antigen is predominantly expressed on the immature cells, and these represent a minority of the cell population.

As immature cells undergo differentiation, the level of expression of this antigen diminishes by at least three orders of magnitude, so among the normal cell complement of bone marrow and peripheral blood there is a heterogeneous population of CD34 positive cells. This highlights one of the technical difficulties in exploiting the CD34 antigen in physical separation procedures, as the strength of binding of CD34+ cells to anti-CD34 MAb coated matrices will reflect the level of expression of the antigen on the cell surface. This implies the risk that positive cells may be lost during washes in the negative fraction by adhering too loosely, or they stick too tightly to the matrix for detachment with the positive fraction. Furthermore, the nature of the anti-CD34 MAb and variations in the structure and accessibility of the epitope affect the antibody-antigen interaction.

Correspondence: Dr. E. Wunder, Institut de Recherche en Hématologie et Transfusion, Hôpital du Hasenrain, 87 Avenue d'Altkirch, 68051 Mulhouse, France.

 ISBN 1-880854 17-1

Nevertheless, over recent years, several systems for positive selection of $CD34^+$ cells have been developed, and these are now commercially available (Table I). They allow easy access to highly enriched immature cell populations and will be discussed individually in the following chapters.

All the systems based on immunoadsorption must be used within a limited time span following their production. So it is recommended that purifications performed within the short-term be carefully planned, and only the calculated numbers of devices ordered. In this way optimal results can be expected and the degradation of these rather expensive materials avoided.

Before starting cell separation, it is worthwhile analyzing the main prerogatives for enriched $CD34^+$ cells, as this may influence the choice of system. Apart from yield and degree of purity, the time needed for the procedure may play a role. By and large, a minimum of three to four hours appears to be necessary for any separation if cell preparation and getting the system ready for use are included. If adjacent purification steps are to be incorporated, such as efficient removal of a particular cell contaminant, this will obviously increase the preparation and separation time.

Immunoadsorptive Systems

Most immunoadsorptive systems are constructed in different sizes; the small devices allow preparation of sufficient hematopoietic cells required for diagnostic or analytical purposes, while the larger devices aim to process whole grafts for transplantation of enriched stem cell fractions. In the case of transplantation, a major concern is that all hematopoietic cells indispensable for complete long-term recovery are retained in the enriched fraction. Here, the yield is the main criterion, while in other separations for specific research investigations, the purity of the collected cells is of paramount importance,

Table I. Different commercially available systems used for enrichment of $CD34^+$ cells

I) Fluorescence activated cell sorting (FACS)
II) Systems based on immunoadsorption
- A) Panning (AIS)
- B) Immune adsorption column chromatography (CellPro)
- C) Immune adsorption on ferromagnetic beads, which are collected by magnets
  - 1) Large beads (near cell size)
    - a) Detachment by competition with nonspecific antibodies (Dynal)
    - b) Enzymatic detachment (Baxter)
  - 2) Middle size beads (Immunotech)
  - 3) Microbeads of submicroscopic size (Miltenyi)

III) Systems based on physical parameters of cells
- A) Density gradient centrifugation (Percoll)
- B) Centrifugal counter flow elutriation (CCE, Beckman)

even on the expense of lower recovery. It is evident then that the criteria for the quality of separated cells will vary according to the purpose for which processed cells will be used.

Fluorescence Activated Cell Sorting (FACS)

Fluorescence activated cell sorting (FACS) is the classical way of collecting cells which appear "CD34$^+$" on cytofluorograms. While these cells show fluorescence intensities above the background level, it must be borne in mind that some nonspecifically labeled cells will be among this "positive" fraction, and an entirely pure population cannot be obtained (see chapter by *Larsen*, pp. 133-140). The same is true for immunoadsorption methods where cells such as monocytes may be nonspecifically labeled with MAb, which is retained on the cell surface by sticking (underlining the necessity for careful washing during purification procedures). Although extremely effective, FACS is relatively slow, so that large-scale purification is not practical. It was mainly for this reason that immunoadsorption systems were developed.

Cytofluorimetric Analysis

Cytofluorimetric analysis is desirable at each step, but this may involve the sacrifice of too many cells in the final enriched fraction (particularly if small immunoadsorption devices have been used). One solution may be to use miniature vials in the cytofluorimeter, which can help to reduce losses; 2 cm plastic tubes with an opening just large enough for the nozzle are useful (supplied f.e. by *Greiner*). Alternative solutions are discussed in the chapter by *de Wynter et al.* (pp. 281-288).

Measurement of CD34$^+$ Cell Enrichment

One fundamental question arises for all of these systems: How can enrichment and loss of certain CD34$^+$ cells be monitored in order to obtain reliable estimates of the separation achieved? Short-term colony assays for colony forming units granulocyte-macrophage (CFU-GM) are most frequently used to monitor progenitors throughout all phases of cell separation, but the results must be interpreted with some caution, as discussed below. In addition, results will only be available one week later, so that evaluation is retrospective.

In order to evaluate the quality of the separation, it is helpful to record the results at each stage of purification, by following a systematic protocol. If the following fundamental definitions are applied universally, results will further on be comparable not only between different laboratories, but also in the literature.

Generally, a mononuclear cell (MNC) fraction is used as the starting material for purification, and this fraction is obtained by a density gradient centrifugation step (usually Ficoll-Hypaque, p = 1.077 g/ml at 20°C). For specific modification in large-scale purification, see *Dr. Lanza's* article dealing with Percoll (pp. 255-270).

Definition of Parameters

MNC are lost during purification, as some cells bind nonspecifically to various surfaces while others are lost during the washing and detachment procedures. The percentage of MNC recovered at each step or at the end of the entire procedure may be calculated as follows:

$$\textbf{\% MNC recovery} = \frac{\text{No. of MNC recovered} \times 100}{\text{Input no. of MNC}}$$

The total number of $CD34^+$ cells in the initial MNC fraction can be calculated using the formula:

$$\textbf{Initial No. of CD34}^{+}\textbf{ cells} = \frac{(\%\ \text{CD34}^{+}\ \text{cells/MNC}) \times (\text{Total initial no. of MNC})}{100}$$

The percentage of $CD34^+$ cells may be obtained from flow cytometry read-outs; if a control antibody is used to determine the nonspecifically stained cells, the percentage of $CD34^+$ cells must be adjusted by subtracting this figure.

Not all $CD34^+$ cells will be recovered after the purification procedure; some may be lost because they detach unduly and therefore show up in the "negative" fraction. Others may not have detached properly, thus reducing the numbers in the "positive" fraction.

Additionally, the "positive" fraction may contain some $CD34^-$ cell contamination. Therefore the yield of $CD34^+$ cells resulting from the purification (usually expressed as a percentage) is calculated as:

$$\textbf{\% Yield of CD34}^{+}\textbf{ cells} = \frac{\text{No. of cells in “positive” final fraction} \times \%\ \text{purity of CD34}^{+}\ \text{cells}}{\text{Initial no. of CD34}^{+}\ \text{cells}}$$

In this equation the purity of the resulting positive fraction may be derived from flow-cytometry results and is defined as follows:

$$\% \textbf{ Purity} = \frac{\text{No. of actual CD34}^{+}\text{ cells in "positive" fraction} \times 100}{\text{Total no. of cells in "positive" fraction}}$$

Cytofluorimetric Evaluation

This evaluation can be most illustrative, and printed out dotplots contain plenty of information. Try to store and save all data in list mode for future analysis. If the standard criteria outlined for enumeration are applied, uniform measurements can be made for the different stages of separation. However, where low numbers of purified cells are available, it may not be practical to sacrifice any for this measurement.

Evaluation of Short-Term Colonies

The conventional method for evaluating enrichment of colony forming cells is to determine the number of CFU-GM in short-term colony assays after stimulation by growth factors. In this method, however, monitoring is restricted to clonogenic cells of the myelomonocytic lineage. Apart from this, another limitation is that as the degree of purification increases the cloning efficiency of progenitor cells in these assays decreases. The stimulatory growth factors being commonly used in this assay, like granulocyte-macrophage colony stimulating factor (GM-CSF) or placental cell conditioned medium, act indirectly on clonogenic progenitors via accessory cells, such as monocytes; when these monocytes are efficiently removed, a dramatic further reduction in cloning efficiency results, as shown in a separation protocol of normal bone marrow (see Table II). The efficiency recovers after reconstitution with purified monocytes, indicating that these cells supply vital cytokines required for stimulation of the colony forming cells [1]. This may explain why sometimes few or no colonies are observed after separation; the purity of $CD34^{+}$ cells may be high, but the indirectly stimulating cytokines cannot act. To overcome this problem, stimulation with a mixture of cytokines, including stem cell factor, is recommended.

Applications for Enriched $CD34^{+}$ Cells

Especially in patients with solid tumors, it is possible to substantially reduce the tumor load of malignant cells in grafts for autologous transplantation by positive selection of $CD34^{+}$ cells. Also, depletion of residual contaminating malignant cells can be accomplished to a much higher degree in enriched $CD34^{+}$ cell fractions than is otherwise possible. By this method, undesirable effects of cytostatic in vitro purging on normal hematopoietic cells are eliminated. A practical advantage of concentrated, enriched stocks of

Table II. Colony yield (CFU-GM) per $CD34^+$ cell content in normal human bone marrow prior to and after cytofluorimetric cell sorting and adjacent monocyte depletion by specific complement lysis.

	%($CD34^+$/MNC)	$CD34^+$/dish	CFU-GM/dish	CFU-GM Enrichment	%(CFU-GM/$CD34^+$)	PSR($CD34^+$/CFU-GM)
Bone Marrow MNC						
Total	1.1	2,200	232	1	10.5	9.5:1
Flow Sorting						
a) fluorescent cell fraction	90	18,000	1,150	50	6.4	15.7:1
b) nonfluorescent cell fraction	0 (3)	–	63	–	–	–
Monoc. Purge*	90-100	18-20,000	4	–	0.02	4,5-5,000:1
Reconst.	1.1	2,200	211	0.9	9.6	10.4:1

MNC after Ficoll separation were specifically stained by FITC-anti $CD34^+$ MAb HPCA (B-D) and flow sorted on a FACStar (B-D). CFU-GM yields and calculated $CD34^+$ cell numbers in total MNC are given for 2×10^5 MNC per dish and accordingly calculated for enriched fractions. “Cloning efficiency” based on CFU-GM per absolute number of $CD34^+$ cells in culture given as % is shown in the former row. The “progenitor stimulation rate” (PSR) contains the same information, but in the more illustrative form of no. of $CD34^+$ cells per CFU-GM. The cells are stimulated with GM-CSF + IL-3, and colonies are read at day 7. For reconstitution, the stained and unstained (corresponding to “positive” and “negative”) cell fractions were mixed in appropriate concentrations in order to reproduce the initial composition.
*After purging, cells were put into culture without further analysis, and the range of $CD34^+$ cells, to which the CFU-GM number corresponds, is indicated.

CD34+ cells is that a reduced and more compact sample can be stored in liquid nitrogen. This is of particular benefit if banks of cord blood stem cells and enriched CD34+ cells from cytapheresis harvests are to be established.

There is an increasing demand for purified populations of CD34+ cells in the fields of cancer research and cell biology, where applications cover a broad spectrum ranging from the identification of the totipotent hematopoietic stem cell to studies on gene transfer into immature cell populations. The CD34+ population is heterogeneous, and rare subsets of these cells can be examined by cytofluorimetry in an enriched fraction more easily than in unpurified MNC fractions, as demonstrated by *Bühring* (pp. 89-97).

For some applications, where the presence of mature cells (e.g., monocytes and T cells) disturbs or interferes with normal functioning of immature hematopoietic cells, uncontaminated immature cells can now be isolated.

Furthermore, the effects of growth factors on individual CD34+ cells, either singly or in combination, can be investigated conveniently by use of modern FACS sorting facilities which distribute target cells automatically into the wells of microtiter plates.

References

1 Wunder E, Thing-Mortensen B, Sovalat H, Hénon P, Charbord P. Role of mononuclear macrophages in the regulation of haemopoiesis: in vitro experiments and observations in vivo. In: Hematopoietic Growth Factors and Mononuclear Macrophages. van Furth R ed., Basel, Switzerland: Karger, 1992:44-53.

Principles, Capacity and Limitations of Immunofluorescent Flow Sorting of Rare Cell Species

Jørgen K. Larsen

Finsen Laboratory, Rigshospitalet, University Hospital, Copenhagen, Denmark

Key Words. Flow cytometry • Fluorescence activated cell sorting • Flow sorting • Rare cells • Hematopoietic stem cells

Introduction

Flow cytometry offers a rapid, objective and quantitative method for analysis and purification of cells in suspension [1-5]. The fundamental concept of flow cytometry is simple. Cells or other particles interact with a light beam as they pass by single-file in a liquid stream. Interaction with the light is generally measured as light scatter and fluorescence according to the staining of the cells. If a fluorochrome is specifically and stoichiometrically bound to a cellular component, the fluorescence intensity will ideally represent the amount of that particular component.

Multiparameter flow cytometry allows one to estimate, with high accuracy, relative quantities of a variety of cell constituents simultaneously. When the measurements are recorded in a list mode, it is possible to attribute each of the several measured features to a particular cell and thus to obtain correlated measurements of these features on a cell by cell basis. Cellular heterogeneity can thus be estimated and cell populations with distinct characteristics can be discriminated. Thus, multiparameter flow cytometry offers improved opportunities to describe the complex relationship between cell activation, proliferation, maturation and differentiation in the heterogeneous populations of, e.g., blood and bone marrow where different differentiation lineages are mixed together or tumors where malignant cells may be discriminated by clonal characteristics.

In a flow sorter [6], individual cells can be physically separated from larger populations, based on a composite of parameters. Any set of criteria derived from the flow cytometric analysis can be used to activate the sorting decision for the single cell. Flow sorting is the only method that separates cells by their quantitative expression of molecules or their combination of predefined properties. On this basis, flow sorting can be used as part of an analytical strategy or for preparative purposes, e.g., in isolation of hematopoietic stem cells.

Correspondence: Jørgen K. Larsen, Finsen Laboratory, Rigshospitalet, Dept. 8621, Strandboulevarden 49, DK-2100 Copenhagen, Denmark.

 ISBN 1-880854 17-1

Instruments

Practically all flow sorting of hematopoietic stem cells has been done using droplet sorters. Individual cells that fulfill the flow cytometrically defined criteria are trapped in microdroplets that are formed further downstream, the transformation of the liquid jet into droplets being stabilized by a piezoelectric crystal. Those individual droplets that contain desired cells are given a positive or negative electrical charge and are electrostatically deflected for separate collection. The physical basis for droplet sorting has been extensively reviewed and discussed by *Lindmo et al.* [6]. Practical instructions in the use of droplet sorters are given elsewhere [2, 3]. Up-to-date commercial instruments are the Becton Dickinson's FACStar and FACS Vantage, in which the cells are illuminated in a liquid jet after its passage through a nozzle; and the Coulter Electronics' EPICS Elite, in which the cells are illuminated inside a quartz flow chamber.

An alternative construction is the fluid switch sorter, where selected cells are separated inside a closed liquid system, thereby reducing potential biohazard risks in work with infectious materials. However, fluid switch sorters have relatively low sorting rates—no more than a few hundred cells/sec. Commercial fluid switch sorters are Partec's PAS II/III and Becton Dickinson's FACSort. Special nozzles and chambers for sorting of very large particles are available with the various instruments. For high-speed flow sorting at rates of approximately 2×10^4 cells/sec, special prototypes have been developed [7, 8].

Limitations and Critical Aspects

In flow sorting, there is a mutual relationship between sorting capacity, efficiency, recovery and purity. Optimization of any of these parameters implies limitations in the other parameters [6]. The comments below refer to commercial droplet sorters.

Capacity

Sorting capacity is defined as the yield of isolated cells per unit of time. Two subpopulations, characterized by two sets of discriminative parameters, can be sorted out simultaneously using positive and negative charging of droplets. The speed of flow sorting is limited principally by electronics dead time, droplet generation time and spatial distribution of cells in flow. Although the electronics, such as amplifiers and analog-to-digital converters, can handle pulse signals of 2-4 μsec, the droplet sorting rate is clearly limited by the droplet frequency. The time needed to deflect a single cell in a single droplet is on the order of 30 μsec. When three droplets per wanted cell are deflected, a cell sorter may check up to five droplets for coincidence. This increases the time to sort a single cell from 30 μsec to 150 μsec, thereby reducing the maximum sorting rate. Sorting of two or three droplets is common practice, as it increases the chance that the desired cell is deflected. Higher frequency requires a smaller nozzle orifice or increased sheath fluid pressure. Nozzles smaller than 50 μm are undesirable because of clogging and damage to the cells. Nozzles of 70-80 μm are generally preferred for sorting hematological cells at droplet frequencies of 20-35 kHz. Sorting at the theoretical maximum speed is not compatible with pure sorting, because of statistical coincidence from unwanted cells in the deflected set of droplets. Sorting of cells from a subpopulation representing >10% is realistic with a rate on the order of 200-500 deflected cells/sec, resulting in collection of 10^6 sorted cells in ½-1½ h. However, for pure sorting of rare cells, such as hematopoietic stem cells, this rate is not realistic. Furthermore, the setup and control procedures are time consuming [2, 3]. The yield of isolated cells depends on sorting efficiency and recovery.

Efficiency

Sorting efficiency is defined as the number of activated sort events, relative to the number of total analyzed cells that belong to the desired category. If it is important to obtain as many desired cells as possible out of a certain sample, sorting should take place at a low input rate, so that rejection rate due to coincidences will be low. The situation will be different, if the objective is to obtain the highest possible rate of sorted cells, as might be the case if there is a sufficient supply of sample and the aim is to reach a certain number of sorted cells in the shortest possible time [6].

Recovery

Sorting recovery is defined as the number of cells actually found in the sorted fraction at the end of a sort run, relative to the number of activated sort events. Sorting recovery may be low for two different reasons: the charged droplet never reached the collection vessel set up for the sorted fraction, or the droplet reached the collection vessel but contained no cell. The latter problem may be helped by adjusting the sort delay and the droplet synchronization, or by increasing the number of droplets to be deflected per activated sort event. Setting the correct sort delay will usually be a two-step procedure: first estimate the delay and then verify the setting by test sorting. Estimating the delay can be done by measuring out the distance from the optical focus along the jet to the droplet break-off point, and determining how many droplet periods this corresponds to by counting the number of droplets over an equally long distance further downstream. The estimated delay is verified by test sorts with easily identifiable particles (e.g., fluorescent beads from Polysciences, Flow Cytometry Standards, or Molecular Probes) for a series of delay settings around the proposed value and using a deflection of only one drop per event [2, 6]. Using the opposite charge for deflection of an internal reference particle onto slides for control in the microscope enables a current control of the sorting recovery without interrupting a long lasting experiment for sorting of a rare cell type.

Low recovery may be due to too small a nozzle orifice or cell aggregates disturbing the drop formation, resulting in "fanning" of the deflection streams. A good result depends on the preparation of monodispersed suspensions of viable cells. Cell aggregates may be eliminated by pretreatment with DNase and filtration of the suspension through nylon gauze (40-50 μm). Before sorting cells for culture experiments, the sheath and sample fluid system must be cleaned by rinsing with disinfectants, e.g., 0.5% sodium hypochloride followed by 0.1% 7X-PF (Flow Laboratories) [2, 3], and anti-bacterial filters must be inserted in the air and sheath fluid supply lines. Repulsion of charged droplets from the collecting vessels due to buildup of static electricity can be avoided by using collection vessels of glass instead of plastic or using a grounding wire. The collecting vessel must be appropriately prepared according to the planned use of the sorted cells, this may include coating with serum to enable later transfer of the cells. Biohazards from infectious material caused by aerosol formation can be prevented by evacuating and filtering the air from the flow chamber [3, 9].

Purity

Sorting purity is defined as the fraction of sorted cells that belong to the desired category, relative to the number of recovered cells. The enrichment rate is defined as (% desired cells after sort/% undesired cells after sort)/(% desired cells before sort/% undesired cells before sort) [10]. Highest purity (>99%) and highest enrichment rate (>10^3) are only obtained, if full coincidence discrimination is used at a low sample input rate and if the cell suspension is perfectly monodispersed without clumps. If electronic thresholds are set to detect undesired as well as desired cell types, decision logics can be enabled to search for unwanted passenger cells within a chosen coincidence checking gate and, in case of coincidence, to then cancel droplet deflection. The coincidence checking gate can be programmed to find unwanted cells within the dead time required to deflect a set of droplets, or when neighboring droplet sets for wanted and unwanted cells would overlap [2, 6]. In sample preparation, measures must be taken to avoid aggregates of loosely adhering cells, as these may be caused to separate by the acceleration forces in the hydrodynamic focusing region of the nozzle, resulting in inclusion of nondetected, unwanted cells in the set of deflected droplets.

Summarizing the critical aspects of flow sorting: good results depend on adequately stained, monodispersed cell suspensions to be run through a clean flow system and collected appropriately. It must be emphasized that it is not possible in a single run to obtain optimal performance with respect to both sorting capacity, efficiency, recovery and purity. It is necessary that the number of deflected cells and the sorting purity, although these data are intentionally indicated by the instrument, be controlled by flow cytometric re-analysis of the sorted fraction or examined by fluorescence microscopy, hemocytometer counts or otherwise.

Rare Cells

Methods for detection of rare cells are needed for progress in areas like detection of residual disease in leukemias and lymphomas, detection of micrometastasis of solid tumors, detection of genetically transfected cells, and characterization and isolation of hematopoietic stem cells [3, 11]. In a model study, *Gross et al.* [12] seeded the pre-B cell line REH into peripheral blood mononuclear cells (PBMC) at concentrations of 10^{-4}-10^{-6} of total cells. By flow cytometry (Becton Dickinson FACScan) they were able to detect the REH cells and found a background of about one event per 10^8 PBMC. This sensitivity was achieved by removing four sources of false positive events: nonspecific immunofluorescence, autofluorescence, background particles from previous experiments and bursts of events during acquisition. To overcome limits to rare event detection imposed by nonspecific staining and autofluorescence, they used positive and negative selection markers for the REH cells. Another fluorochrome was added to stain the background cells and particles. In order to remove particles and background from previous experiments, a cleaning technique was developed and event bursts were removed from the analysis by developing an algorithm that screened the list mode data for events that were not Poisson distributed.

Single Cell Sorting

For most droplet sorters, special devices allow sorting of a single cell per well in a culture tray. This enables characterization of the phenotype of self renewing pluripotent hematopoietic stem cells. *Huang* and *Terstappen* [13] report on new formation of a hematopoietic microenvironment as well as hematopoietic stem cells in cultures of single cells sorted from human bone marrow according to the combined phenotypic criteria $CD34^{+}HLA\text{-}DR^{-}CD38^{-}$. These data, based on the flow sorting of single cells, probably represent the first identification of a single cell capable of reconstituting the hematopoietic cells and their associated bone marrow microenvironment.

Preparative Sorting

If a large number of cells have to be sorted it may be efficient to use the flow sorter twice: at a high rate in a first run, yielding many coincident unwanted passengers, and subsequently using the collected suspension for a second run at low sample pressure and full coincidence discrimination [14, 15]. However, alternative methods of cell separation—e.g., using methods based on immunomagnetic beads (Dynal's Dynabeads, Immunotech's IO-beads, MACS-beads, Baxter-beads), avidin-coated beads (CellPro), or panning (Applied Immune Sciences' Cellector)—do offer advantages of simplicity and yields, and may be more cost and time effective than flow sorting when large numbers of cells are to be separated and when purity is not critical.

Strategies for enrichment of hematopoietic stem cells have recently been reviewed by *Watt* and *Visser* [15-18]. Rapid enrichment using a univariate bulk technique, followed by multivariate flow sorting, seems optimal for the purification of hematopoietic stem cells. Purification of $CD34^+$ cells from human peripheral blood, from a level of 0.2% to more than 98% purity, has recently been reported by *Kato* and *Radbruch* [10]. This was achieved by using positive selection with biotinylated anti-CD34 antibody and streptavidin-coated magnetic beads (MACS) in a first step. In a second step, the cells were flow sorted in a FACStar Plus, using sorting gates in forward and sideward light scatter and according to positive staining with CD34 antibody and negative staining with propidium iodide, to exclude dead cells.

References

1 Melamed MR, Lindmo T, Mendelsohn ML, eds. Flow cytometry and sorting. 2nd ed, New York: Wiley-Liss, 1990.

2 Ormerod MG, ed. Flow cytometry. A practical approach. Oxford: IRL Press, 1990.

3 Radbruch A, ed. Flow cytometry and cell sorting. Berlin: Springer Verlag, 1992.

4 Darzynkiewicz Z, Crissman HA, eds. Flow cytometry. Methods Cell Biol 1990;33.

5 Larsen JK. Cell proliferation: analysis by flow cytometry. Nouv Rev Fr Hematol 1992;34:317-335.

6 Lindmo T, Peters DC, Sweet RG. Flow sorters for biological cells. In: Melamed MR, Lindmo T, Mendelsohn ML, eds. Flow cytometry and sorting, 2nd edition. New York: Wiley-Liss, 1990:145-169.

7 Peters D, Branscomb E, Dean P, Merrill T, Pinkel D, Van Dilla M, Gray JW. The LLNL high-speed sorter: design features, operational characteristics, and biological utility. Cytometry 1985;6:290-301.

8 Herweijer H, Stokdijk W, Visser JWM. High-speed photodamage cell selection using bromodeoxyuridine/Hoechst 33342 photosensitized cell killing. Cytometry 1988;9:143-149.

9 Merrill JT. Evaluation of selected aerosol-control measures on flow sorters. Cytometry 1981;1:342-345.

10 Kato K, Radbruch A. Isolation and characterization of $CD34^+$ hematopoietic stem cells from human peripheral blood by high-gradient magnetic cell sorting. Cytometry 1993;14:384-392.

11 DeJongh MO, Rozemuller H, Bauman JGJ, Visser JWM. Use of biotin-labelled growth factors for receptor studies. In: Jacquemin-Sablon A, ed. Flow cytometry—New developments. Berlin: Springer-Verlag, 1993:219-225.

12 Gross H-J, Verwer B, Houck D, Recktenwald D. Detection of rare cells at a frequency of one per million by flow cytometry. Cytometry 1993;14:519-526.

13 Huang S, Terstappen LW. Formation of haematopoietic microenvironment and haematopoietic stem cells from single human bone marrow stem cells. Nature 1992;360:745-749.

14 McCoy JPJ, Chambers WH, Lakomy R, Campbell JA, Stewart CC. Sorting minor subpopulations of cells: use of fluorescence as the triggering signal. Cytometry 1991;12:268-274.

15 Visser JW, de Vries P. Identification and purification of murine hematopoietic stem cells by flow cytometry. Methods Cell Biol 1990;33:451-468.

16 Watt SM, Visser JWM. Recent advances in the growth and isolation of primitive human haemopoietic progenitor cells. Cell Prolif 1992;25:263-297.

17 Visser JWM. Isolation and biological characterization of bone marrow stem cells and progenitor cells. In: Laerum OD, Bjerknes R, eds. Flow cytometry in hematology. London: Academic Press, 1992:9-30.

18 Visser JWM, Hogeweg-Platenburg MGC. Identification and isolation of bone marrow stem cells. In: Jacquemin-Sablon A, ed. Flow cytometry—New developments. Berlin: Springer-Verlag, 1993:141-154.

Suppliers of Instruments and Reagents

Flow Cytometers and Cell Sorters

1 Becton Dickinson Immunocytometry Systems, 2350 Qume Drive, San José, CA 95131-1807, U.S.A.; Phone: 1-800-223-8226/1-800-448-BDIS; Fax: 1-408-954-BDIS (FACScan, FACSort, FACStar, FACS Vantage).

2 Coulter Electronics, Inc., P.O. Box 4486, Hialeah, FL 33014, U.S.A.; Phone: 1-800-633-7427, ext. 4866; Fax: 1-305-883-6805 (EPICS Elite).

3 Partec GmbH, Otto-Hahn-Strasse 32, D-4400 Münster, Germany; Phone: +49-2534-5270; Fax: +49-2534-8588 (PAS II/III).

Immunomagnetic Beads

1 Miltenyi Biotec GmbH, Friedrich-Ebert-Strasse 68, D-5060 Bergisch Gladbach 1, Germany; Phone: +49-2204-8096; Fax: +49-2204-85197 (MACS-beads).

2 Dynal AS., P.O. Box 158, Skoyen N-0212, Oslo 2, Norway; Phone: +47-472-529000; Fax: +47-472-507015 (Dynabeads).

3 Immunotech S.A., 130 Av. J. de Lattre de Tassigny, F-13009 Marseille, France; Phone: +33-91172700; Fax: +33-91412794 (IObeads).

4 Baxter Healthcare Corp., Fenwal Biomedical Therapy Systems, 3015 South Daimler, Santa Ana, CA 92705, U.S.A.

Other Separation Systems

1 Applied Immune Sciences, Inc., 5301 Patrick Henry Drive, Santa Clara, California 95054-1114, U.S.A.; Phone: 1-408-492-9200; Fax: 1-408-980-5888 (Cellector).

2 CellPro, Inc., 22322 – 20th Avenue S.E., Suite #100, Bothel, WA 98021, U.S.A.; Phone: 1-800-221-2778; Fax: 1-206-485-4787.

Fluorescence Standards (Microsphere/Fluorochrome)

1 Flow Cytometry Standards Corporation, P.O. Box 12621, Research Triangle Park, NC 27709, U.S.A.; Phone: 1-800-227-8143/1-919-967-9345; Telex: 4944413 WDL.

2 Polysciences, Inc., 400 Valley Road, Warrington, PA 18976-2590, U.S.A.; Phone: 1-215-343-6484/1-800-523-2575; Fax: 1-215-343-0214.

3 Molecular Probes, Inc., P.O. Box 22010, 4849 Pitchford Avenue, Eugene, OR 97402-0414, U.S.A.; Phone: 1-503-465-8300; Fax: 1-503-344-6504.

Other Reagents

1 Flow Laboratories Inc., 7655 Old Springhouse Road, McLean, VA 22102, U.S.A.; Phone: 1-703-893-5925; Fax: 1-703-356-0774 (7X-PF surfactant).

Immunomagnetic Isolation of CD34+ Cells: Methodology and Monoclonal Antibodies

Torstein Egeland, Gustav Gaudernack
Institute of Transplantation Immunology, Rikshospitalet, The National Hospital, Oslo, Norway

Key Words. CD34+ cells • Immunomagnetic isolation • Monoclonal antibodies CD34 molecule • Glycosylation • Lymphohematopoietic progenitors • Stem cell transplantation

Introduction

Immunohematopoietic stem cells can be isolated with monoclonal antibodies (MAbs) against the cell surface molecule CD34 by flow cytometry sorting or by different immunosorbent techniques including affinity chromatography [1], panning [2] and immunomagnetic separation (IMS) [3]. All methods are critically dependent upon the affinity of the CD34-specific MAb, the distribution of the CD34 epitope on the different maturation stages of the stem cells, and the efficiency of detachment of isolated cells from the absorbent matrix. Several issues have been addressed thoroughly elsewhere in relation to IMS technology [3-6].

The core protein of the CD34 molecule contains a large number of O- and N-glycosylation sites that give rise to a series of different glycosylation-dependent epitopes [7]. These epitopes have been classified according to sensitivity to different glycoproteases [8]. The expression of the epitopes is dependent upon the glycosyltransferase activity of the cell. The regulation of these enzymes and their relationship to maturation of the cells and to the function of the CD34 molecule is not known.

A recent study shows that two forms of CD34 messenger RNA (mRNA) can be generated by alternative splicing. The amount of the two alternative forms of mRNA varies according to maturation [9]. It is possible that these two forms also contribute to the heterogeneity of the CD34 epitopes.

Different CD34-specific MAbs react with different epitopes on the CD34 molecule. The distribution of these epitopes on normal and leukemic CD34+ cells and their reactivity with CD34-specific MAbs are matters of great interest for characterization and isolation of CD34+ cells for stem cell transplantation, stem cell transfection, and in vitro studies of early events in immunohematopoiesis.

Correspondence: Dr. Torstein Egeland, Associate Professor, Institute of Transplantation Immunology, Rikshospitalet, The National Hospital, N-0027 Oslo, Norway.

©AlphaMed Press ISBN 1-880854 17-1

Immunomagnetic Separation (IMS) of CD34$^+$ Cells

Paramagnetic, monosized M450 beads (Dynal, Oslo, Norway) can be reproducibly used for high purity and high recovery isolation of CD34$^+$ cells from bone marrow [3-6], umbilical cord blood (*Steen et al.,* unpublished), and probably also peripheral blood cells after bone marrow cell mobilization. The CD34$^+$ cells, being 1-2% of bone marrow and umbilical cord mononuclear cells (MNC), can be isolated without pre-enrichment of the target cells.

In short, the procedure is as follows: MNC and antibody-coupled paramagnetic beads are mixed to allow CD34$^+$ cells to make rosettes, and the rosette-forming cells are separated from non-rosetting cells by application of a magnetic field. This first step is followed by detachment of the beads used for isolation (Fig. 1). The rosettes formed during mixing of MNC and beads can be formed either by an indirect or a direct technique. In the indirect technique, CD34$^+$ cells are sensitized with an anti-CD34 MAb followed by incubation with beads coupled with a secondary antibody directed against the MAb used for sensitization. In the direct technique, CD34$^+$ cells can be incubated with

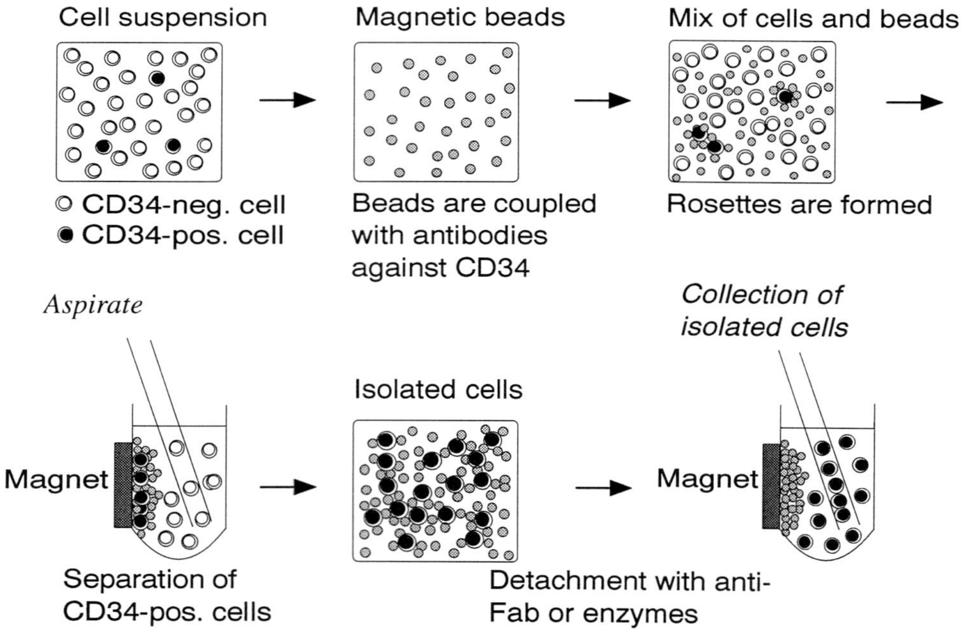

Fig. 1. The principles of immunomagnetic isolation (IMS) of CD34$^+$ cells, utilizing paramagnetic beads coupled with a monoclonal antibody against CD34. Detachment of beads from isolated cells is performed by a polyclonal antibody against murine Fab fragments or enzymes that degrade the CD34 epitope used.

beads precoated with an anti-CD34 MAb. After careful mixing of beads and MNC in a ratio of approximately 1:1 under cold conditions, the beads quickly form rosettes with $CD34^+$ cells. DNase should be present throughout the whole procedure to reduce nonspecific rosette formation that would otherwise cause impaired purity after the isolation.

After rosette formation, detachment of the beads from the isolated cells can efficiently occur either by enzymatic treatment [10] or incubation with a polyclonal antibody against mouse Fab fragments (DETACHaBEAD®; Dynal) [4-6]. In both instances, the MAb used for isolation is also effectively removed from the cell surface [4]. By enzymatic treatment, some CD34 epitopes are left undigested while other epitopes, as well as other cell surface molecules, are digested and need 1-3 days in culture to recover. With detachment based on the anti-Fab antibody interaction, the CD34 as well as all other cell surface molecules are left intact on the cell surface. The advantage of this technique is that important homing and growth factor receptors are probably not affected, and immunophenotypic analyses of the isolated cells can take place immediately after isolation. However, it cannot be excluded that small conformational changes of some CD34 epitopes might occur.

Generally, the recovery after IMS treatment is 60-95% of the target cells or approximately 1% of bone marrow MNC. With a given MAb and the same batch of beads, the recovery is fairly constant from experiment to experiment. The recovery of the whole $CD34^+$ cell population might be substantially lower if the MAb used for isolation reacts with an epitope expressed only by a small subset of cells.

The ability to pull out $CD34^+$ cells from MNC is another way to evaluate the efficiency of the IMS technology. The efficiency can be tested by enumerating the number of remaining clonogenic and repopulating cells in MNC after isolation. With the most efficient MAbs, more than 90% of colony forming units-granulocyte-macrophage (CFU-GM) and burst forming units-erythroid (BFU-E) are removed. However, this may not correlate to the final recovery, since the ability to detach cells from the absorbent matrix used for isolation is another critical parameter.

On forward and side scatter flow cytometry analyses, bone marrow $CD34^+$ cells typically constitute two distinct populations (Fig. 2). If MNC are stained with a fluorochrome-conjugated anti-CD34 MAb, and positively stained cells defined by a forward scatter versus fluorescence intensity dot plot (Fig. 2B) are gated and transferred to a forward versus side scatter dot plot (Fig. 2C), a "CD34 gate" can be drawn consisting of two regions that can be labeled R1 and R2 cells (Fig. 2C). The majority of the cells within the R1 and R2 regions

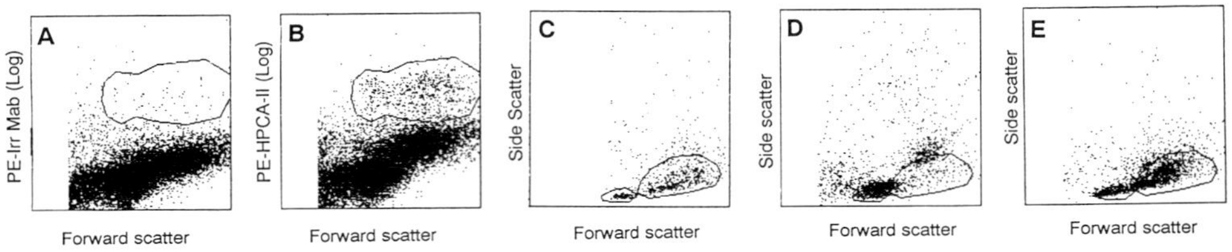

Fig. 2. A-E. Staining of bone marrow mononuclear cells (MNC) depleted of mature B and T cells for CD34 to define the "CD34 gate". A) Side scatter vs. fluorescence dot plot of a negative control with PE-conjugated irrelevant monoclonal antibody. B) Positive staining with PE-conjugated HPCA-II (8G12; Becton Dickinson, Mountain View, CA). The positively stained cells are within the R3 region. C) Forward and side scatter dot plot of events from the R3 region of dot plot B. Based on these events, regions R1 and R2, i.e., the "CD34 gate", can be drawn. D) The localization of the "CD34 gate" compared to ungated events of bone marrow MNC. For better visualization of the gate relative to the lymphocyte and monocyte populations, only 2,000 events are shown. E) Forward and side scatter dot plot of all collected events from analysis of immunomagnetically isolated bone marrow CD34$^+$ cells. The isolated cells fall within the "CD34" gate" defined above.

have lower granularity, i.e., side scatter profile, than lymphocytes and monocytes (Fig. 2D). The R1 cells are typically located in the lymphocyte gate, while the R2 cells are located below and in the lower part of the monocyte gate. Bone marrow CD34$^+$ cells in the R1 region constitute immature B cells, i.e., CD34$^+$CD19$^+$CD37$^-$ cells, while the CD34$^+$ cells in the R2 region are mainly pluripotent cells (to the left in the region) and various myeloid and T cell precursors [11]. Further, isolated CD34$^+$ cells (Fig. 2E) fall within the "CD34 gate" defined in Figure 2C.

For purity assessment of isolated CD34$^+$ cells, the selection of MAb is critical. The MAb has to react with an epitope expressed in high amounts of all CD34$^+$ cells, and the structure of the epitope must not be altered by the isolation procedure. To reduce background staining, we recommend to use directly conjugated MAbs and an excess of human immunoglobulin (Ig)G to block Fc receptors. Purity assessment is still difficult because the number of CD34 molecules is low on a large proportion of the cells, making it difficult to separate negative and positive populations. Nevertheless, it can be argued that the purity after isolation with BI3C5-coupled M450 beads is regularly 80-95% [4, 6]. Contaminating cells are almost exclusively mature B cells, i.e., CD34$^-$CD19$^+$CD37$^+$ cells, found in the R1 region. These cells can efficiently be removed by purging with paramagnetic beads coupled with a MAb against CD37 or against other molecules confined to mature B cells, resulting in a purity of 98-99%. Purity varies between different MAbs used for isolation. With a new anti-CD34 IgG2a MAb labeled 561 (see below), exceptionally high purity and recovery are reproducibly obtained in the single step IMS procedure.

Viability is unaffected by the IMS procedure, and the cells function normally in clonogenic and repopulating assays. The number of CFU-GM and BFU-E in $CD34^+$ cells is enriched by a factor of approximately 2 log compared to MNC [12].

Monoclonal Antibodies Against CD34

A number of MAbs against CD34 exist. Several of these are being used for positive selection of $CD34^+$ cells by different methods or for immunofluorescence and flow cytometry. There is a common observation that certain MAbs are better than others with respect to both isolation and immunofluorescence. This might be due to differences in affinity or to different distribution of the relevant CD34 epitope.

We have generated thirteen new anti-CD34 MAbs after immunization of mice with the cell line KG1A (*Gaudernack et al.*, manuscript in preparation). These MAbs have been designated by numbers ranging from 547 to 581. Epitope mapping of several of these and many reference MAbs has been performed (Fig. 3), and distinct epitopes can be identified both at the molecular

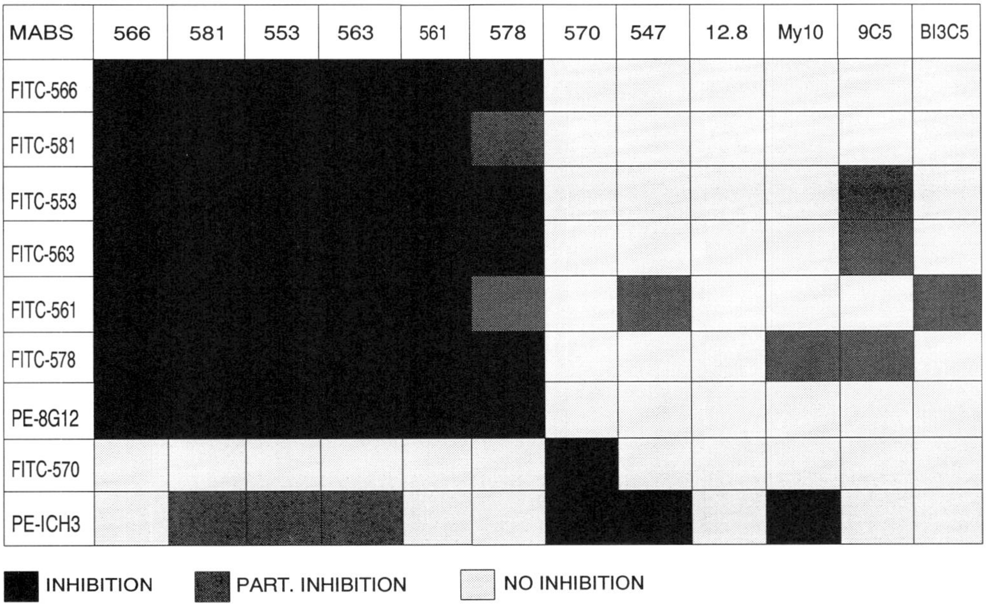

Fig. 3. Epitope mapping shown by blocking experiments of several monoclonal antibodies (MAbs) against CD34. The $CD34^+$ cell line KG1A was used in the study. Blocking MAbs are indicated horizontally.

level and at the cell subset level. Further, some anti-CD34 MAbs react with reduced numbers of normal bone marrow CD34⁺ cells (data not shown), indicating that the expression of certain epitopes is restricted to an as yet undefined subpopulation of stem cells. This observation illustrates the necessity of selecting the right MAb for stem cell studies or transplantation.

In an attempt to define the expression of certain epitopes as a function of maturation and/or lineage commitment, the reactivity of 18 anti-CD34 MAbs on leukemic cells was studied (*Egeland et al.,* in preparation). Figure 4 shows that the MAbs studied can be divided into two groups: group I represents MAbs reactive with leukemic cells from patients with CD34⁺ acute leukemia while group II MAbs are sometimes or frequently non-reactive with cells from the same patients. Typically, some of the group II MAbs tend to react with more immature cells from acute myelogenic leukemia patients. This might reflect a preferential expression of certain group II-assigned epitopes on more immature normal cells. On the other side, preliminary data suggest that a group II MAb like 570 also binds a large number of mature CD34⁺ cells positive for the monocytic marker CD14.

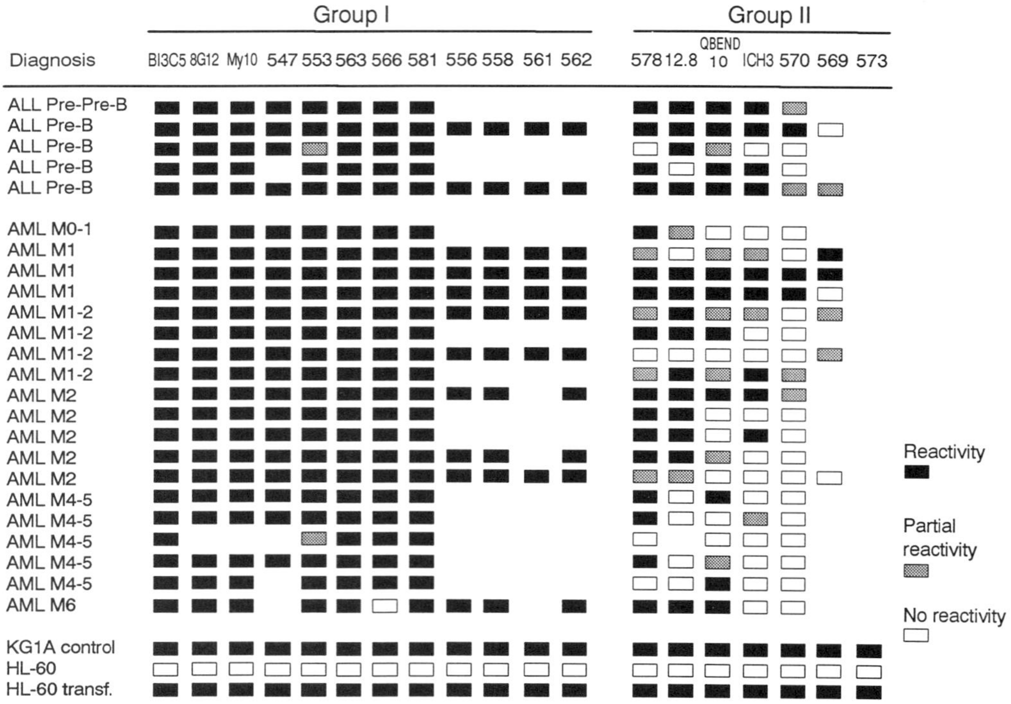

Fig. 4. The reactivity of different monoclonal antibodies against CD34 with cells from patients with CD34⁺ acute leukemia. The leukemia patients were selected based on their leukemic cells' reactivity with the monoclonal antibody BI3C5. The cell lines KG1A and HL-60, the latter with or without transfection of the CD34 gene, were used as controls. Open areas = not tested.

Since the group I MAbs also react with the majority of normal CD34$^+$ cells, they are candidates for positive selection for stem cell transplantation. However, different affinity and detachment properties favor certain MAbs, at least for IMS technology. In particular, the use of the MAb 561 has revealed high purity and recovery in multiple experiments.

When patients with CD34$^+$ leukemias are in remission, the use of group II MAbs may permit isolation of non-leukemic, i.e., potentially normal, CD34$^+$ cells for autologous stem cell transplantation. This can be performed by selecting MAbs that were screened as non-reactive with the CD34$^+$ leukemic cells.

Conclusion

Technology and a series of different MAbs against CD34 exist which allow purification of CD34$^+$ cells that can be used for stem cell transplantation, gene transfection and in vitro studies of hematopoiesis. In addition, the MAbs can be used to study subsets of CD34$^+$ cells as defined by their expression of distinct glycosylation epitopes and possibly to subclassify CD34$^+$ leukemias. Today, there is virtually no knowledge of the characteristics and clinical significance of the different subsets of CD34$^+$ cells. The present panel of CD34-specific MAbs will permit such studies to be performed.

Acknowledgments

Eva Boretti and *Rannveig Østrem* are acknowledged for their technical assistance. The work was supported by grants from The Norwegian Cancer Society, The Royal Norwegian Council for Scientific and Industrial Research, and Dynal. The monoclonal antibodies were kindly obtained from *R.G. Andrews, I.D. Bernstein, C.I. Civin,* and Dynal AS, or were purchased from Becton Dickinson and Caltag.

References

1 Berensen RJ, Andrews RG, Bensinger WI, Kalamasz D, Knitter G, Buckner CD, Bernstein ID. CD34$^+$ marrow cells engraft lethally irradiated baboons. J Clin Invest 1988;81:951-955.

2 Saeland S, Caux C, Favre C, Aubry JP, Mannoni P, Pebusque MJ, Gentilhomme O, Otsuka T, Yokota T, Arai N, Arai K, Banchereau J, de Vries JE. Effects of recombinant human interleukin-3 on CD34-enriched normal hematopoietic progenitors and on myeloblastic leukemia cells. Blood 1988;72:1580-1588.

3 Egeland T. Stem cell isolation and purification. In: Kemshead JT, ed. Magnetic Separation Techniques Applied to Cellular and Molecular Biology. Sommerset: Wordsmith's Conf Publ, 1991:135-142.

4 Smeland EB, Funderud S, Kvalheim G, Gaudernack G, Rasmussen A-M, Rusten L, Wang Y, Tindle R, Kiil Blomhoff H, Egeland T. Isolation and characterization of human hematopoietic

progenitor cells: an effective method for positive selection of CD34+ cells. Leukemia 1992;6:845-852.

5 Smeland EB, Funderud S, Kvalheim G, Egeland T. Effective isolation of human hematopoietic progenitor cells; a new method for detachment of immunomagnetic beads from positively selected CD34+ cells. Int J Cell Cloning 1992;10(suppl 1):108-110.

6 Egeland T, Tjønnfjord G, Steen R, Gaudernack G, Thorsby E. Positive selection of bone marrow-derived CD34 positive cells for possible stem cell transplantation. Proceed Transpl Soc 1993;25:1261-1263.

7 Greaves MF, Brown J, Molgaard HV, Spurr NK, Robertson D, Delia D, Sutherland DR. Molecular features of CD34: A hematopoietic progenitor cell-associated molecule. Leukemia 1992;6:31-36.

8 Sutherland DR, Marsh JCW, Davidson J, Baker MA, Keating A, Mellors A. Differential sensitivity of CD34 epitopes to cleave *Pasteurella haemolytica* glycoprotease: implications for purification of CD34-positive progenitor cells. Exp Hematol 1992;20:590-599.

9 Nakamura Y, Komano H, Nakauchi H. Two alternative forms of cDNA encoding CD34. Exp Hematol 1993;21:236-242.

10 Civin CI, Strauss LC, Fackler MJ, Trischmann TM, Wiley JM, Loken MR. Positive stem cell selection—basic science. Progr Clin Biol Research 1990;333:387-410.

11 Tjønnfjord GE, Veiby O-P, Steen R, Egeland T. T-lymphocyte differentiation in vitro from adult human prethymic CD34+ bone marrow cells. J Exp Med 1993;177:1531-1539.

12 Egeland T, Steen R, Quarsten H, Gaudernack G, Yang Y-C, Thorsby E. Myeloid differentiation of purified CD34+ cells after stimulation with recombinant human GM-CSF, G-CSF, M-CSF and IL-3. Blood 1991;78:3192-3199.

Immunomagnetic Separation of Hematopoietic Progenitor Cells Using Dynabeads® CD34 and DETACHaBEAD®

B.V. Herikstad, E. Lien

Dynal A.S., Skoyen, Oslo, Norway

Key Words. Immunomagnetic separation • Bead detachment system • Cell separation • Hematopoietic progenitor cells • CD34 antigen expression • CD34 positive cells • Stem cells • Stem cell transplantation

Introduction

For both basic and clinical research, a reproducible method for isolation of high purity $CD34^+$ hematopoietic cells from different sources is demanded. We have developed a positive selection system which provides high purity $CD34^+$ cells with unchanged antigen expression, meaning no remaining mouse antibodies on the cell's surface and intact surface antigens.

Immunomagnetic cell isolation with Dynabeads® CD34 provides a fast and reliable method for positive selection of $CD34^+$ cells. Cells can be isolated from a suspension of mononuclear cells (MNC) as obtained by density gradient centrifugation of bone marrow or from mobilized peripheral blood. During a short incubation period, the $CD34^+$ cells bind to Dynabeads CD34, and the rosetted cells can be isolated and washed by simply placing the tube in a magnet (Dynal MPC®). Subsequently, Dynabeads CD34 may be removed from the selected cells by a short incubation with DETACHaBEAD®. The isolated cells are pure (>90% $CD34^+$), show high viability (>95%), have apparently unperturbed antigen expression and are significantly enriched for colony forming cells as demonstrated in different in vitro assays [1].

DETACHaBEAD is a preparation of polyclonal antibodies produced in sheep or goats, with affinity for the Fab part of mouse immunoglobulin (Ig)G molecules. Addition of these antibodies in excess to the positively selected stem cells releases the binding between CD34 antibody coated Dynabeads and CD34 antigens on target cells. Dynabeads CD34 can easily be removed from the cells by a magnet after a short incubation.

The average yield of isolated $CD34^+$ cells from human bone marrow in 26 successive experiments was 1.5% of bone marrow mononuclear cells. This corresponds to an average recovery of 64% [1].

Correspondence: Dr. B.V. Herikstad, Dynal A.S., P.O. Box 158, Skoyen, 0212 Oslo, Norway.

Materials and Methodology

Materials that are not included, but are needed to perform cell isolation with Dynabeads CD34 and DETACHaBEAD:

- Magnetic separation device (for all work with Dynabeads, Dynal recommends the use of a Dynal Magnetic Particle Concentrator, DYNAL MPC®-1/DYNAL MPC®-6).
- Apparatus allowing both tilting and rotation of test tubes (e.g., Dynal Sample Mixer).
- Test tubes (use round bottom tubes for best mixing of cells and Dynabeads during incubation), glassware, pipettes and pipettors.
- Buffers/Solutions.
- Lymphocyte separation medium (Isopaque-Ficoll, e.g., Lymphoprep™, Nycomed, Oslo, Norway).
- Culture media.
- Growth factors, cytokines, etc.

Reagent Preparation

- Phosphate buffered saline (PBS) pH 7.4

$NaH_2PO_4 \cdot H_2O$	1.57 g
$Na_2HPO_4 \cdot 12\ H_2O$	19.80 g
NaCl	81.00 g
Distilled water to	10 L

or alternatively

$NaH_2PO_4 \cdot H_2O$	1.57 g
$Na_2HPO_4 \cdot 7\ H_2O$	14.82 g
NaCl	81.00 g
Distilled water to	10 L

- PBS/FCS: Add 2% fetal calf serum (final concentration) to PBS.
- PBS/HSA: Add 0.3% human serum albumin (final concentration) to PBS.
- PS (penicillin - streptomycin) solution: 5,000 IU/ml penicillin, 5,000 IU/ml streptomycin.
- RPMI/PS: Add 10 ml PS solution to 500 ml RPMI.

- RPMI/Heparin: Add 1.25 ml (1,000 IU/ml) heparin to 50 ml RPMI/PS.
- RPMI/10% FCS: Add 50 ml FCS to 450 ml RPMI/PS.
- DNAse: 10 mg/ml DNAse (e.g., Sigma D4527, 1910 units/mg solid) in RPMI, sterility filtered.
- Citrate phosphate dextrose (CPD) solution: (Baxter Fenwal, 93B17BW).
- PBS/2%HSA, 10%CPD:

PBS (pH 7.4)	400 ml
CPD solution	50 ml
Human serum albumin (HSA) 20%	50 ml
PS (penicillin - streptomycin)	10 ml

All reagents should be analytical grade. The fetal calf serum should be heat inactivated for 30 min at 56°C and tested for cytotoxicity before use.

Instructions for Use

Positive selection of CD34⁺ cells from human bone marrow

For positive selection of $CD34^+$ cells, Dynal recommends a Dynabeads CD34 to cell ratio of 1:1 relative to the total number of MNC as obtained by density gradient centrifugation of bone marrow. In addition, the concentration of Dynabeads during incubation should be equal to or higher than 5×10^7 beads/ml to obtain a sufficient reaction kinetics. The reaction volume should be adjusted to obtain such conditions.

A. Preparation of Dynabeads CD34

1 Resuspend Dynabeads M-450 CD34 in the vial.

2 Transfer the volume of beads needed for an experiment to a tube.

3 Place the tube on a magnetic particle concentrator (Dynal-MPC) for 60 seconds and pipette off the fluid.

4 Remove the tube from the Dynal MPC, and add 2 ml of PBS/FCS.

5 Repeat steps 3 and 4 and resuspend the washed Dynabeads CD34 in a volume of PBS/FCS equal to that originally transferred from the vial.

6 Remove PBS/FCS from the beads immediately before cells are added.

B. Preparation of cells

All culture media referred to under steps 1-5 below should be at room temperature. DNAse should be added immediately before use. RPMI/Heparin and RPMI/10% FCS may be replaced by PBS/2%HSA, 10%CPD if use of FCS is undesirable.

This protocol is optimized for isolation of $CD34^+$ cells from a suspension of 5-20 × 10^7 MNC as obtained from approximately 50 ml of normal bone marrow. Use fresh samples of bone marrow.

1 Dilute the aspirated bone marrow 1:5 in RPMI/Heparin with 10 μg/ml DNAse and mix thoroughly.

2 Layer 25 ml of this cell suspension onto 15 ml Isopaque-Ficoll in a 50 ml tube, and centrifuge at 975 *g* for 20 min.

3 Aspirate the density gradient separated cells and transfer them to a new 50 ml tube. Add 50 μl DNAse and fill the tube with RPMI/Heparin. Centrifuge at 500 *g* for 20 min. Remove the supernatant.

4 Resuspend the pellets and collect the cells from all tubes in one new 50 ml tube. Add 50 μl DNAse and fill the tube with RPMI/Heparin and centrifuge at 300 *g* for 20 min.

5 Resuspend the final cell pellet in 1 ml RPMI/10% FCS, with 10 μg/ml DNAse. Count the cells. Recommended cell concentration is 5-20 × 10^7 cells/ml. Use round bottom tubes to facilitate optimal mixing during incubation with Dynabeads CD34 and DETACHaBEAD.

C. Incubation of cells with Dynabeads CD34

1 Leave the cell suspension at room temperature for 5 min and put on ice briefly (5 min).

2 Transfer the cell suspension to the washed Dynabeads CD34, (Section A, Steps 1-6). The number of Dynabeads CD34 should be the same as number of MNC in the sample, (Section B, Step 5). Final volume during incubation should be 1-1.5 ml, and the Dynabeads CD34 concentration 5-20 × 10^7 beads/ml.

The table below gives examples of volumes of Dynabeads CD34 required, relative to number of MNC in the starting material. The calculated volumes should be aspirated from the Dynabeads CD34 vial and prepared as described in Section A:

# MNC in the sample	5 × 10^7	10 × 10^7	15 × 10^7	20 × 10^7
Dynabeads CD34 vol.:	360 μl	720 μl	1,100 μl (= 1.1 ml)	1,450 μl (= 1.45 ml)
Dynabeads CD34 have a concentration of 1.4 × 10^8 beads/ml				

3 Resuspend the cell-Dynabeads CD34 mixture well by pipetting up and down 15-20 times before incubation for 45 min at 4°C with gentle tilt rotation (e.g., Dynal Sample Mixer) at approximately 10 rpm. Make sure the Dynabeads are kept in suspension during incubation. The tube may be raised at the cap-end to avoid loss of cells in the tube cap.

D. Magnetic separation of rosetted cells

1 Place the tube in a Dynal MPC to allow the Dynabeads CD34 and rosetted cells to migrate toward the magnet. Allow 2 min for the beads/rosettes to accumulate on the tube wall.

2 Withdraw the non-targeted cells while the tube is still exposed to the magnet.

E. Washing the rosettes

Use culture media at room temperature

1 Remove the tube from the Dynal MPC and carefully add 5-10 ml RPMI/10% FCS containing 10 μg/ml DNAse at room temperature.

2 Resuspend the rosettes carefully, and then expose the tube to the Dynal MPC for 2 min, and remove the supernatant with the non-rosetted cells.

3 Repeat steps 1-2 six additional times for a total of seven washes.

4 After the final washing, resuspend the rosettes in 100 μl RPMI/10% FCS.

Usually 70-80% of the $CD34^+$ cells in a normal bone marrow are rosetted by Dynabeads CD34.

F. Detachment of Dynabeads CD34 from selected cells

Efficient detachment (60-80%) of Dynabeads CD34 from the positively isolated cells is obtained using DETACHaBEAD.

1 Add one unit (10 μl) DETACHaBEAD per 1×10^7 Dynabeads CD34 used for rosetting to the isolated cells resuspended in 100 μl RPMI/10% FCS (Section E, Step 4). However, to keep a sufficient concentration, do not use less than 100 μl DETACHaBEAD.

2 Resuspend the suspension by pipetting up and down 20 times to facilitate an optimal initial distribution of DETACHaBEAD.

3 Incubate at room temperature with tilt rotation (e.g., Dynal Sample Mixer) at approximately 18 rpm for 45-60 min. Make sure the cell-bead rosettes are kept in suspension during incubation. Due to the relatively small sample volumes, care should be taken that the cells remain in the bottom of the tube during the incubation to avoid loss of cells.

4 After incubation, add 1 ml RPMI/10% FCS to the tube, and resuspend the sample thoroughly by pipetting up and down 20 times to enhance detachment of Dynabeads CD34 from the cells. Avoid foaming.

5 Place the tube in a Dynal MPC and allow the Dynabeads CD34 to accumulate on the tube wall (2 min).

6 Aspirate the released cells and transfer to a new tube.

G. Washing the detached Dynabeads CD34

1 Add 1 ml of RPMI/10% FCS to the tube with the remaining Dynabeads CD34 and mix by pipetting.

2 Put the tube on a Dynal MPC and allow the Dynabeads CD34 to migrate toward the magnet for 1 minute. Aspirate the supernatant to collect residual cells and transfer to the isolated cells (Section F, Step 6).

3 Repeat steps 1-2 one additional time.

H. Washing the positive selected CD34$^+$ cells

1 Place the tube with the selected cells (Section F, Step 6) once more in a Dynal MPC to remove any residual Dynabeads CD34. Allow the beads to accumulate on the tube wall for 2-3 min. It is important that all beads are removed, as residual beads can form new rosettes during centrifugation.

2 Aspirate the supernatant and transfer to a new tube.

3 Add 10 ml RPMI/10% FCS to the tube and centrifuge the cells at 300 *g* for 10 min. Remove the supernatant.

4 Repeat step 3 one more time and resuspend the final cell pellet in 1 ml RPMI/10% FCS and count the cells.

Recovery of CD34$^+$ cells is normally in the range of 50-75% of the initial number of CD34$^+$ cells in the marrow sample, as measured by flow cytometry.

I. Adjustment of the bone marrow protocol for separation of CD34$^+$ cells from samples containing less than 5 × 10^7 MNC

The following adjustments enable separation from samples containing 1-5 × 10^7 MNC:

Preparation of tubes with blocking proteins

1 Use a small tube (e.g., 2 ml NUNC cryo tube) for rosetting and a 5 ml tube (e.g., Falcon) for detachment.

2 Fill both tubes with FCS and incubate at room temperature for 30 min prior to use, to minimize non-specific attachment of cells to the tube wall.

Incubation of cells with Dynabeads CD34

3 Positive selection is performed in a total volume of 100 μl in the small tube.

4 Use the same ratio of Dynabeads CD34, and number of MNC per test as recommended in the bone marrow protocol (Section C, Step 2). Optimal Dynabeads CD34 concentration is 5-20 × 10^7 beads/ml.

The table below gives examples of volumes of Dynabeads CD34 required, relative to number of MNC in the starting material. The calculated volumes should be aspirated from the Dynabeads CD34 vial and prepared as described in Section A:

# MNC in the sample	1×10^7	2.5×10^7	5×10^7
Dynabeads CD34 volume	70 μl	180 μl	360 μl
Dynabeads CD34 have a concentration of 1.4×10^8 beads/ml.			

5 After incubation, add 1 ml RPMI/10% FCS, 10 μg DNAse/ml and transfer the suspension to the 5 ml tube. Make sure that nothing is left in the small tube.

Washing the rosettes

6 Place the 5 ml tube on a Dynal MPC and allow the rosetted cells to migrate toward the magnet (2 min). Aspirate and remove the supernatant.

7 Remove the tube from the magnet and resuspend the rosetted cells in 4 ml RPMI/10% FCS, 10 μg DNAse/ml.

8 Repeat steps 2-3 three times for a total of four washes. Resuspend the rosetted cells after the final wash in 50 μl RPMI/10% FCS, 10 μg DNAse/ml.

Detachment of Dynabeads CD34 from selected cells

9 Add 50 μl DETACHaBEAD and proceed according to the protocol as described in Section F, Step 2 through Section H.

Adjustment of the bone marrow protocol for isolation of CD34$^+$ cells from mobilized peripheral blood—proposed protocol:

Peripheral blood collected by apheresis procedures from patients mobilized by growth factors (with or without chemotherapy) has a higher than normal proportion of immature hematopoietic cells. The stage of maturation of the CD34$^+$ cells in the apheresis product depends on the time lapse from initial mobilization to apheresis.

Experiments have shown that gradient centrifugation using Isopaque-Ficoll may not be necessary for isolation of CD34$^+$ from mobilized peripheral blood. However, to increase the purity of isolated cells, a pre-depletion step consisting of incubation with Dynabeads directly coated with a B cell antibody (Dynabeads M-450 CD19) has been beneficial. Following this predepletion procedure, mature B cells as well as cells which nonspecifically associate with Dynabeads are removed before positive selection with Dynabeads CD34 is performed.

Positive selection of $CD34^+$ cells from mobilized peripheral blood is performed according to the bone marrow protocol, following pre-depletion.

It should be noted that when mobilized peripheral blood is the starting material, we recommend replacing RPMI/Heparin and RPMI/10% FCS with PBS/2% HSA, 10% CPD, since this has been shown to reduce phagocytosis of Dynabeads. This solution is prepared as described above.

J. Preparation of Dynabeads M-450 CD19

Prepare the Dynabeads CD19 as described for Dynabeads CD34 in Section A, Steps 1-6. (PBS/2% HSA, 10% CPD, may replace PBS/FCS).

K. Preparation of cells

This protocol has been developed for isolation of $CD34^+$ cells from mobilized peripheral blood containing $1\text{-}5 \times 10^8$ low density cells (LDC).

Adjust the concentration of LDC from apheresis to 1×10^8 cells/ml in PBS/2% HSA, 10% CPD.

L. Incubation of cells with Dynabeads CD19

1 Add Dynabeads CD19 to obtain a ratio of Dynabeads to total LDC of 1:2; the final concentration of Dynabeads CD19 is now 5×10^7 beads/ml.

The table below gives examples of volumes of Dynabeads CD19 required, relative to number of LDC in the starting material. The calculated volumes should be aspirated from the Dynabeads CD19 vial and prepared as described in Section J:

# LDC in the sample	1×10^8	2.5×10^8	5×10^8
Dynabeads CD19 volumes	125 μl	313 μl	625 μl
Dynabeads CD19 have a concentration of 4×10^8 beads/ml.			

2 Incubate at room temperature for 30 min with tilt rotation (e.g., Dynal Sample Mixer) approximately 10 rpm.

M. Magnetic separation/depletion of $CD19^+$ cells

1 Conclude the incubation by filling the tube with PBS/2% HSA, 10% CPD. Rosetted cells are collected by exposing the tube to a magnet (Dynal MPC) for 2 min.

2 Aspirate the non-rosetted cells and transfer them to a new tube (50 ml).

3 Wash the cell-bead rosettes still attached to the Dynal MPC by gently adding 5-10 ml PBS/2% HSA, 10% CPD to the tube.

4 Aspirate the supernatant and combine with the non-rosetted cells (Step 2).

N. Preparation of cells for positive selection of CD34⁺ cells

1. Centrifuge the cell suspension (Section M, Step 2) at 300 *g* for 10 min and remove the supernatant.

2. Resuspend the cell pellet to a concentration of 1×10^8 cells/ml in PBS/2% HSA, 10% CPD.

O. Positive selection of CD34⁺ cells

Positive selection of CD34⁺ cells from pre-depleted mobilized peripheral blood (Section N, Step 2) is now carried out according to the protocol for positive selection of CD34⁺ cells from bone marrow (Instructions for Use, above).

Make sure that the concentration of Dynabeads CD34 is kept at 1×10^8 beads/ml during incubation.

Note also the replacement of RPMI/Heparin and RPMI/10% FCS by PBS/ 2% HSA, 10% CPD, which may be beneficial for the isolation procedure.

Issues of importance for an optimal positive selection with Dynabeads CD34 and DETACHaBEAD:

- Start with fresh sample material.
- Establish the separation technique according to the presented protocols before any individual adjustments are performed.
- Use round bottom tubes to facilitate optimal sample mixing.
- Use the recommended Dynabeads CD34 concentration during rosetting.
- Use the recommended DETACHaBEAD concentration during detachment.
- Remove all free Dynabeads CD34 from the isolated cells, as remaining beads may form new rosettes.
- Wash the selected cells properly to remove DETACHaBEAD.
- Store the selected cells in culture medium containing FCS.

Troubleshooting

P. Low recovery of CD34⁺ cells

1. Use the recommended number of MNC/LDC as described in the protocol. If the sample contains less than 5×10^7 MNC, make the adjustments as described in Section I.
2. Use fresh sample material. If bone marrow has to be stored overnight prior to isolation of CD34⁺ cells, isolate the MNC fraction and store it at 4°C in RPMI containing 10% FCS.

3 Resuspend the MNC fraction well before addition of Dynabeads CD34.

4 During incubation of cells with Dynabeads CD34, the following should be avoided:

- end to end rotation of the tube
- fast rotation leading to foam in the tube
- slow rotation leading to sedimentation of Dynabeads CD34
- use of conical tubes.

5 Physically disturb the binding between cells and Dynabeads CD34 before and after incubation with DETACHaBEAD by pipetting up and down as described in Section F.

6 Take care during incubation with DETACHaBEAD to keep the mixture in the bottom of the tube to avoid loss of cells.

7 Make sure the rosetted cells and non-rosetted Dynabeads CD34 are kept in suspension during incubation with DETACHaBEAD.

Q. Low purity

1 Wash the positive selected cells after detachment as described to remove any remaining DETACHaBEAD. The presence of soluble anti-Fab antibodies may inhibit the binding of labeled CD34 antibodies used for staining.

2 As in Section P, Points 2 and 3.

3 Check the quality of labeled CD34 antibody used for staining.

4 Remove as much fat as possible from within the bone marrow prior to incubation with Dynabeads CD34.

5 Wash rosetted cells according to protocol prior to detachment to remove any non-specific attached cells.

6 Use pre-depletion as described in Sections J-M when isolation is performed from mobilized peripheral blood.

R. Low yield measured by flow cytometry but acceptable enrichment of colony forming cells as measured by in vitro assays

As in Section Q, Point 1.

Cell Characterization

Flow cytometry

Human progenitor cells positively selected from human bone marrow with Dynabeads® CD34 and DETACHaBEAD® have been analyzed by flow cytometry using fluorescence labeled antibodies. Subpopulations of the cells expressed myeloid markers (CD13, CD33 and to a lesser extent CD14, CD15) or early B lineage markers (CD19 and CD10). In general, cells with low forward scatter expressed B lineage markers. Only a small fraction of the cells (1-2%) were positively stained with an antibody against a T lineage marker (CD2). Most of the cells expressed CD38 and a majority of them also expressed CD41b. No signs of activation of the cells were observed. In addition, the cells could be restained with a number of CD34 monoclonal antibodies, indicating that DETACHaBEAD removes the Dynabeads CD34 without affecting the expression of the CD34 antigen [1].

Colony assays

$CD34^+$ progenitor cells isolated from human bone marrow with Dynabeads CD34 have been evaluated in several in vitro growth and differentiation assays. They responded strongly to various cytokines such as interleukin (IL)-3, granulocyte-macrophage-colony stimulating factor (GM-CSF), mast cell growth factor (MGF) and G-CSF alone or in combinations as measured by ^3H-thymidine incorporation.

The selected $CD34^+$ cells were enriched for colony forming units-granulocyte-macrophage (CFU-GM) whereas the CD34 negative cells were significantly depleted of cells capable of generating CFU-GM, as compared to bone marrow MNC.

The $CD34^+$ cells were also enriched for primitive hematopoietic progenitors on a stromal feeder layer, as examined by the capacity of forming blast colonies. The CD34 negative cell fraction however, was significantly depleted as compared to bone marrow MNC.

References and Selected Readings

1 Smeland EB, Funderud S, Kvalheim G, Gaudernack G, Rasmussen AM, Rusten L, Wang MY, Blomhoff HK, Tindle RW, Egeland T. Isolation and characterization of human hematopoietic progenitor cells: An effective method for positive selection of $CD34^+$ cells. Leukemia 1992;6(8):845-852.

2 Tindle RW, Nichols RAB, Chan L, Campana D, Catovsky D, Birnie GD. A novel monoclonal antibody BI-3C5 recognises myeloblasts and non-B non-T lymphoblasts in acute leukaemias and CGL blast crises, and reacts with immature cells in normal bone marrow. Leukemia Research 1985;9(1):1-9.

3 Smeland EB, Funderud S, Kvalheim G, Egeland T. Effective isolation of human progenitor cells: A new method for detachment of immunomagnetic beads from positively selected $CD34^+$ cells. Int J of Cell Cloning 1992;10(suppl 1):108-110.

4 Egeland T, Quarsten H, Gaudernack G. Effect of recombinant stem cell growth factors on immunomagnetically isolated $CD34^+$ cells. Int J of Cell Cloning 1992;10(suppl 1):53-55.

5 Egeland T, Tjønnfjord GE, Steen R, Gaudernack G, Thorsby E. Positive selection of bone marrow derived $CD34^+$ cells for possible stem cell transplantation. Proceed Transpl Soc 1993;25:1261-1263.

6 Tjønnfjord GE, Veiby O-P, Steen R, Egeland T. T lymphocyte differentiation in vitro from adult prethymic $CD34^+$ bone marrow cells. J Exp Med 1993;177(6):1531-1539.

Product and ordering information

Dynal International, Dynal AS, P.O. Box 158, Skoyen 0212, Oslo, Norway
TEL: + 47-22-529450, FAX: + 47-22-507015, TLX: 79133 DYNAL N

USA/Canada: Dynal Inc., 5 Delaware Drive, Lake Success, NY 11042, USA
TEL: 800-638-9416, FAX: 516-326-3298

UK/Ireland: Dynal UK, 26 Grove Street, New Ferry, Wirral, L62 5AZ UK
TEL: 051-644-6555, FAX: 051-645-2094

Germany/Austria: Deutsche Dynal GmbH, Postfach 11 19 65, D-20419 Hamburg
TEL: 040-366811, FAX: 040-366040

France: Dynal France S.A., Contre de Transfort de, 1 U.T.C., 66 Av. de Londshut, 60200 Compiegne
TEL: 44-23-45-95, FAX: 44-23-16-14

Japan: Nihon Dynal K.K., Champion Bldg., 1-1-9, Atago, Minato-Ku, Tokyo 105
TEL: 03-3435-1558, FAX: 03-3435-1526

For information on Dynal distributors worldwide, please contact Dynal AS, Oslo, Norway.

CD34+ Cell Purification by Immunomagnetic Beads/Chymopapain System from Normal and Myeloid Leukemias, Bone Marrow and Peripheral Blood for Research Use

Federico Silvestri

Chair of Hematology, Department of Medical and Morphological Researches, Udine University School of Medicine, Udine, Italy

Key Words. CD34+ cells • Purification • Immunomagnetic beads • Chymopapain

Introduction

The progenitors of all hemolymphopoietic lineages [1, 2], and clonogenic cells of most of the patients with acute non-lymphocytic leukemia (ANLL) and chronic myeloid leukemia (CML) [3-5] express on their surface the antigen CD34, while the more mature cells are CD34−. This knowledge has made their selective separation possible.

Taking advantage of the availability of many CD34 antibodies [1, 2], several methods of positive immunoselection like flow-cytometric cell-sorting, panning, avidin-biotin immunoadsorption on column and immunomagnetic beads have been developed in the last few years.

The immunomagnetic beads cell separation, employing the enzyme chymopapain to detach the isolated cells from the beads, was developed by *Civin et al.* [6] and applied for isolating CD34+ cells from normal bone marrow [6, 7]. In this paper we describe the application of this same method for selecting CD34+ cells from bone marrow (BM) and peripheral blood (PB) samples of patients with ANLL and CML, in addition to that from normal bone marrow.

Materials and Methodologies

Samples

After an informed consent was given, six BM samples (two normal, one CML and three ANLL) and ten PB samples (two CML and eight ANLL) were obtained from two healthy volunteers, three patients with CML and nine with ANLL.

Cell Preparation

NB: all media were kept at 4°C unless otherwise specified.

Correspondence: Dr. Federico Silvestri, Cattedra di Ematologia, Policlinico dell'Università di Udine, P.le S. Maria della Misericordia, 33100 Udine, Italy.

 ISBN 1-880854 17-1

1 Heparinized BM or PB samples were collected.

2 Low density mononuclear cells (LDMNC) were prepared by density cut centrifugation on Ficoll-Paque (d = 1.077 g/cm^3) (25 min at 1,000 rpm, 4°C) in a 50 ml tube (15 ml Ficoll + 35 ml BM or PB).

3 LDMNC were collected and washed twice with 20 ml of RPMI-1640 medium (RPMI) (10 min at 1,000 rpm, 4°C).

4 The washed cells were resuspended in 5 ml of RPMI and a cell count was done. Cells (2×10^6) were taken for immunofluorescence and colony assays (unseparated fraction).

5 The cells were then spun and resuspended in RPMI brought to 10% with fetal calf serum (RPMI-10% FCS) at a final concentration of 10×10^6 cells/ml.

Sensitization

NB: from now on a 14 ml tube was used if total number of LDMNC was < 150 × 10^6 or a 50 ml tube was used if cells numbered > 150 × 10^6.

6 The cells were incubated with My10 antibody (1 μg/10^6 cells) for 30 min, at 4°C in a blood mixer (4 rpm).

7 After incubation the cells were spun and washed twice with 15 ml of RPMI-10% FCS (10 min at 1,000 rpm, 4°C) to remove unbound antibody.

8 The washed cells were then resuspended in RPMI-10% FCS at a concentration of 10×10^6 cells/ml and a cell count was repeated.

Separation Procedure

9 The sensitized cells were incubated with sheep anti-mouse immunoglobulin G^1 (IgG1)-coated beads at a ratio of 0.5 beads/cell for 30-40 min, at 4°C, in a blood mixer (4 rpm).

10 The tube was then exposed to the magnet for 2 min to hold beads/rosettes on the tube wall.

11 With the magnet in place, the supernatant was poured off in a 50 ml tube (CD34$^-$ fraction).

12 The beads/rosettes were then resuspended in 7 ml of RPMI-10% FCS and mixed again in a blood mixer for 5 min.

13 The tube was re-exposed to the magnet (2 min) and step 11 was repeated.

14 The CD34$^-$ fraction was then spun and resuspended in 5 ml of RPMI-10% FCS. Cell count and viability were done and 2×10^6 cells were taken for immunofluorescence and colony assays (negative fraction).

15 The beads/rosettes were resuspended in 7 ml of plain RPMI and gently mixed by hand for 30 seconds.

16 Once again the tube was exposed to the magnet (2 min).

17 The supernatant was discarded.

18 Steps 15 to 17 were repeated once more.

19 The beads/rosettes were resuspended in 4.5 ml of plain RPMI kept at room temperature.

Release

NB: from now on a 14 ml tube was used.

20 The beads/rosettes were incubated with 0.5 ml of a 2,000 U/ml solution of chymopapain (final concentration 200 U/ml) for 15 min in a 37°C water bath.

21 After 15 min the cells were mixed with 3 ml of cold (4°C) RPMI-10% FCS to stop the reaction.

22 The tube was then exposed to the magnet (2 min) to retain the beads on the tube wall.

23 With the magnet in place, the supernatant was poured off in another 14 ml tube ($CD34^+$ fraction).

24 The beads were resuspended once more in 5 ml of RPMI-10% FCS and the tube re-exposed to the magnet (2 min). Step 23 was repeated.

25 The $CD34^+$ fraction was spun and resuspended in 2 ml of RPMI-10% FCS and the tube exposed to the magnet (2 min) to remove the last remaining beads.

26 With the magnet in place, the cell suspension was then pipetted off in a 6 ml tube and cell count and viability (Trypan-Blue dye exclusion method) were done.

The purified $CD34^+$ cells were then used for further studies.

Immunofluorescence Assay

The percentage of $CD34^+$ cells in each cell fraction before and after separation was evaluated by indirect or direct immunofluorescence according to standard methods (see other chapters in this book). My10 antibody (Ab) was used to detect the percentage of $CD34^+$ cells in the unseparated and negative fractions, while for the positive fraction 8G12 Ab (or other class III CD34 Abs, such as TuK3) was used because the epitope detected by My10 Ab is lost after chymopapain treatment [6, 8], while the one recognized by class III Abs is retained.

Semisolid Culture of Progenitor Cells

The frequency of clonogenic cells was evaluated by plating 5×10^3 cells from the $CD34^+$ fractions and 1 to 2×10^5 cells from the unseparated and $CD34^-$ fractions in a total volume of 1 ml of Iscove's modified Dulbecco's medium (IMDM) brought to 25% with FCS and supplemented with 10% v/v of phytohemagglutinin stimulated leukocyte-conditioned medium and 0.8% methylcellulose in 35 mm tissue culture dishes.

Chymopapain Toxicity

In order to evaluate the toxicity of chymopapain to the clonogenic cells, the unseparated marrow cells from one ANLL patient, three CML patients and two normal bone marrows were plated, under the same conditions described above, before and after incubation with the enzyme.

Definitions

a) CD34 positivity or purity: the percentage of $CD34^+$ cells in a given sample or fraction.

b) Recovery: the percentage recovery of $CD34^+$ cells in the isolated positive fraction, which is calculated as follows:

$$R = \frac{\text{\% positive cells in isolated positive fraction} \times \text{total number of cells isolated}}{\text{\% positive cells in unseparated fraction} \times \text{total number of starting cells}} \times 100$$

c) Enrichment: the fold enrichment of $CD34^+$ cells in the isolated positive fraction, which is calculated as follows:

$$E = \frac{\text{\% positive cells in the isolated positive fraction}}{\text{\% positive cells in the unseparated fraction}}$$

Statistical Analysis

Student's *t*-test was used to test the probability of significant differences among groups. Data are presented as mean ± SD.

Results and Discussion

The results of the separation experiments and the cloning data are reported in Table I, while in Figure 1 a representative experiment is shown.

For research use, the method here described is very useful for obtaining $CD34^+$ cells in numbers sufficient to perform several biological studies. In fact with a mean (± SD) number of starting LDMNC of $101.8 \pm 44.8 \times 10^6$ (range 11.5 to 203.0), $10.9 \pm 12.1 \times 10^6$ cells (range 1.1 to 44.2) were obtained in the positive fractions. The maximum number of cells processed in our experiments was 203×10^6 LDMNC, but this can be scaled up to 500×10^6 without losing efficiency (*Egeland,* personal communication).

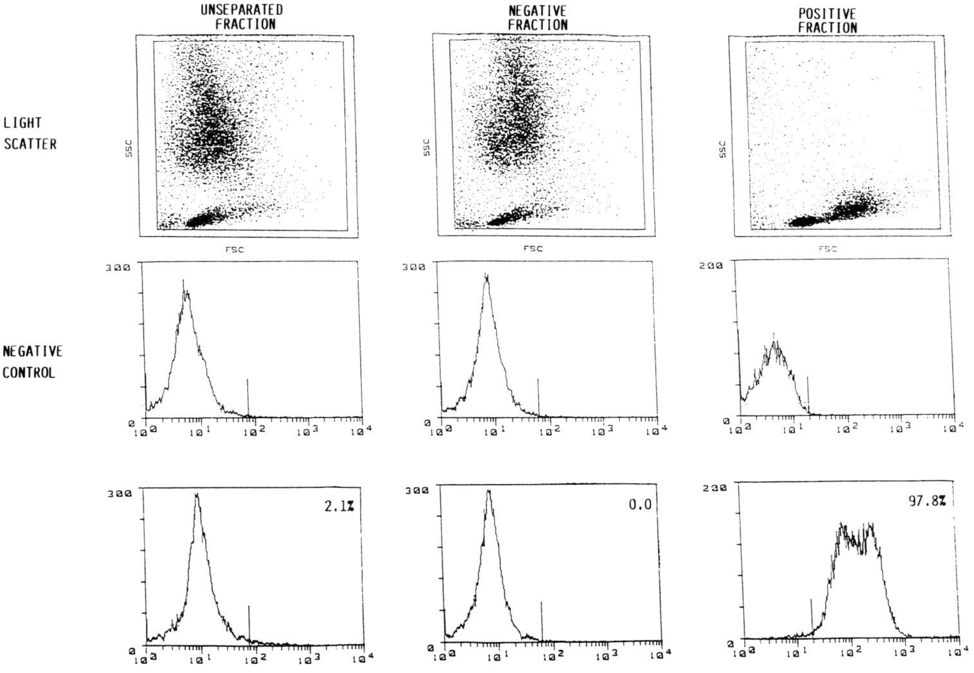

Fig. 1. Normal bone marrow, sample #2. Light scatter (upper line) and histograms (second and third lines) of unseparated (left), negative (middle) and positive (right) fractions. The percent of CD34+ cells in the unseparated fraction was 2.1% and reached 97.8% in the isolated positive fraction.

The mean percentage of CD34+ cells in the unseparated samples was 24.3 ± 28.1 and reached 85.0 ± 10.6% in the isolated positive fractions, with a mean CD34+ cell recovery of 64.0 ± 22.0%. The method is also very efficient when initial CD34 positivity is very low (i.e., < 5%). For example, in samples #1 to 5, 9, 11 and 16, starting CD34 positivity was only 2.1 ± 1.7% but reached 84.6 ± 8.9% in the isolated positive fractions, with a mean recovery of 72.2 ± 25.4%.

The frequency of CD34+ cells in the negative fractions was only 2.7 ± 6.6%. In particular, only two ANLL samples [#8, 10] showed a significant amount of CD34+ cells in this fraction; a negligible amount of CD34+ cells was found in two different ANLL samples [#6, 7] where the initial CD34 positivity was >39%, while in the other samples CD34+ cells were completely removed from the negative fractions. These data could be important in that this separation method allows the study of phenotypic characteristics and cloning efficiency of a cell population depleted of CD34+ cells.

Because My10 Ab and beads/cells ratio were titrated on normal bone marrow, it might be possible that a higher beads/cells ratio in the specimens with a high

Table I. Results of experiments and cloning data

Sample	Diagnosis	% CD34 Cells			CD34⁺ Cells	Colonies/10^5 cells plated		
		Unsep.	Neg.	Pos.	Recovery %	Unsep.	Neg.	Pos.
1	NBM	3.8	0	86	30	117	0	800
2	NBM	2.1	0	97	97	146	0	3,707
3	CML	0.5	0	68	99	5	1	30
4	CML	0.4	0	81	40	20	0	5,100
5	CML	0.6	0	87	73	ND	ND	ND
6	ANLL	39	1.5	80	32	265	16	950
7	ANLL	40	1.2	94	67	12	0	290
8	ANLL	66	21	98	52	107	4	897
9	ANLL	4	0.2	93	91	NG	NG	NG
10	ANLL	72	19	99	78	28	NG	NG
11	ANLL	0.7	0	75	56	6	0	307
12	ANLL	89	0	96	49	33	NG	NG
13	ANLL	22	0	73	44	NG	NG	NG
14	ANLL	20	0	77	67	0	0	250
15	ANLL	23	0	66	58	844	95	1,455
16	ANLL	5	0	90	92	NG	NG	NG

NBM = normal bone marrow; CML = chronic myeloid leukemia; ANLL = acute non-lymphocytic leukemia; NG = no growth; ND = not done percentage of starting CD34$^+$ cells (as in most ANLL) could allow a better depletion of CD34$^+$ cells from the negative fractions, but we do not know what the impact of this would be on the purity of the isolated positive fractions (decreased, due to nonspecific binding?). On the other hand, 1 μg/10^6 cells of My10 Ab should be enough in specimens very rich in CD34$^+$ cells as well; in fact recently the use of 0.5 μg/10^6 cells was proposed for samples with a low percentage of CD34$^+$ cells [9].

According to the separation of CD34$^+$ cells in different fractions, the great majority of clonogenic cells was separated in the CD34$^+$ fractions and depleted in the CD34$^-$ ones, showing that also in myeloid leukemias, as in normal BM, clonogenic potential in vitro is restricted to cells expressing the CD34 antigen [3-5].

Some technical maneuvers of the separation procedure need to be underlined. Washing the samples has to be performed very carefully without losing cells or beads/rosettes in the tube caps or along the tube walls; in particular, steps 12 to 18 are very important to remove all the CD34$^-$ cells trapped in between the beads/rosettes on the tube wall. It is better to repeat these steps once more (CD34$^+$ cells are not lost because they are strongly attached to the beads) than once less! Mixing must be performed very carefully (using a slow-speed blood mixer or hand mixing) as well as centrifugations (gentle, 1,000 rpm). Two minutes exposure to the magnet is an absolutely sufficient time, because migration of beads or beads/rosettes to the tube wall on the magnet requires only a few seconds.

Another critical point is the release reaction; chymopapain hydrolyzes aspecifically all proteic substrates (but the hydrolysis of native immunoglobulins is limited), and the reaction works better at 37°C [10, 11]. For these reasons it is important to use plain RPMI (without FCS) from step 15 on and to use room temperature RPMI in step 19, just before adding the enzyme and putting the tube in the 37°C water bath. Because more than 15 min exposure to the enzyme has been shown to be slightly toxic to the cells [6], chymopapain activity needs to be diluted and the reaction stopped rapidly by adding cold RPMI supplemented with 10% FCS. Recently the release reaction was also performed successfully at room temperature [9].

When employed as described above, chymopapain proved to be non-toxic to the clonogenic cells; in fact the number of colonies grown by plating six unseparated marrows before and after incubation with the enzyme was similar (41.5 ± 54.6 versus 44.9 ± 79.7, $p = 0.80$). That CD34$^+$ cells obtained with this technique also retain their marrow repopulating potential was recently shown in vivo in a murine autologous transplantation model [6, 7] and in a human-to-fetal sheep allogeneic transplantation model [12].

We confirmed [8] the previous report by *Civin et al.* [6] that the CD34 epitope detected by the My10 antibody is lost from KG1a and human cells after treatment with chymopapain, whereas the epitopes detected by other class III CD34 Abs (such as 8G12 or TuK3) are retained, thereby permitting estimation of the purity of the $CD34^+$ cell population isolated by the enzyme. This is another important point to be kept in mind because the use of the wrong antibody does not allow detection of the real percentage of $CD34^+$ cells in the positive fraction. The use of phycoerythrin-conjugated preparations of antibodies offers a better resolution index over the fluorescein isothiocyanate (FITC)-conjugated or the unconjugated ones, especially in the unseparated fractions with low CD34 positivity [13].

In conclusion we showed that positive immunoselection using My10 antibody, immunomagnetic beads and chymopapain is a suitable method for isolating almost pure progenitors from the BM and the PB of both normal healthy subjects and patients with myeloid leukemias.

Advantages over other methods include the technical simplicity of the method which can be easily learned and performed, the short execution time (about three hours) and the knowledge that, since $CD34^+$ cell recovery is always more than 30%, one can easily calculate in advance how many cells are required to begin the experiment to obtain the number of pure progenitors needed to perform other assays.

Materials

How to get in materials used in this study.

1 Ficoll-Paque, catalog # 17-0840-02 was purchased from Pharmacia Biotech SpA, via Alessandro Volta 16, 20093 Cologno Monzese (MI), Tel. 02-273221, Fax 02-27302212.

2 Magnetic beads (Dynal, Dynabeads M-450 coated with sheep anti-mouse IgG1) cat. # D11003; Magnet (Dynal, Magnetic Particle Concentrator MPC1) cat. # D12001; Blood Mixer (Robbins) cat. # RS100A; and Fetal Calf Serum (Imperial laboratories) cat. # IL004 were purchased from Unipath SpA, Via Montenero 180, 20024 Garbagnate Milanese (MI), Tel. 02-9955651, Fax 02-9958260.

3 Methylcellulose cat. # M7027; Phytohemagglutinin cat. # L9132; Iscove's modified Dulbecco's medium (IMDM) cat. # I4136; and RPMI-1640 medium cat. # R7880; were purchased from Sigma Chimica, via Gallarate 154, 20151 Milano, Tel. 02-33417310 or 1678-27018, Fax 02-38010737.

4 Chymopapain (Chymodiactin) was kindly provided by Boots Pharmaceuticals Inc., 300 Tri State International Center, Lincolnshire, IL 60069, USA, Tel. 708-405-7400, Fax 708-405-7505; it can be purchased in Italy from Sigma Chimica (see above address), cat. # C8526.

5 My10 and 8G12 antibodies were kindly provided respectively by *Dr. C. Civin,* Johns Hopkins Oncology Center, Baltimore, MD, USA and *Dr. P. Lansdorp,* Terry Fox Laboratories, Vancouver, BC, Canada; they can be purchased in Italy from Becton Dickinson Italia SpA, Via Coldera 21, 20153 Milano, Tel. 02-452401, Fax 02-48204775: My10 (HPCA-1) cat. # 347660; 8G12 (HPCA-2) cat. # 348050/53/57.

6 Tubes (Falcon): 6 ml (cat. # 2063), 14 ml (cat. # 2059) and 50 ml (cat. # 2070) and Culture Petri dishes 35 mm (cat. # 1008) were purchased from Sacco Srl, Via Manzoni 29/A, 22071 Cadorago (Como), Tel. 031-904443, Fax 031-904596.

References

1 Silvestri F, Banavali S, Baccarani M, Preisler HD. The CD34 hemopoietic progenitor cell associated antigen: biology and clinical applications. Haematologica 1992;77:265-272.

2 Silvestri F, Bruno G, Virgolini L, Damiani D, Tozzoli R, Baccarani M. Phenotypic characterization of hemopoietic progenitor and stem cells. Eur J Lab Med 1993;1:87-92.

3 Silvestri F, Banavali S, Yin M, Hulette B, Gopal V, Civin CI, Baccarani M, Preisler HD. CD34 antigen expression of acute myeloid leukemia-colony forming cells. Int J Cell Clon 1992;10(suppl 1):98-100.

4 Yin M, Silvestri F, Banavali S, Gopal V, Hulette B, Kuvelkar R, Young A, Mayers G, Preisler HD. Clonogenic potential in vitro is restricted to myeloid leukemia cells expressing the CD34 antigen. Eur J Cancer 1993 (in press).

5 Silvestri F, Banavali SD, Hulette BC, Civin CI, Preisler HD. Isolation and characterization of the $CD34^+$ hematopoietic progenitor cells from the peripheral blood of patients with chronic myeloid leukemia. Int J Cell Clon 1991;9:474-490.

6 Civin CI, Strauss LC, Fackler MJ, Trischmann TM, Wiley JM, Loken MR. Positive stem cell selection: basic science. In: Gross S, Gee A, Worthington-White D, eds. Bone Marrow Purging and Processing. New York: Wiley-Liss, 1990:387-402.

7 Strauss LC, Trischmann TM, Rowley SD, Wiley JM, Civin CI. Selection of normal human hematopoietic stem cells for bone marrow transplantation using immunomagnetic microspheres and CD34 antibody. Am J Pediatric Hematol Oncol 1991;13:217-221.

8 Silvestri F, Banavali S, Yin M, Gopal V, Savignano C, Baccarani M, Preisler HD. CD34-positive cell selection by immunomagnetic beads and chymopapain. Haematologica 1992;77:307-310.

9 Law P, Ishizawa L, van de Ven C, Burgess J, Hardwick A, Plunkett M, Gee A, Cairo M. Immunomagnetic positive selection and colony culture of $CD34^+$ cells from cord blood. J Hematother 1993 (in press).

10 The Merck Index. Budavari S, ed. Rahway, NJ: Merck and Co. Inc. 1989:351.

11 Methods of Enzymatic Analysis. Vol II. Bergmeyer HU, Bergmeyer J, GraBl M, eds. Weinheim, Germany: VCH Verlagsgesellschaft. 1988:263-265.

12 Traycoff C, Zanjani ED, Gee A, Law P, Ishizawa L, Mansour V, Abboud MR, Laver J, Hoffman R, Srour EF. Hematopoietic engraftment of sheep transplanted in utero with adult human bone marrow and umbilical cord blood $CD34^+$ cells isolated by immunomagnetic separation. 34th Annual American Society of Hematology Meeting. Anaheim, CA, December 4-8, 1992. Blood 1992;80(suppl 1):233a.

13 Silvestri F, Fritsch G, Serke S, Sovalat H, Wunder E. Comparison of two monoclonal antibodies (8G12 and QBEND10) in detecting peripheral blood circulating $CD34^+$ cells. Eur J Lab Med 1993 (in press).

Selection of Human CD34+ Cells Using Indirect Immunomagnetic Procedures and a Magnetic Cell Separation System

Lori Ishizawa,[a] Julie Burgess,[a] Alan Hardwick,[a] Giao Hangoc,[a] Adrian Gee,[b] Ping Law[a]

[a]Baxter Healthcare Corporation, Immunotherapy Division, Santa Ana, California, USA; [b]Division of Transplantation Medicine, Department of Medicine, University of South Carolina, Columbia, South Carolina, USA

Key Words. Positive selection • CD34+ cells • Immunomagnetic beads • Cell separation system

Introduction

Human hematopoietic CD34+ cells can be enriched from human marrow, cord blood and mobilized peripheral blood. Using anti-CD34 antibody, immunomagnetic beads and chymopapain, a final cell product containing ≥ 90% CD34+ cells can be separated from human marrow. In this method, the target CD34+ cells are sensitized by monoclonal antibody, rosetted with paramagnetic microspheres, and the rosetted cells are released from the magnetic beads by incubation with chymopapain. Previously, laboratory scale selections, using centrifuge tubes and hand-held magnets, had been described to enrich up to 2 $\times 10^6$ CD34+ cells from 1×10^8 low density mononuclear cells. Larger quantities of highly purified cells would facilitate studies of growth factor mediated stem cell/progenitor cell expansion, and introduction of genetic material into stem cells/progenitor cells. In this report, a magnetic cell separation system, capable of processing 5 to 25×10^8 cells, is described.

Materials

1. Flow Chart for Indirect Immunomagnetic Selection of CD34+ Cells (Fig. 1)

There are three major steps in the separation process. Low density mononuclear cells (MNC) obtained by Ficoll-Paque centrifugation are used as the starting cell population. Procedures for the processing of mobilized peripheral blood samples are described later. In step 1, the target CD34+ cells are sensitized with mouse monoclonal anti-CD34 antibody and unbound antibody is removed by washing. In step 2, sensitized cells are rosetted with Dynal paramagnetic beads coated with sheep anti-mouse immunoglobulin (Ig)G1 (Fc) antibody. The beads/rosettes are collected using an array of permanent magnets and the non-rosetted cells are removed by washing. In the final step, the CD34+ cells are released by incubation of the beads/rosettes with chymopapain. These steps are described in detail in the Methodology section.

Correspondence: Dr. Ping Law, Baxter Healthcare Corporation, Immunotherapy Division, 3015 South Daimler Street, Santa Ana, CA 92705, USA.

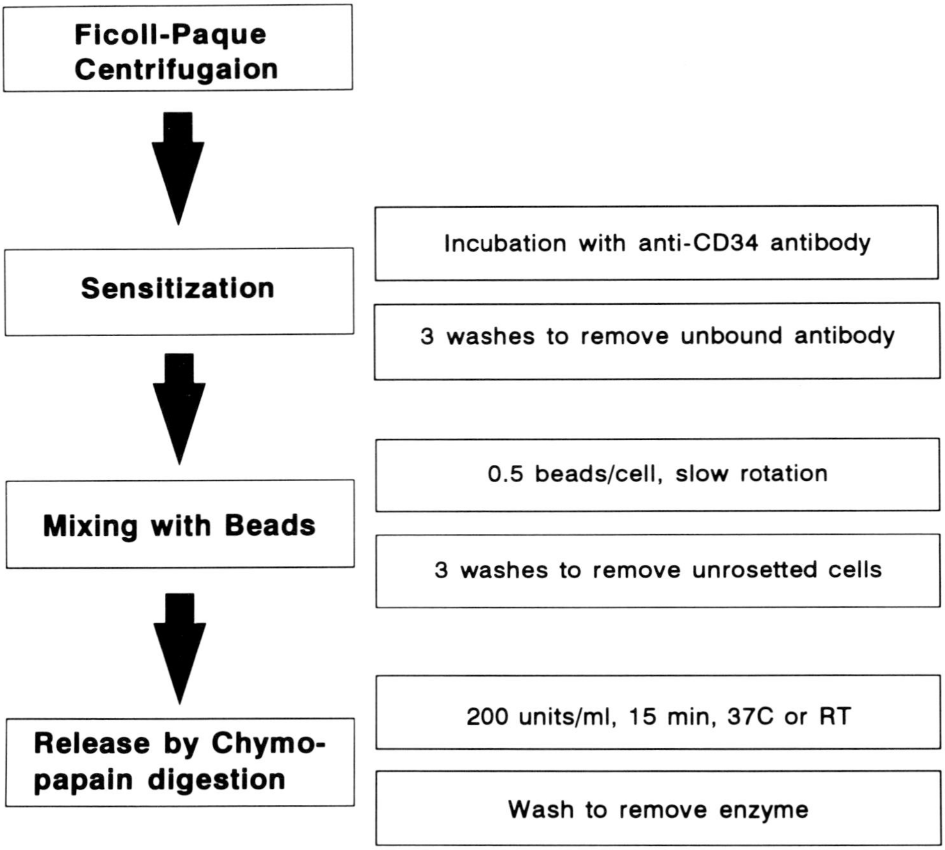

Fig. 1. Flow diagram of indirect immunomagnetic selection.

2. Reagents

Magnetic Cell Separation Reagent Kit

Baxter Product Code 4R5470. The kit contains 1 vial of 9C5 anti-CD34 antibody (1 mg in 2 ml buffer), 1 vial of Dynal paramagnetic beads coated with sheep anti-mouse IgG1 (Fc) antibody (SAM beads) (1×10^9 beads in 2.5 ml), 2 vials of lyophilized chymopapain (ChymoCell-R) (500 units [pKats]/vial), and 1 vial of sterile water for reconstituting the enzyme.

Additional Reagents Required

RPMI 1640: GIBCO-BRL (Grand Island, NY, USA) or equivalent. Human Serum Albumin (HSA): Baxter/Hyland Product Code 060-010 (Glendale, CA, USA). Human Immune Globulin or Gammagard (IG): Baxter/Hyland Product Code 060-322.

3. Magnetic Cell Separation System (Fig. 2)

Magnetic Cell Separator
ISOLEX-50: Baxter Healthcare Corporation, Deerfield, IL, USA, product code 4R4519. The cell separator consists of an array of permanent magnets mounted on a sliding mechanism, a stand to hold the disposable chamber and an adjustable solution pole to hold the washing buffer.

Disposable set
Product code 4R5402. The disposable set contains a sterile rigid chamber for mixing the antibody-sensitized cells and beads. A septum and an air vent are provided at the top of the chamber to facilitate introduction of cells and beads. Inlet and outlet tubing are provided for the various washing steps.

4. Additional Equipment

Rotator: Capable of slow rotation (~4 rpm) for mixing.

Hand-held magnetic separator (Dynal MPC-1): for preparing the beads before adding to the sensitized cells.

Centrifuge: For preparing MNC (Ficoll-Paque centrifugation and washes), and washing a) the sensitized cells to remove unbound antibodies, and b) the final cell product to remove chymopapain.

Pipettors (1000, 100, 20 and 10 μl sizes).

5. Supplies (sterile if the cells are to be cultured after separation)

Pipettes, centrifuge tubes (15-ml and 50-ml), syringes (1 ml, 10 ml and 20 ml) and needles (16 or 18 gauge).

Methodology

1. Preparation of Buffers and Media

RPMI containing 1% HSA (RPMI/HSA): for washing of cells and beads/rosettes. Part of the solution (~200 ml) can be introduced into a transfer pack (Baxter/Fenwal 4R2023) and kept on ice to be used later to wash the beads/rosettes.

RPMI/HSA containing 0.5% IG (RPMI/HSA/IG): for mixing sensitized cells with magnetic beads. Stock IG is prepared as 5% solution according to package instructions, and diluted 1:10 using RPMI/HSA.

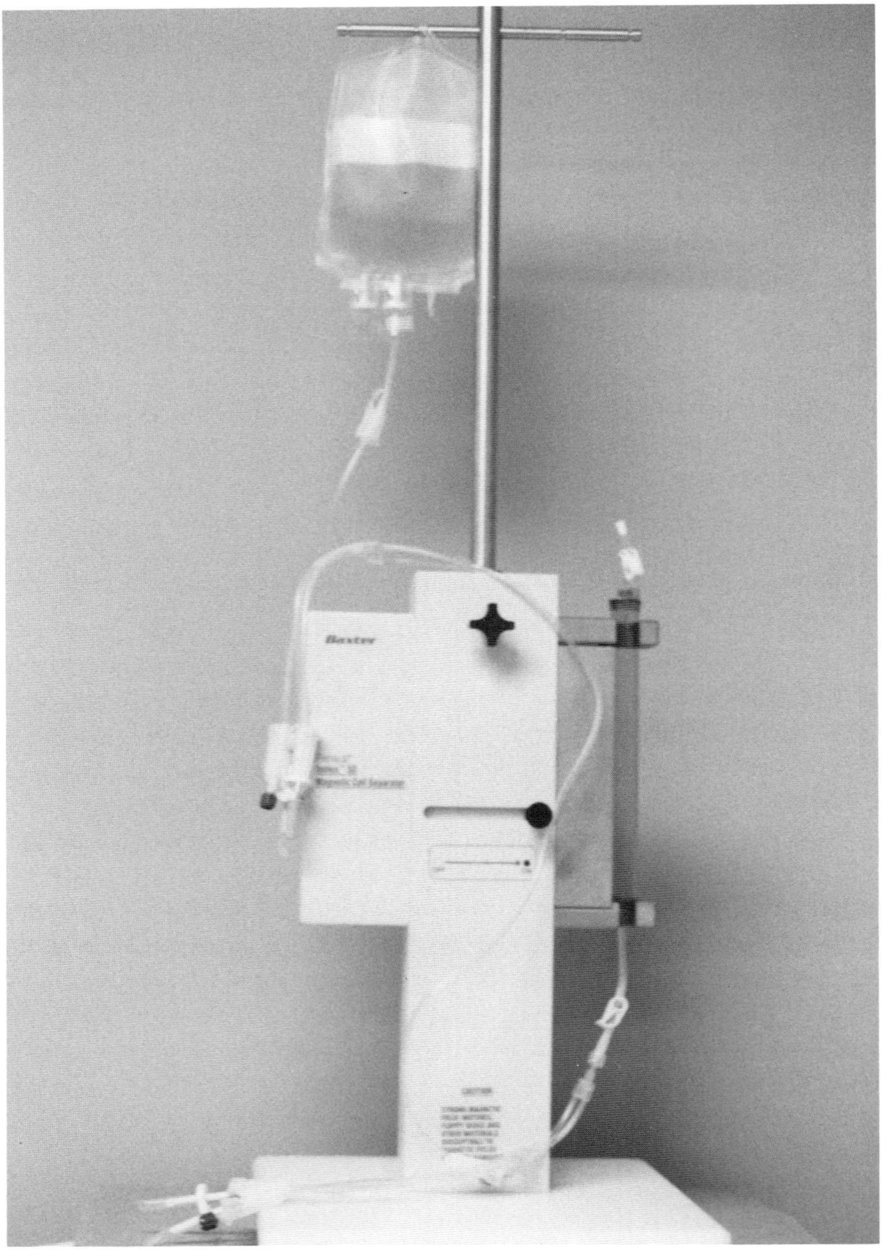

Fig. 2. The ISOLEX-50 Magnetic Cell Separation System. The system consists of a Magnetic Cell Separation System and a sterile rigid plastic chamber (50 ml) with inlet and outlet tubing. The components and the operating procedures are described in the materials section.

Chymopapain: Prepared by injecting 0.25 ml of sterile water into a vial of ChymoCell-R. The stock concentration is 2000 units/ml. *ChymoCell-R should be reconstituted immediately before use.*

2. Preparation of Cells

Low density MNC are separated from fresh human marrow or cord blood using standard procedures with Ficoll-Paque or Ficoll-Hypaque. The interface cells are washed 2 to 3 times (low speed centrifugation, 200 *g*, at room temperature) to remove residual density gradient material and platelets. The final cell pellet is resuspended in RPMI/HSA. The nucleated cell concentration is determined using an electronic particle counter or an equivalent manual method, and adjusted to 1 to 5 × 10^7/ml in RPMI/HSA.

3. Preparation of Beads

Dynal paramagnetic beads are supplied in a buffer containing 0.02% sodium azide. An appropriate number of beads (sufficient to provide 0.5 beads/nucleated cell, using the total number of cells determined above) are washed 3 × in a 15-ml tube, using the MPC-1 magnetic separator for bead collection. Each wash consists of ≥ 5 ml of RPMI/HSA, and the beads are collected by exposure to the magnet for 2 min. Washed beads are resuspended in 1 ml of RPMI/HSA/IG and used immediately (kept on ice until sensitized cells are ready). Fresh beads should be prepared during the sensitization step for each experiment.

4. Sensitization of Cells

Target $CD34^+$ cells within the MNC are sensitized with mouse antibody 9C5 (provided in the reagent kit) at 0.5 μg/10^6 cells for 30 min at 4°C. Lower concentrations of antibody (< 0.5 μg/10^6 cells) have been shown to produce inferior selection results. The cell concentration is maintained at 1 to 5 × 10^7 cells/ml in RPMI/HSA either in a centrifuge tube (15-ml or 50-ml) or in a transfer pack. Mixing is provided by slow (~4 rpm) end-over-end rotation. Unbound antibody is then removed by three washes (centrifugation at 400 *g* for 5 min at 4°C) in RPMI/HSA. The final pellet is resuspended in RPMI/HSA/IG at 2 to 5 × 10^7 cells/ml. Other anti-CD34 antibodies, which react with chymopapain-sensitive epitopes such as My-10 (HPCA-1) (Becton Dickinson; B-D), can be used at the same concentration for sensitization.

5. Mixing of Sensitized Cells with Beads

Sensitized cells and washed beads are introduced into the disposable chamber through the septum using a syringe and needle. The air vent must be open before injection and then closed prior to mixing. Mixing of cells and beads is accomplished by slow (~4 rpm) end-over-end rotation at 4°C for 30 min. The chamber is then mounted on the Magnetic Cell Separator and the array of magnets is moved into contact ("ON" position) with the chamber to collect the beads/rosettes (a 2-min exposure to the magnets is sufficient). While the beads/rosettes are migrating toward the magnets, the tubing set is connected to the chamber and the inlet tubing is attached to the bag of RPMI/HSA (prepared in step 1). The non-rosetted cells are then drained through the outlet tubing into a collection bag or tube (the appropriate clamps and the air vent must be open).

Some non-rosetted cells will be trapped in the beads/rosettes fraction collected on the side of the chamber. These are removed by washing 3 × with RPMI/HSA. The wash buffer (~20 ml of RPMI/HSA) is introduced into the chamber via the inlet tubing by opening the inlet clamp and air vent, while the beads/rosettes are held against the chamber wall by the magnets ("ON" position). If the beads/rosettes are free (magnets in "OFF" position) when the chamber is filling, some beads/rosettes may fall into the tubing. All clamps are then closed and the chamber is removed from the Magnetic Cell Separator. Beads/rosettes are gently mixed by inverting the chamber a few times until resuspended. The wash buffer is then drained as described above and the washing process is repeated two additional times. The non-rosetted cells may be collected, counted and analyzed for $CD34^+$ cell content and colony formation, for measuring capture (or rosetting) efficiency.

6. Incubation with Chymopapain

After the final wash, the beads/rosettes are resuspended in 1 ml (for $\leq 5 \times 10^8$ starting MNC) or 2 ml ($5 - 10 \times 10^8$ MNC) of RPMI/HSA, which is injected into the chamber through the septum. Freshly reconstituted ChymoCell-R (0.125 ml for each ml of RPMI/HSA; final enzyme concentration is 200 units/ml) is added, and the chamber is rotated (~4 rpm) at room temperature for 15 min. Cold RPMI/HSA (~20 ml) is then added to slow the enzymatic reaction and the chamber is mounted onto the Magnetic Cell Separator to collect the beads (2 min exposure as described above). The released cells are harvested and the beads are gently washed once with 20 ml of RPMI/HSA to rinse out any trapped cells. Residual enzyme is removed by centrifugation (400 *g* for 5 min at 4°C) and the cells are resuspended in a small volume (~ 2 ml) of RPMI/HSA (or medium suitable for later studies), and counted. Unused ChymoCell-R should be stored immediately at –20°C or –80°C. Thawed ChymoCell-R may be substituted for fresh enzyme in a later experiment if used immediately after thawing. Repeated freeze-thaw of ChymoCell-R is not recommended.

7. Flow Cytometry

The content of $CD34^+$ cells is determined by flow cytometric procedures as outlined by other authors of this special issue. A directly-conjugated antibody, such as 8G12 (HPCA2-fluorescein isothiocyanate (FITC) or HPCA2-phycoerythrin (PE)) (Becton Dickinson), which recognizes a chymopapain-resistant epitope on the CD34 antigen can be used to measure the $CD34^+$ cells before and after selection. Selected cells can be stained immediately, post-selection culture is *not* required. The results reported in this manuscript were determined as % of $CD34^+$ events with low side scatter within the total leukocyte population (defined using anti-CD45 antibody).

8. Selection of $CD34^+$ Cells from Other Sources

Screen Marrow

Cells non-specifically trapped on the screens used to filter marrow during harvest for transplantation are a rich source of hematopoietic cells suitable for laboratory studies. MNC can be obtained from material washed from the screens. An additional step, however, is required to improve selection efficiency, since the screens also trap other undesirable elements, e.g., bone chips, etc. The step, referred to as pre-depletion, consists of incubating MNC with uncoated magnetic beads (Dynal 14002) (0.5 beads/cell at 1 to 5 × 10^7 cells/ml in RPMI/HSA for 30 min at 25°C to 37°C) and removing cells associated with the beads prior to sensitization of the remaining cells with anti-CD34 antibody. Cellular elements and debris which might interfere with the rosetting and release processes are removed by their interaction with the uncoated beads. MNC, after pre-depletion, are treated as described above for selection. Since the pre-depletion step removes cells that interact non-specifically with the magnetic beads, IG (Gammagard) is not required in the buffer during mixing of sensitized cells with SAM beads.

Mobilized Peripheral Blood Samples

The procedures for selecting $CD34^+$ cells from mobilized blood samples collected by apheresis are slightly different from those described for marrow aspirates and cord blood. Ficoll-Paque separation of low density MNC is not necessary, and may result in substantial loss of $CD34^+$ cells. Before sensitization, platelets in the blood sample are reduced by low speed centrifugation and washing (200 *g* for 10 min at room temperature, 2 to 3 ×). A pre-depletion step, similar to that described for screen marrow cells (except that the uncoated beads are used at 1 bead/cell and incubation is performed at 37°C), is also required to increase the selection efficiency. The method therefore consists of the following: a) washes to remove platelets, b) pre-depletion with uncoated beads (1 bead/cell), c) sensitization with anti-CD34 antibody, d) rosetting with SAM beads (IG not required in the mixing buffer) and e) release by incubation with chymopapain.

Discussion

Summary of Selection Results

High purity $CD34^+$ cells have been isolated using the procedures described (Fig. 3). Starting from marrow and cord blood MNC containing, respectively,

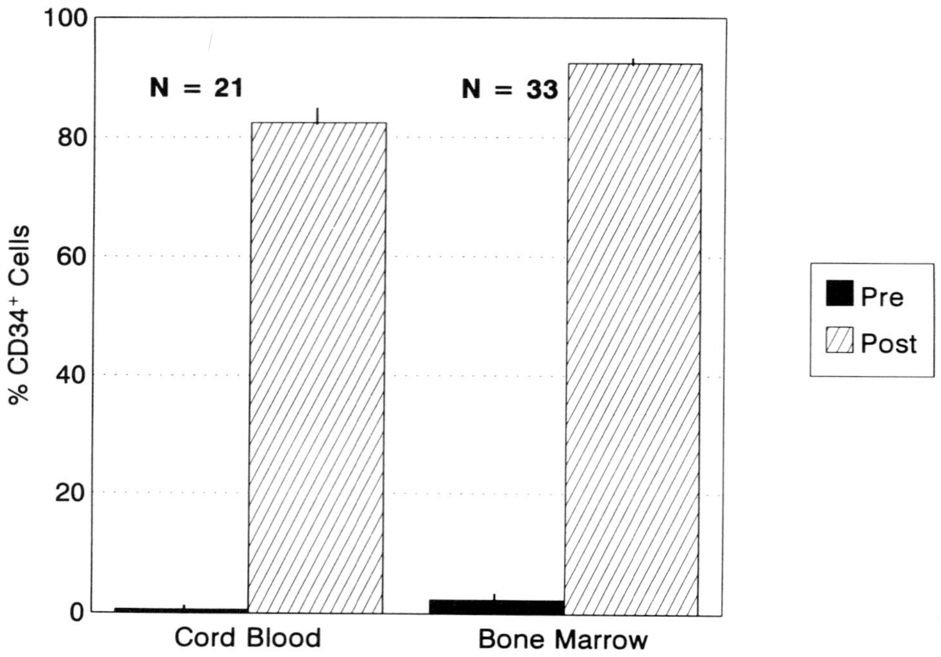

Fig. 3. Marrow and cord blood CD34+ cell separation. The fractions of CD34+ cells (and the total number of experiments, N) in marrow and cord blood MNC are shown before and after immunomagnetic selection.

2.3 ± 0.2% (mean ± SE, N = 33) and 0.6 ± 0.1% (N = 21) CD34+ cells, the final cell products averaged 92.4 ± 1.1% (range: 69.4 to 97.7%) and 82.4 ± 2.3% (range: 43.4 to 94.7%) CD34+ cells. Average enrichment can be calculated to be 54-fold (± 5, for marrow) and 169-fold (± 17, for cord blood). Similar enrichment in colony forming cells (78-fold and 106-fold, for marrow and cord blood, respectively) were achieved using conditioned media and erythropoietin as colony stimulating factors. Selection efficiency was not compromised when the cell concentration during the rosetting step was as high as 5×10^7/ml. Since 50 ml of cells and beads can be effectively mixed in the disposable chamber, the system can process up to 2.5×10^9 cells in a single experiment.

Selection of CD34+ cells from marrow screen samples is shown in Figure 4. The addition of the pre-depletion step (using uncoated beads prior to sensitization) resulted in the final purity increasing from 40.2 ± 2.2% to 78.6 ± 2.2%. Pre-depletion nucleated cell recovery averaged 70.6% and CD34+ cell yield was 73.4%, while 72.6% of the monocytes (CD14+) were removed.

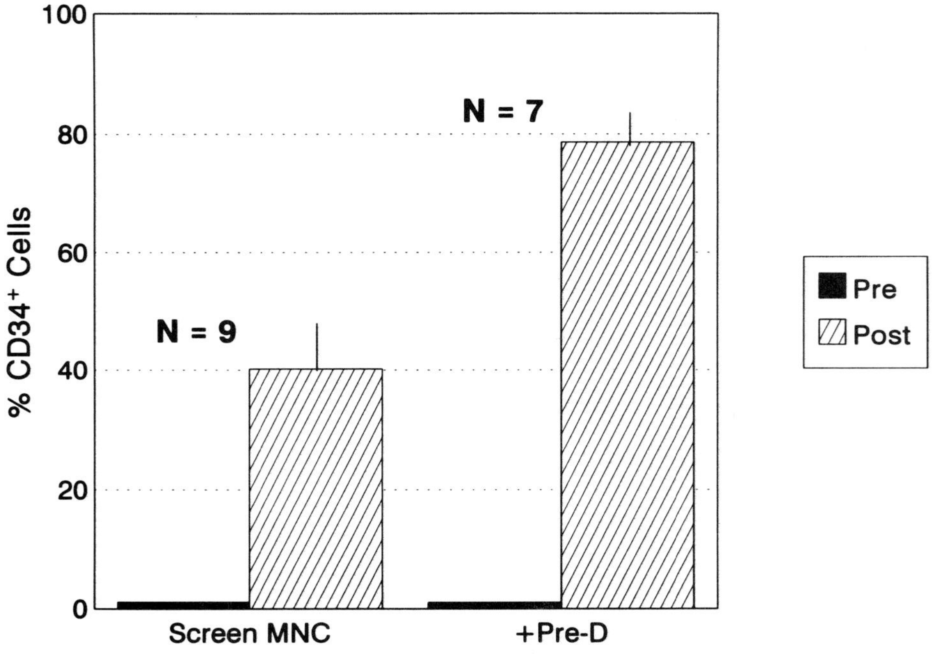

Fig. 4. Separation of CD34+ cells from marrow screens. The selection results using marrow screen MNC with and without pre-depletion are shown. The improvement of final purity is statistically significant (Student's t test, $p \leq 0.05$).

Figure 5 shows the results of selecting CD34+ cells from mobilized blood samples using different combinations of pre-treatment methods. MNC isolation by Ficoll-Paque centrifugation is not recommended, as the process led to a substantial loss (48.8%) of CD34+ cells. Using the pre-depletion step alone, the final purity was comparable to that using Ficoll and pre-depletion (78.8 ± 1.1%, range: 57.5 to 96.0%; versus 76.4 ± 8.4%). Nucleated cell recovery during the pre-depletion was 61.8%, CD34+ cell yield was 74.4%, and 69.0% of the monocytes were removed.

Modifications to the Selection Procedures

The selection procedures have not been completely optimized. Experiments are currently underway to determine whether a) the time for selection can be shortened, b) the rosetting step can be performed at room temperature, or c) the pre-depletion step for mobilized peripheral blood selection can be replaced by other procedure(s). Updates of the selection method will be available from the corresponding author.

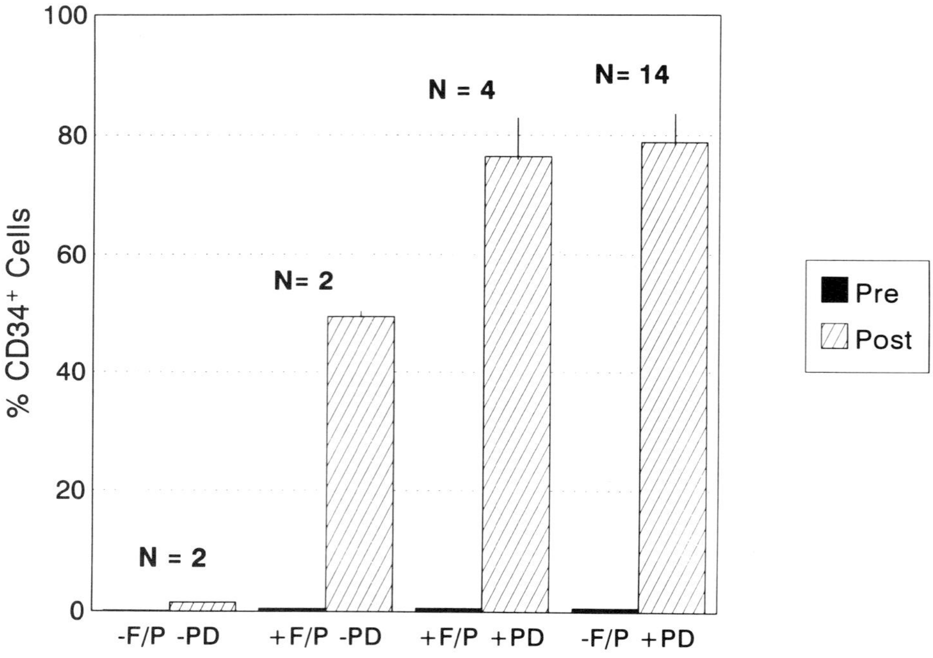

Fig. 5. Separation of CD34+ cells from mobilized blood. Mobilized blood samples were washed to reduce platelets before selection (except for Ficoll-Paque experiments, where platelet-washes were performed after density gradient centrifugation). Selection results using different pre-treatment methods were shown. F/P = Ficoll-Paque density gradient separation of MNC, and PD = pre-depletion with uncoated beads.

Calculation of Yield

The yield of the selection experiments, defined as the % of CD34+ cells recovered from the total number of CD34+ cells applied, was 34.9 ± 2.5% for marrow and 63.6 ± 6.6% for cord blood. Calculations and comparisons of yield are complicated by the fact that a) the cells do not maintain a homogeneous expression of the CD34 antigen (cells with high expression are preferentially selected), and b) that different methods are used at different institutions for the measurement of CD34+ cells (e.g., use of different anti-CD34 antibodies, lysis of red cells, direct versus indirect staining, analysis using total leukocyte gate or lymphocyte gate, etc.). Small differences in quantitating the initial CD34+ cell content, especially in cord blood MNC and mobilized blood samples where low numbers of CD34+ cells (≤ 0.5%) are not uncommon, can result in large variations in the estimates of yield. Calculations of yield are useful when different selection procedures are compared using identical starting material.

Small Scale Experiments

The ISOLEX-50 system can be used for selecting CD34+ cells from 2×10^8 to 2.5×10^9 starting nucleated cells. When lower cell numbers are encountered, the entire selection procedure can be performed in polypropylene tubes (10-ml or 15-ml). The immunomagnetic procedures described work equally well in the small scale settings, although manipulation of cells after release (washing, counting, staining, etc.) may, however, become difficult because of the small numbers.

Chymopapain Incubation

Other Sources of the Enzyme
Purified chymopapain (ChymoCell-R in the reagent kit) is manufactured by Boots Pharmaceuticals (Nottingham, England). Other sources of chymopapain have been evaluated and the selection results were unsatisfactory.

Use of HSA
Inclusion of HSA in the buffer for the washing of beads/rosettes and the chymopapain incubation produced no decrease in release efficiency. Preliminary experiments comparing washing and incubation in protein-free versus protein containing buffer, showed that cell clumping was reduced by using HSA in RPMI.

Temperature
Early immunomagnetic separation procedures were carried out with the chymopapain incubation at 37°C. Preliminary experiments comparing room temperature versus 37°C incubation showed that release efficiencies at both temperatures were identical.

CD34 Epitopes Affected by Chymopapain
Epitope(s) on the CD34 antigen recognized by 9C5 and My-10 are modified by chymopapain. When the selected $CD34^+$ cells were cultured in medium containing fetal bovine serum (no growth factors were used, to avoid differentiation), significant re-expression of the epitope was detected after overnight incubation (≥ 90% of the 8G12-positive cells could be stained with 9C5 or My-10, with lower fluorescent intensity compared to the base-line value of the untreated control stained with the same antibodies). Re-expression appeared to be completed after 48 h of culture, as measured by the 9C5 or My-10 fluorescence intensity.

Toxicity of the Selection System
Each component of the selection system (exposure to antibody, magnetic field, beads, and chymopapain) was tested for effects on colony formation. No effects on colony forming units-granulocyte-macrophage (CFU-GM), burst forming units-erythroid (BFU-E) and CFU-Mix were detected.

Selected Readings

1 Cairo MS, Law P, van de Ven C, Plunkett JM, Williams D, Ishizawa L, Gee AP. The in vitro effects of stem cell factor and PIXY321 on myeloid progenitor formation (CFU-GM) from immunomagnetic separated $CD34^+$ cord blood. Pediat Res 1992;32:277-281.

2 Strauss LC, Trischmann TM, Rowley SD, Wiley JM, Civin CI. Selection of normal human hematopoietic stem cells for bone marrow transplantation using immunomagnetic microspheres and CD34 antibody. Amer J Pediat Hematol Oncol 1991;2:217-221.

3 Srour EF, Zanjani ED, Brandt JE, Leemhuis T, Briddell RA, Heerema NA, Hoffman R. Sustained human hematopoiesis in sheep transplanted *in utero* during early gestation with fractionated adult human bone marrow cells. Blood 1992;79:1404-1412.

4 Hardwick A, Law P, Mansour V, Kulcinski D, Ishizawa L, Gee AP. Development of a large-scale immunomagnetic separation system for harvesting CD34-positive cells from bone marrow. In: Worthington-White DA, Gee AP, Gross S, eds. Advances in Bone Marrow Purging and Processing. New York: Wiley-Liss, 1992;583-589.

5 Hardwick A, Kulcinski D, Mansour V, Ishizawa L, Law P, Gee AP. Design of large-scale separation systems for positive and negative immunomagnetic selection of cells using superparamagnetic microspheres. J Hematotherapy 1992;1:379-386.

6 Saeland S, Duvert V, Caux C, Pandrau D, Favre C, Valle A, Durand I, Charbord P, deVries J, Banchereau J. Distribution of surface-membrane bound molecules on bone marrow and cord blood $CD34^+$ hematopoietic cells. Exp Hematol 1992;20:24-33.

7 Bender JG, Unverzagt KL, Walker DE, Lee W, van Epps DE, Smith DH, Stewart CC, To LB. Identification and comparison of CD34-positive cells and their subpopulations from normal peripheral blood and bone marrow using multicolor flow cytometry. Blood 1991;77:2591-2596.

Antibody-Coated Magnetic Particles for CD34⁺ Cell Separation

Nathalie Debernardi, Christophe Camilla, Yves Traore, Joëlle Hirn
Immunotech SA, Department of Monoclonal Antibodies, Marseille, France

Key Words. CD34⁺ • Magnetic particles • Positive selection • Hematopoietic progenitor cells • Colony forming cells • Bone marrow • Cord blood • Cultures • Proliferation • Differentiation

Introduction

A newly developed immunomagnetic procedure in which CD34 positive cells are bound to antibody-coated magnetic beads can be used efficiently for positive stem cell selection after a simple passage through a magnetic field.

These magnetic beads are magnetic latexes which have the appearance of a dark brown liquid, the intensity of brown varying with the iron oxide content of the particles. Each particle encloses very finely dispersed iron oxide, uniformly distributed in the polystyrene matrix, and has a mean diameter of 1 μm. The particles are superparamagnetic, i.e., the magnetization of the beads increases with the applied magnetic field but falls back to zero when the field is removed.

Reactive CD34 magnetic beads are obtained by directly grafting a high-affinity monoclonal antibody (MAb), Immu-133 [1], using an avidin-biotin system. Such positive selection has the advantage that CD34 cells with a high degree of purity are obtained. This method also results in good recovery of CD34 cells in a viable and functional state as assessed by progenitor cell assay systems.

Unlike in commonly used immunomagnetic bead approaches, the selected CD34 cells are cultivated directly with the beads still bound without affecting proliferation and differentiation.

Materials

Equipment

- Laminar flow hood
- 7.5% CO_2 humidified incubator
- Flow cytometer
- Inverted microscope

Correspondence: Dr. Joëlle Hirn, Immunotech SA, Department of Monoclonal Antibodies, 130 avenue de Lattre de Tassigny, BP 177, 13276 Marseille, Cedex 9, France.

©AlphaMed Press ISBN 1-880854 17-1

- Vortex
- Centrifuge
- Plasticware for cell separation:
  - 50 ml polypropylene tube (e.g., Falcon #2098)
  - 50 ml Leucosep TM tube (Esquire Chemic AG, Obere Zaune 12, P.O. Box 315-CH-8025 Zurich/Switzerland-Phone: 41-1-259-82-96 Fax: 41-1-259-21-77). Optional.
  - 5 ml polystyrene tube (e.g., Falcon #2052)
- Plasticware for cell culture:
  - 12-well plates (e.g., Falcon #3043)
  - 25 cm^2 tissue culture flasks (e.g., Falcon #3082)
  - 75 cm^2 tissue culture flasks (e.g., Falcon #3084)

Magnetic Beads and MAbs

- CD34-coated magnetic beads (Immunotech SA, #1177)
- Sheep anti-mouse immunoglobulin G (IgG)-coated magnetic beads, SaMIg beads (Immunotech SA, Marseille, France, #1181). Optional
- Magnetic holders (Immunotech SA, #0564 or #1057, for 1 or 4 × 5 ml hemolytic tubes, respectively). For larger tubes, other magnetic separation apparatus may also be used.
- Basic panel of MAbs for $CD34^+$ cell phenotyping (Immunotech SA, see catalog for immunology).

Culture Media and Chemicals

- Lymphoprep™ (Nycomed Pharma, #221 366).
- Iscove's modified Dulbecco's medium (IMDM) 25 mM Hepes (Biowhittaker, M12.726 B)
- L-glutamine (Sigma, St. Louis, MO, G7513)
- Nonessential amino acids (Sigma, N7145)
- Sodium pyruvate (Sigma, S8636)
- Fetal calf serum (FCS)
- Penicillin-streptomycin (Sigma, P0781)
- Hydrocortisone (Sigma, H0888)
- 2-mercaptoethanol (Sigma, M7522)
- Interleukin 3, human (rhIL-3) (Boehringer Mannheim, #1 381 547)
- Granulocyte macrophage colony stimulating factor, human (rhGM-CSF) (Boehringer Mannheim #1087 762)
- Human bone marrow stem cell proliferation kit (GIBCO BRL, Grand Island, NY, #680-3826 SA), with addition of rhIL-3 (30 U/ml), and rhGM-CSF (30 U/ml)

Preparation of Culture Media

- IMDM, 20% FCS, consists of IMDM supplemented with:
  - 2 mM L-glutamine
  - 1 mM sodium pyruvate
  - 100 U/ml penicillin-streptomycin
  - 20% FCS, heat-inactivated at 56°C for 30 min

- IMDM, 15% FCS (for liquid culture)
  - 2 mM L-glutamine
  - 1 mM sodium pyruvate
  - 100 U/ml penicillin-streptomycin
  - 15% FCS, heat-inactivated at 56°C for 30 min
  - 5 ng/ml hydrocortisone
  - 5×10^{-5} M 2-mercaptoethanol
  - 500 U/ml rhIL-3
  - 200 U/ml rhGM-CSF

Methodology: $CD34^+$ Cell Isolation

The following procedures have been established for initial samples of 20 ml (umbilical cord blood, bone marrow). Larger volumes may be processed by taking care to adjust the proportions of media and magnetic beads. All manipulations should be performed under sterile conditions.

Isolation of Mononuclear Cells (MNC) by Ficoll-Hypaque Gradient Centrifugation

- This step may be performed according to the regular method.
- For faster separation, it is convenient to use the LeucoSep tubes, consisting of two compartments separated by a specially designed porous barrier:

  Add 15 ml of Ficoll-Hypaque (Lymphoprep) in a 50 ml LeucoSep tube. Take two tubes for an initial sample of 20 ml.

  Centrifuge for 30 sec at 800 *g*.

  Layer 20 ml of sample, diluted in an equal volume of room-temperature IMDM without any supplements, over the disk.

  Centrifuge for 10 min at 800 *g*, 20°C.

  Discard plasma.

  Transfer the MNC layer from each tube to another tube. Centrifuge tube (Falcon, 50 ml).

  Wash cells by adding excess IMDM (approximately three times the volume of the MNC layer).

  Centrifuge for 10 min at 400 *g*, 20°C.

  Remove supernatant, resuspend cells in IMDM and repeat the wash once.

  Resuspend cell pellet in IMDM, 20% FCS.

  Count cells and determine viability by Trypan-Blue exclusion.

  Pipette an aliquot for:

  1) determination of $CD34^+$ cells by flow cytometry

  2) colony assays

  Adjust to 1×10^7 cells/ml (for 20 ml umbilical cord blood or bone marrow sample; this should be of the order of 15-20 ml).

  Isolating MNC takes 30 min to 1 h. This is dependent on the initial volume of sample obtained.

Depletion of Monocytes

Depletion of monocytes from MNC suspension improves $CD34^+$ cell isolation in terms of recovery and purity.

Depletion of Monocytes by Adherence to Plastic:

Centrifuge MNC for 10 min at 400 *g*.

Remove supernatant and resuspend cell pellet in IMDM, 20% FCS, to a final concentration of 2×10^6 cell/ml.

Transfer 50 ml cell suspension to a 75 cm^2 tissue culture flask.

Incubate horizontally, overnight, in a 37°C, 7.5% CO_2 humidified incubator.

Decant cells in suspension into a centrifuge tube.

Rinse tissue culture flask with 37°C IMDM, 20% FCS.

Add this wash to the centrifuge tube.

Centrifuge for 10 min at 400 *g*.

Discard supernatant.

Resuspend cells in IMDM, 20% FCS at 1×10^7 cells/ml.

Count cells and check viability by Trypan-Blue exclusion.

Pipette an aliquot for:

1) analysis of the MNC population by flow cytometry to assess purity: dual color analysis with CD45/CD14 antibodies should give $CD45^+/CD14^-$ MNC population (80%)
2) determination of $CD34^+$ cells by flow cytometry.

Depletion of Monocytes by $CD14^-$ Magnetic Beads

This procedure is advantageous since it avoids the adherence step.

CD14 Magnetic Bead Preparation

This preparation is performed under sterile conditions. SaMIg-beads should be complexed with the CD14 MAb (Immunotech SA, #0643) prior to use with cell suspension. SaMIg-beads are supplied as a 20 mg sterile suspension in 2 ml of phosphate buffered saline (PBS: 10 mM sodium phosphate, 0.1 M NaCl, pH 7.2), without any preservative.

- After brief vortexing, the bead suspension is homogeneous and can be pipetted as a solution. In a polystyrene sterile tube, dilute beads to 1/20 in PBS, 0.2% bovine serum albumin (BSA).
- Separation of the beads from the buffer solution is achieved in 5 min by contact with a magnet. Supernatant becomes clear and can be discarded.
- Complex the CD14 antibody to beads by adding 5 μg of antibody per mg of beads (100 ml). Adjust the volume to 200 ml with PBS, 0.2% BSA. Mix gently and incubate for at least 15 min at room temperature.
- Add 2 ml of PBS, 0.2% BSA, and place the tube in contact with the magnet for 5 min. Discard the supernatant and repeat once in order to eliminate any unbound antibody.
- The CD14 magnetic beads are now ready for use. The preparation should keep for 3-4 weeks at 4°C.

Depletion of Monocytes

- Use 1 mg (100 μl) of CD14 magnetic beads for 1×10^7 MNC in 1 ml of IMDM, 20% FCS.
- It is recommended to wash the beads with IMDM, 20% FCS, once just prior to use with cell suspension.
- In a tube (5 ml Falcon #2052), one can incubate at most 4 ml of MNC suspension (1×10^7 cells/ml) with 400 μl (4 mg) of CD14 beads.

For processing 15-20 ml MNC suspension, 4 to 5 tubes are necessary. However, a single larger tube may be used with a suitable magnet.

- Mix gently with manual shaking or by slight vortexing. Incubate the mixture for 15 min at 4°C and gently mix every 5 min. CD14 magnetic beads will bind to target cells and form rosettes with monocytes.
- Place the tube in contact with the magnet for 10 min. Do not remove the tube from the magnet.
- Carefully collect the monocyte-free cell suspension and pool suspensions if several tubes have been used.

  The positive fraction, i.e., beads bound to monocytes, has to be eliminated.

  Count cells and check viability by Trypan-Blue exclusion.

  Approximately 70% of MNC are recovered.

  Adjust MNC suspension to 1×10^7 cells/ml with IMDM, 20% FCS.

  Pipette an aliquot for:

  1) analysis of the MNC population by flow cytometry to assess purity; a dual color analysis with CD45/CD14 antibodies should give $CD45^+/CD14^-$ MNC population (>95%).
  2) determination of $CD34^+$ cells by flow cytometry.

  Time required is approximately 30 min for depletion of monocytes with $CD14^-$ beads.

Isolation of $CD34^+$ Cells

- CD34 magnetic beads are supplied as a 20 mg sterile suspension in 2 ml of PBS, without any preservative.
- Washing: after brief vortexing, the bead suspension is homogeneous and can be pipetted as a solution. In a polystyrene sterile tube, dilute beads to 1/20 in IMDM, 20% FCS.
- Bead separation from the medium is achieved in 5 min with a magnet. Supernatant becomes clear and should be discarded. The CD34 beads are resuspended in the initial volume of buffer (1 mg/100 μl) in IMDM, 20% FCS.
- It is necessary to wash beads before use to remove any residual unbound antibody.
- Use 1 mg (100 μl) of CD34 magnetic beads for 1×10^7 MNC free of monocytes in 1 ml of IMDM, 20% FCS. In a tube (5 ml Falcon #2052), one can incubate at most 4 ml MNC suspension (1×10^7 cells/ml) with 400 μl (4 mg) of CD34 beads.
- For processing 15-20 ml of MNC suspension, 4 tubes are necessary. However, a single larger tube may be used with a suitable magnet.

  Mix gently with manual shaking or by slight vortexing. Incubate for 15 min at 4°C and mix gently every 5 min.

Place the tube on the magnet for 10 min. Do not remove tube from the magnet while removing the negative fraction (free of beads). Collect the negative fractions in the same tube if more than one tube has been used for the separation.

Remove the tube from the magnet.

Resuspend the positive fraction (rosetted cells) in excess IMDM, 20% FCS. Wash the positive fraction twice again using the magnet device to recover the rosetted cells.

Pool the positive fractions if more than one tube has been used for the separation. Resuspend the final positive fraction in IMDM, 20% FCS (20% to 30% of the initial volume used for the incubation).

Count cells and rosetted cells, respectively, in the negative and the positive fractions. Viability of rosetted cells is determined with acridine orange-ethidium bromide.

Expected results: in optimal conditions, 5×10^5 $CD34^+$ cells are isolated from 1×10^7 MNC with 1 mg $CD34^-$ magnetic beads.

Time consideration: approximately 30 min for isolation of $CD34^+$ cells.

Yield and Purity

Definition of Terminology

$$\% \text{ MNC recovery} = \frac{\text{no. of MNC recovered}}{\text{no. of input MNC}} \times 100$$

Initial no. of CD34 = % $CD34^+$ cells × total initial no. of MNC.

The % $CD34^+$ is obtained from analysis by flow cytometer.

$$\text{Yield of } CD34^+ (\%) = \frac{\text{no. of cells in ``positive'' final fraction} \times \% \text{ purity of } CD34^+ \text{ cells}}{\text{initial no. of } CD34^+ \text{ cells}} \times 100$$

$$\% \text{ purity} = \frac{\text{no. of actual } CD34^+ \text{ cells in ``positive'' fraction}}{\text{Total no. of cells in ``positive'' fraction}} \times 100$$

Determination of $CD34^+$ Cells by Flow Cytometry

This evaluation is performed on the MNC suspension, before and/or after monocyte depletion, on the negative fraction after isolation of $CD34^+$ cells. Due to the small size of beads, the positive fraction may be analyzed also on a flow cytometer.

The samples are analyzed on the FACScan flow cytometer. Data acquisition and analysis is done with the Lysis II software. Any other flow cytometer may also be used.

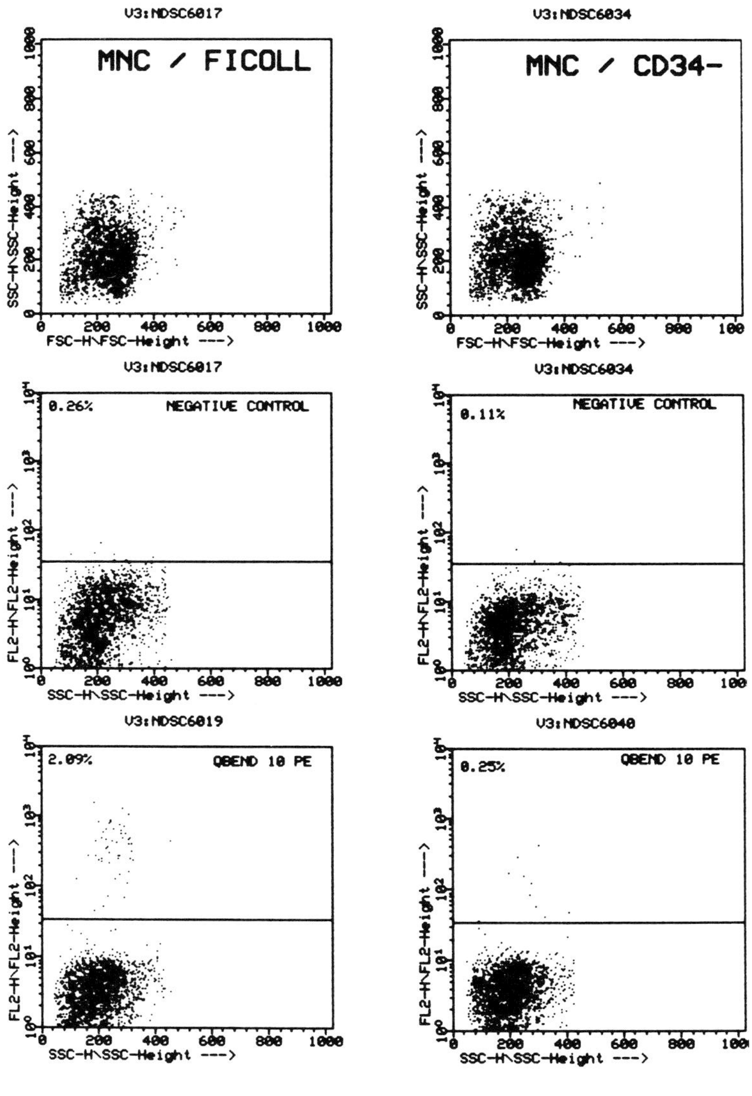

Fig. 1. Flow cytometric analysis of CD34+ cells in the MNC suspension and in the negative fraction before and after isolation with CD34− magnetic beads, respectively. Forward and side scatter dot plot shows gating for cells that are analyzed in FL2 and side scatter dot plot after excluding CD2 and glycophorin A-positive events. Cells are stained with QBend 10 PE (vertical axis). As a negative control, cells are stained with isotype-matched MAb.

For determining number of CD34+ cells in the MNC suspension and in the negative fraction, the following procedure allows the visualization of a low percentage of CD34+ (Fig. 1):

- CD34− cells (such as CD2+ lymphocytes and erythroblasts) can be excluded from acquisition of events:

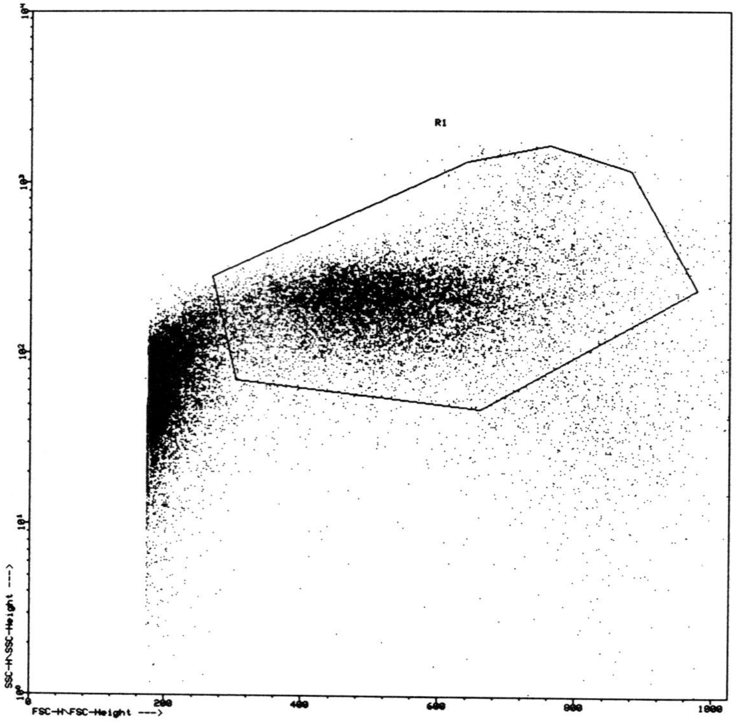

Fig. 2. Flow cytometric analysis of CD34+ rosetted cells, illustrating light-scatter properties (dot representation) of free beads to be excluded from analysis and of rosetted cells (R1).

CD2+ lymphocytes are labeled with an anti-CD2 fluorescein isothiocyanate (FITC), and erythroblasts with an anti-glycophorin A FITC. CD34+ cells are labeled with an anti-CD34 phycoerythrin. Appropriate isotype-matched control antibodies are used.

A side scatter (SSC) versus FL1 dot plot is displayed, and a gate is set (R1) to exclude CD2 and glycophorin-labeled cells.

2×10^4 or, preferably, 5×10^4 events, selected according to gate R1 are acquired.

For positive fractions (rosettes), a SSC log scale is necessary: the presence of beads on the cell surface induces higher side scatter (Fig. 2):

- The FCS versus SSC dot plot is displayed and a gate is set (R1) to exclude free beads.
- The PMT voltage of the fluorescence parameters and the fluorescence compensation have to be adapted to the higher autofluorescence exhibited by rosetted cells.
- Rosettes should be labeled with an anti-CD34 antibody, whose epitope is different from that of Immu-133 (MAb coated on magnetic beads) (Fig. 3). An overnight incubation of rosettes in culture medium at 37°C in a 7.5% CO_2 incubator, induces a partial detachment of beads. As a result, CD34 epitopes are more accessible, thus enhancing the labeling of cells with anti-CD34 MAbs.
- It has to be noted that this difficulty is not encountered with MAbs of different specificity from that of CD34.

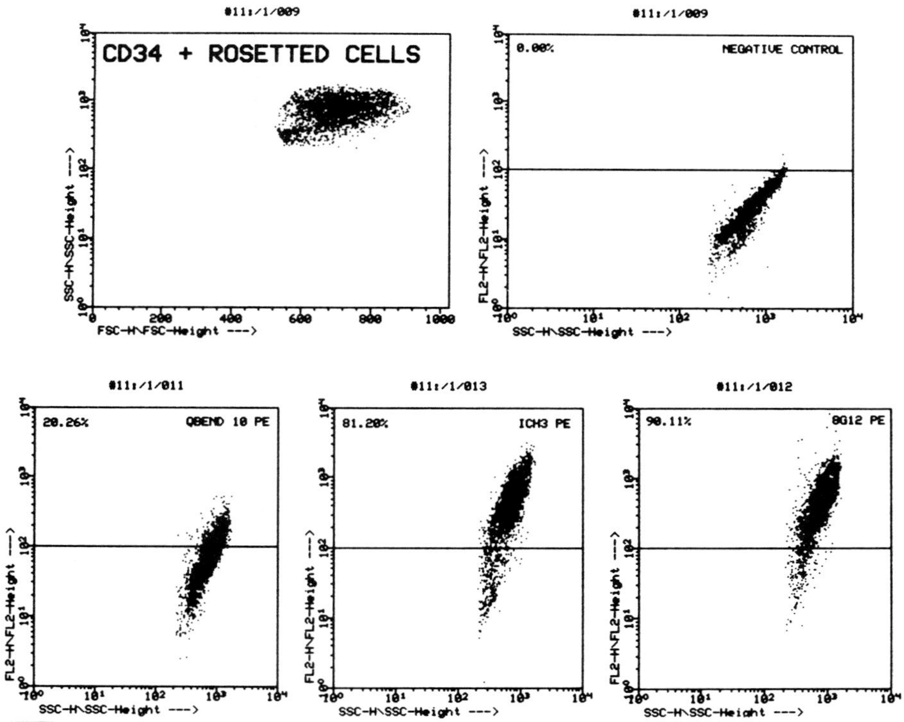

Fig. 3. Flow cytometric analysis of CD34⁺ rosetted cells: dot plot correlating SSC with FL2 (CD34 MAb-PE) and illustrating the importance of the CD34 MAb used for assessing the degree of purity of CD34⁺ rosetted cells.

Some Representative Results

Table I shows typical results of $CD34^+$ cell purifications from initial 20 ml cord blood and bone marrow samples collected.

The use of CD34 magnetic beads ensures:
1) cell viability >95%
2) average yield 80%
3) cell purity 80% to 90%.

Clonogenic Assay of $CD34^+$ Cells

Procedure

Differentiated colony formation is assessed with the GIBCO BRL human bone marrow stem cell proliferation kit that allows the reproducible growth of pluripotent stem cells into hematopoietic colonies: colony forming units

Table I. Purification of human CD34+ cells

Sample CB = cord blood BM = bone marrow	MNC/Ficoll ($\times 10^8$)	% CD34+	CD34− fraction ($\times 10^8$)	% CD34+	CD34+ rosetted cells	% CD34+	Yield of CD34+ (%)
CB1	1.7	0.63	1.56	0.12	1×10^6	0.64	81
CB2	1.44	2.72	1.36	0.10	4×10^6	2.85	85.30
CB3	2	2.18	0.8	0.40	4×10^6	4.76	74
CB4	2	1.81	1	0.53	2.8×10^6	2.72	71.25
CB5	2.4	2.75	0.9	0.76	3×10^6	3.22	73
CB6	1	2.09	0.9	0.25	2.7×10^6	2.17	88
BM	1.44	2.88	0.54	1.55	3.6×10^6	6.25	72
Mean ± SD	1.71 ± 0.45	2.15 ± 0.72	1 ± 0.32	0.53 ± 0.47	3×10^6 ± 0.96	3.23 ± 1.67	78 ± 6.5

Table II. Colony formation before and after CD34 magnetic bead separation

Sample	Total colonies/3×10^4 MNC Ficoll plated		Total colonies/3×10^4 CD34− cells plated		Total colonies/3×10^4 CD34+ cells plated	
	Day 7	Day 14	Day 7	Day 14	Day 7	Day 14
CB1	440 ± 40	1750 ± 22	40 ± 12	606 ± 6	1000 ± 50	3310 ± 510
CB2	192 ± 20	3846 ± 680	74 ± 10	2356 ± 248	836 ± 76	Over
CB3	138 ± 47	3684 ± 316	10 ± 8	1125 ± 274	476 ± 68	Over
CB4	24 ± 0	704 ± 96	2 ± 2	236 ± 88	164 ± 36	3981 ± 614
BM	1022 ± 90	2700 ± 75	240 ± 16	485 ± 25	2634 ± 174	5946 ± 210

Means ± SD quadruplicate plates.
Colonies (>50 cells) plus clusters (<50 cells).
Over = no distinct colonies, many cells dispersed throughout the culture.

granulocyte-macrophage (CFU-GM), burst forming units erythroid (BFU-E) and colony forming units granulocyte, erythrocyte, monocyte, megakaryocyte (CFU-GEMM).

The clonogenic assay was performed according to kit instructions, with the addition of rhIL-3 (30 U/ml) and rhGM-CSF (30 U/ml). Cord blood and bone marrow samples are tested at the following steps:

- after Ficoll isolation: MNC suspension
- after separation of $CD34^+$ cells: negative and positive fraction.

The three cell suspensions are resuspended to 5×10^5 cells/ml and plated, after mixing with dilution medium and stem cell growth medium to 3×10^4 cells per well in a 12-well tissue culture plate.

The positive fraction, e.g., $CD34^+$ rosetted cells, is incubated without detachment of beads from cells.

- To adjust the cell density of the $CD34^+$ rosetted cells, place the tube in contact with the magnet for 10 min.
- Remove the medium and replace it with a suitable volume of dilution medium.
- The colonies are scored after 7 and 14 days of culture in a humidified incubator at 37°C and 7.5% CO_2.

Some Representative Results

As may be seen from Table II, the total colony frequency is the highest in the $CD34^+$ rosetted cells fraction which is consistent with a stem cell enrichment in this fraction. By contrast, in the negative fraction, the clonogenic assay shows depletion of the most immature cells. However it has to be noted that there is not a strong correlation between the number of isolated $CD34^+$ cells (Table I) and the number of colonies.

Figures 4 and 5 illustrate typical morphology of stem cell colonies grown from an umbilical cord blood sample, after 7 days and 14 days, respectively, of culture. The $CD34^+$ fraction is characterized mainly by the formation of large white colonies. By contrast, the $CD34^-$ fraction forms small and large hemoglobinized colonies. The same pattern is seen in all tested culture samples.

Expansion of $CD34^+$ Cells in Liquid Culture

Procedure

Suspension cultures of $CD34^+$ rosetted cells and $CD34^-$ fraction are established in complete medium, IMDM, 15% FCS. The cell density should be 3×10^5 to 5×10^5 cells/ml. In the case of the CD34 rosetted cells, beads are left attached to the cells. This suspension culture comprises both rosetted cells and free beads.

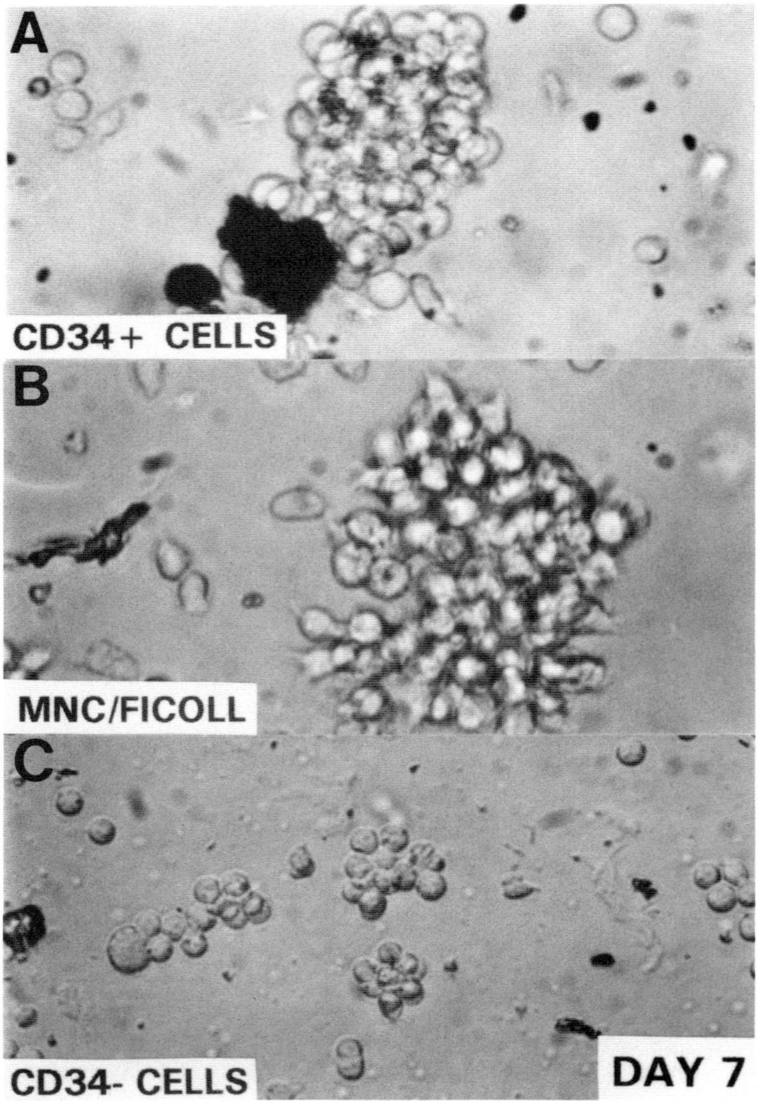

Fig. 4. Typical morphology of stem cell colonies after 7 days of culture of a cord blood sample in the GIBCO BRL human bone marrow stem cell proliferation kit. (A) $CD34^+$ rosetted cells with white colony emerging from rosettes. (B) MNC/Ficoll (unsorted MNC) as a control. (C) $CD34^-$ cells with small colonies.

To adjust the cell density of the CD34 rosetted cells, place the tube in contact with the magnet for 10 min. Remove the medium and replace it by a suitable volume of IMDM, 15% FCS.

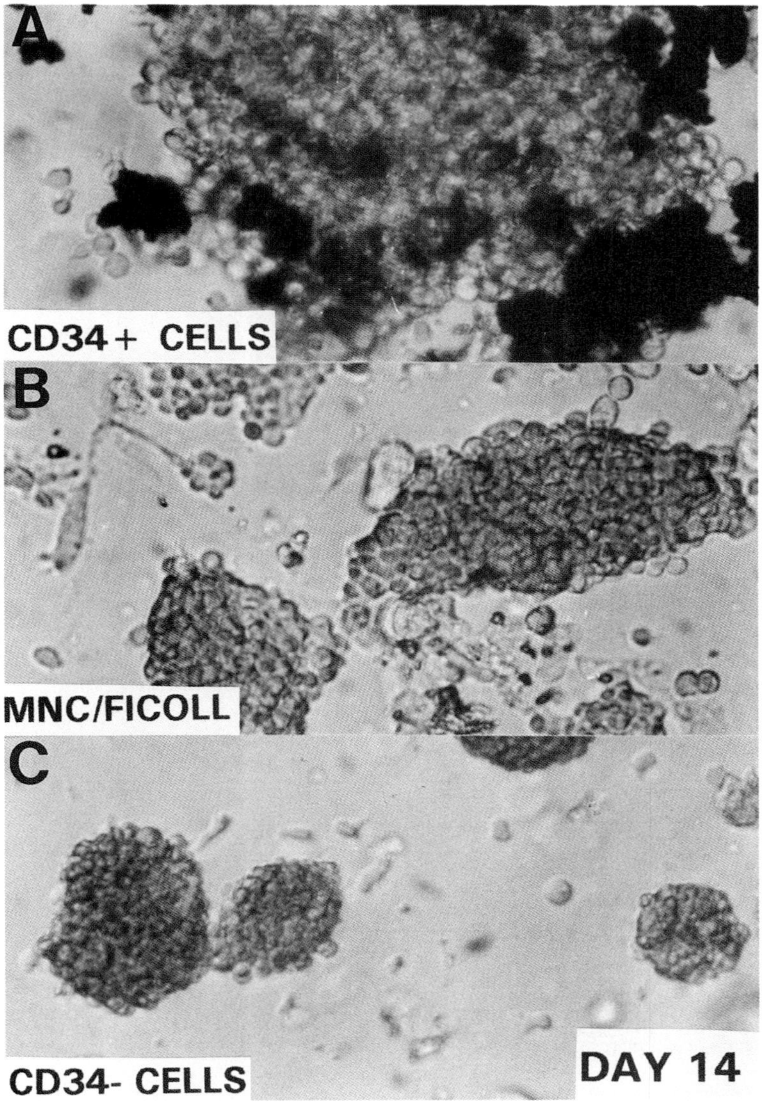

Fig. 5. Typical morphology of stem cell colonies after 14 days of culture (identical sample as described in Fig. 4). (A) $CD34^+$ rosetted cells with very large white colonies emerging from rosettes. (B) MNC/Ficoll (unsorted MNC) as a control. (C) $CD34^-$ cells with erythroid colonies.

The minimal volume of culture is 1 ml per well (12-well plates). A most effective approach for more extensive characterization is to start from at least 10 ml of culture in a 25 cm^2 tissue culture flask. Cultures are incubated horizontally at 37°C in a 7.5% CO_2 humidified incubator. Inspect the cultures the following day (day 1) with an inverted microscope, preferably equipped with phase-contrast optics.

The CD34+ rosetted cell culture appears brown and crowded due to the presence of an excess of free beads. However, it should be possible to begin to see cells partially or totally free of beads.

Between 1-3 days, count cells (rosetted cells and free cells). Cells are diluted 50% with more fresh medium. From 5-6 days, free cells and emerging colonies should be clearly visible. The propagation of cells occurs by successive splitting with 37°C medium twice a week or more frequently if necessary, according to the number of cells. Generally, after 6-10 days of culture, a heterogeneous monolayer is readily observed. These adherent cells are covered with magnetic beads, whereas cells in suspension are free of beads.

At times it may be informative to determine cell morphology as well as to evaluate some phenotypic properties. After a month of culture, growth of cells in suspension will slow progressively. From this point on, most cells are adherent. Signs of deterioration of the culture may occur after two months of culture.

Failure with no or little growth: this probably means that the starting material had very few stem cells or that the selected CD34+ cells were already committed to a lineage. At the same time, clonogenic assays performed on the same material (MNC and CD34 rosetted cells) show a low number of colonies. No or slow growth of CD34+ cells may also reflect the use of FCS incapable of supporting growth. As a control, the CD34− fraction is cultivated in parallel with the CD34+ fraction. After 10 days of culture, an increase of dead cells should be observed in the CD34− culture, followed by fast extinction of this culture.

Some Representative Results

Follow-up of a Culture of CD34+ Rosetted Cells

Table III shows an example of the growth of CD34+ rosetted cells after isolation from a cord blood sample. After 14 days of culture, a 20-fold increase over the input number was obtained. Figure 6 illustrates representative growth of a CD34+ rosetted cell culture. Similar expansion may be obtained with CD34+ rosetted cells isolated from a bone marrow sample.

Example of a Phenotypic Analysis of CD34+ Rosetted Cells after 14 Days of Culture

- On day 14, 83% of cells in suspension, thus free of beads, still express CD34. As shown in Figure 7, this expression is found to be heterogeneous; 50% of the cell population expresses a low level of CD34 and 50% a high level.

Table III. Follow-up of a culture of CD34⁺ cells

D0	3 × 10^5 rosetted $CD34^+$ cells in 1 ml of IMDM, 15% FCS	
D6	1 × 10^6 cells in 12 ml 25% rosetted cells + 75% free cells (from this day on presence of adherent cells with beads)	0% dead cells
D10	2 × 10^6 cells in 12 ml	
D14	5 × 10^6 cells in 20 ml 10% rosetted cells + 90% free cells + 1 × 10^6 adherent cells Phenotyping analysis 2.5 × 10^5 cells in suspension are maintained in culture	0% dead cells

The expression of antigens associated with T, B and myeloid-lineage cells (CD7, CD19 and CD33, respectively) was found to occur at different levels. The CD34 antigen is found on the $CD34^-$ cells in culture, but in contrast to the positive fraction, the majority of these cells express low levels of CD34.

A phenotypic characterization of the adherent layer may also be performed by flow cytometry. Figure 8 shows the identification of endothelial cells, for example. It has to be noted that culture of the $CD34^-$ fraction does not induce adherent cells. This protocol may permit a further optimization of ex vivo culture and a more extensive characterization of the cells generated.

Discussion

The immunomagnetic bead approach presented here is relatively easy to apply in any laboratory with limited expense and laboratory time, if the procedure is followed carefully step by step.

A few practical points need attention:

- It is obvious that the results depend on the quality of the initial sample.
- Moreover, the depletion of monocytes with $CD14^-$ magnetic beads is an alternative to the adherence procedure; we observe regularly better growth of CD34 cells in culture when using the magnetic bead procedure. The adherence method may induce a substantial loss of the cells of interest.
- This enrichment procedure can be used only for research purposes. However, once the feasibility of scaled-up ex vivo culture of $CD34^+$ cells for clinical applications is demonstrated, the magnetic separation approach may provide a richer source of $CD34^+$ cells than any other procedure [2].

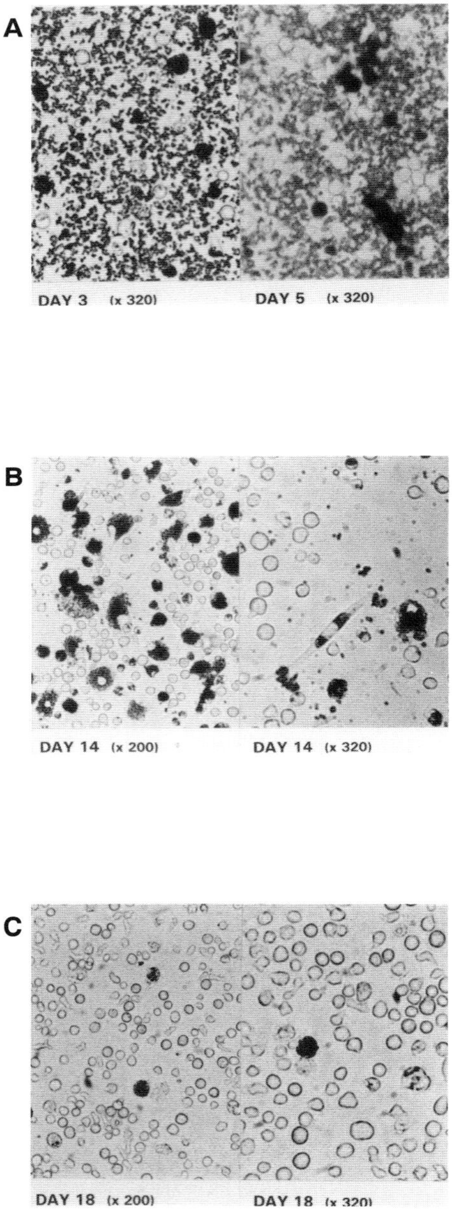

Fig. 6. Growth of a CD34+ rosetted cell isolated from a cord blood sample from day 3 to day 18 of culture (identical cord blood sample illustrated in Fig. 5). (A) Small black points are free beads. Large black points are CD34+ rosetted cells. Cells free of beads appear clearly among beads and rosettes. (B) Day 14 culture: cells free of beads grow in suspension. Black cells (cells covered with beads) are adherent cells with, in some cases, a fibroblast-like morphology. (C) Day 18 culture: after successive splittings of culture, most cells (in suspension and adherent layer) are free of beads.

- The detachment of beads from CD34⁺ cells may be necessary under certain circumstances, but this is not the general rule. The magnetic particles described offer the advantage that they can usually be left on the cells without affecting function, proliferation and differentiation. Other analogous systems using beads without the need for detachment from the cells of interest have already been described [3-5].
- The culture medium used for expansion of CD34⁺ cell cultures may be modified by adding certain factors in various combinations, allowing for creative experimentation. In all cases, a highly effective FCS is required for optimal cell growth. A serum-free medium would be more convenient.

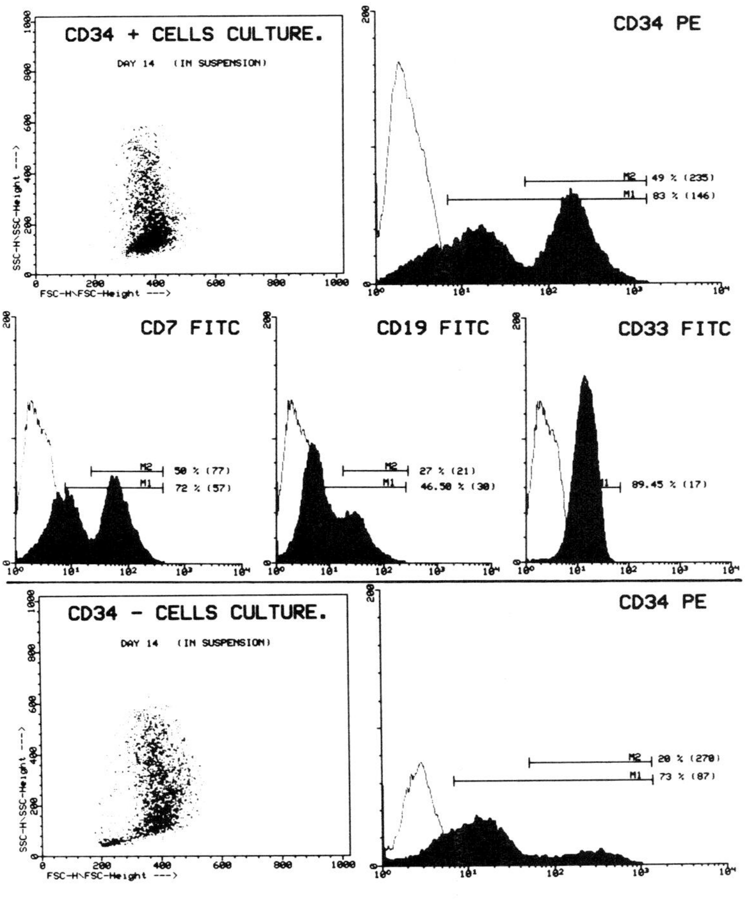

Fig. 7. Flow cytometric analysis of CD34⁺ cells in suspension after 14 days of culture (identical cord blood sample as shown in Figs. 5 and 6), illustrating light-scatter properties (dot plot representation) and expression of CD34, CD7, CD19 and CD33 antigens (fluorescence histograms). As a comparison, flow cytometric analysis of CD34⁻ cells after 14 days of culture illustrating light-scatter properties (dot plot representation) and expression of CD34 antigen (fluorescence histograms). Cells are stained with QBend 10-PE for CD34 expression. As a negative control, isotype-matched MAb is used.

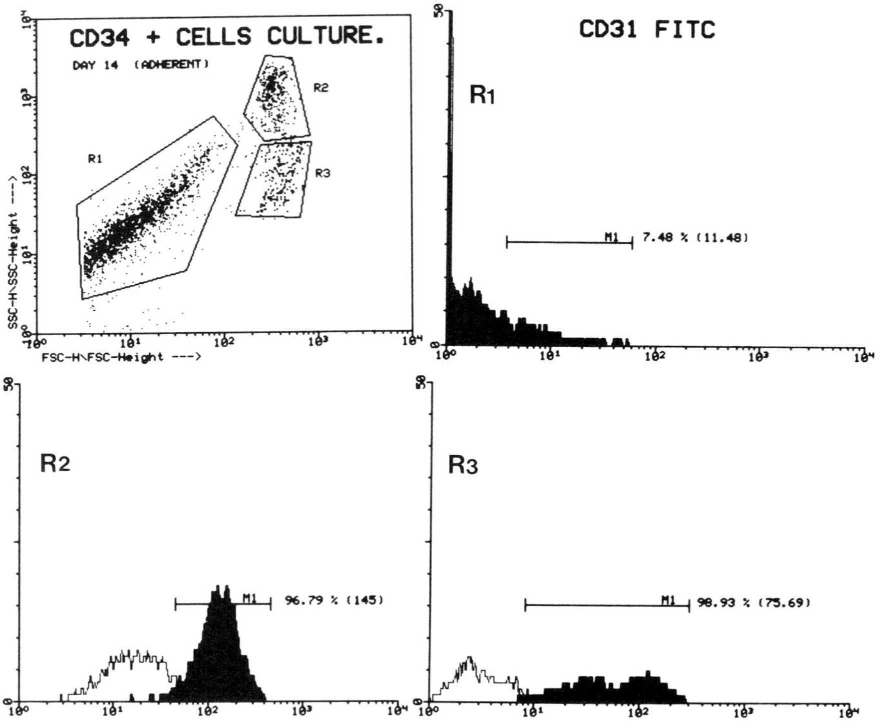

Fig. 8. Flow cytometric analysis of adherent cells from the CD34+ culture after 14 days of culture (identical cord blood sample as shown in Fig. 6), illustrating light-scatter properties (dot plot representation, FSC/SSC in log scale) and expression of a specific endothelial antigen (fluorescence histograms).

References

1 Barrande C, Traore Y, Szekeres G, Hirn J. Isolation and characterization of two new monoclonal antibodies against the CD34 molecule. Hybridoma 1993;12:203-213.

2 Haylock DN, To LB, Dowse TL, Juttner CA, Simmons PJ. Ex vivo expansion and maturation of peripheral blood CD34+ cells into the myeloid lineage. Blood 1992;80:1405-1412.

3 Handgretinger R, Dopfer R, Hammer S, Lang P, Daurer B, Kimmig A, Siedner R, Jalowy B, Treuner J, Neithammer D. The efficiency of a new cell separation technique in bone marrow purging without damaging the purged tumor cells. Prog Clin Biol Res 1990;333:303-309.

4 Schroder U, Pero RW, Sjogren HO. Magnetically tagged subsets of human lymphocytes for assays with laboratory robotic. Clin Chem 1990;36:1282-1287.

5 Horton JK, Evans OM, Swann K, Swinburne S. A new and rapid method for the selection and cloning of antigen-specific hybridomas with magnetic microspheres. J Immunol Methods 1989;124:225-230.

Isolation of CD34+ Hematopoietic Progenitor Cells by High-Gradient Magnetic Cell Sorting (MACS)

Stefan Miltenyi,[a] *Simone Guth,*[a] *Andreas Radbruch,*[b] *Eckhard Pflüger,*[a] *Andreas Thiel*[b]

[a]Miltenyi Biotec GmbH, Bergisch Gladbach, Germany; [b]Institute for Genetics, University of Cologne, Cologne, Germany

Key Words. Magnetic cell separation • Rare-cell sorting • Hematopoietic stem cells • CD34 • Cell-separation-methods • Monoclonal antibody (HPCA-2; QBEND10)

Introduction

The isolation of pure hematopoietic stem cells and progenitor cells is of experimental and clinical importance. CD34 is a highly glycosylated 115 kD type I integral membrane protein of unknown function [1-6]. CD34 is expressed on hematopoietic progenitor cells with a frequency of 1-4% of normal bone marrow cells and less than 0.2% of peripheral blood leukocytes [1-5, 7], on subsets of bone marrow stromal cells [8] and on small vessel endothelium of various tissues [5, 7, 9].

Most methods described for the isolation of $CD34^+$ human hematopoietic cells are based on the separation of target cells on macroscopic immunospecific surfaces: isolation using plastic plates [10], columns or macroscopic magnetic beads [11, 12, 13], all methods employing large surfaces for binding the target cells. Direct and indirect immunospecific labeling techniques are used to capture the cells onto the surfaces.

Several difficulties are associated with the separation of cells according to CD34 expression:

- The CD34 molecule is expressed in low copy numbers in comparison to other cell surface markers.
- CD34 antibodies available often show low affinity [14].
- $CD34^+$ cells are rare cells in a heterogeneous cell background.

Designing a rare cell selection system based on immunoaffinity surfaces is difficult because large surfaces tend to bind cells nonspecifically. Cells do not diffuse well to the binding surface because of their large size, but once bound are difficult to release due to multivalent binding.

Correspondence: Stefan Miltenyi, Miltenyi Biotec GmbH, Friedrich-Ebert-Strasse 68, 51429 Bergisch Gladbach, Germany.

The magnetic cell sorting (MACS) system (Miltenyi Biotec [15]) uses a different concept of "magnetic antibodies" for labeling and active magnetic separation of the target cells. Cells are labeled with very small superparamagnetic microbeads (diameter approximately 60 nm), which show extremely low nonspecific binding combined with fast attachment to the target cells. Separation is done on high gradient magnetic separation columns, retaining the cells which are magnetically labeled. This system avoids the problems associated with surface based separation systems.

The conventional MACS system has been used for CD34 cell enrichment in combination with the CD34 antibody HPCA-2 (fluorescein isothiocyanate [FITC]-conjugated), and MACS rat-anti-mouse IgG1 microbeads. The isolation of subpopulations of the rare CD34 cells from normal peripheral blood has been demonstrated using a combination of MACS and fluorescent activated cell sorting (FACS) [16], employing biotinylated CD34 antibody (QBEND10) and MACS streptavidin microbeads.

We have developed a new improved magnetic labeling and separation technique for fast and efficient isolation of $CD34^+$ progenitor cells. Cells are labeled with a chemically modified CD34 antibody and stained magnetically using specific submicroscopic MACS microbeads. Then, cells are magnetically separated using the MACS or MiniMACS separation system. The benefits of this method, specifically designed for the CD34 cell isolation, are short processing time (1 h), excellent recovery (>75%) and highest purity (for definitions see the chapter by *Wunder* and *deWynter,* pp. 125-131). For the isolated CD34 cells, enrichment rates of about 10,000-fold result in typically 95% to >99% purity from bone marrow and cord blood and 80% from normal peripheral blood mononuclear cells (PBMC).

Materials and Methodology

Sample Preparation

Bone Marrow

Collect bone marrow in 50 ml tubes containing 5 ml PBS-5 mM ethylenediaminetetraacetate (EDTA)-200 units/ml heparin and store before fractionation at 4°C.

For release of the cells, dilute in 10-fold excess of RPMI 1640 (GIBCO)-0.02% collagenase B (Boehringer-Mannheim)-100 units/ml DNAse (Calbiochem) and shake gently at room temperature for 45 min.

Remove clumps by filtering through 50 μm nylon mesh.

Overlay 35 ml of cell suspension on 15 ml Ficoll-Paque (Pharmacia), and centrifuge for 35 min at 400 *g*.

Collect interfaces and wash cells two times in Hank's balanced salt solution (HBSS, GIBCO)-100 units/ml DNAse (Calbiochem). Centrifuge at 300 *g* for 10 min.

Count cells and resuspend them in 300 μl of PBS-0.5% BSA-5 mM EDTA per 10^8 cells. For fewer cells take 300 μl.

Proceed to cell labeling.

NB:

- If cells cannot be separated at the day of harvest, store cells at 4°C. (Storage at higher temperature could result in activation and nonspecific binding of cell subpopulations).
- Remove all clumps during the cell preparation.

Cord Blood

Dilute anticoagulated cord blood 1:4 with PBS-5 mM EDTA and overlay 35 ml on 15 ml Ficoll-Paque.

Spin for 35 min at 400 *g*.

Collect interfaces and wash two times in PBS-5 mM EDTA. Centrifuge at 200 *g* for 10 min.

Count cells and resuspend them carefully in 300 μl of PBS-0.5% BSA-5 mM EDTA per 10^8 cells. For fewer cells take 300 μl.

Proceed to cell labeling.

NB:

- Do not use cord blood older than 4 h at the time of Ficoll separation.
- Blood should be drawn directly into a 50 ml tube containing 5 ml PBS-5 mM EDTA-200 units/ml heparin
- The blood should be stored at 4°C prior to separation.

Peripheral Blood

Overlay with 35 ml of anticoagulated blood (diluted 1:2 with PBS-5 mM EDTA) on 15 ml Ficoll-Paque.

Spin for 35 min at 400 *g*.

Collect interfaces and proceed to washing and counting.

(Start here if you use buffy coat.)

Dilute buffy coat 1:4 with PBS-5 mM EDTA and overlay 35 ml on 15 ml Ficoll-Paque.

Spin for 35 min at 400 *g*.

Collect interfaces.

Washing and counting:

1 wash: Dilute with PBS-5 mM EDTA and spin for 10 min at 300 *g*.

2 wash: Dilute with PBS-5 mM EDTA and spin for 15 min at 200 *g*.

3 wash: Dilute with PBS-5 mM EDTA-0.5% BSA, count cells and spin for 15 min at 200 *g*.

Resuspend cell pellet in 300 μl PBS-5 mM EDTA-0.5% BSA per 10^8 total cells.

Cells may be stored at this point overnight at 4°C in PBS containing 10% autologous serum.

NB:

- The peripheral blood or buffy coat should not be older than 8 h and well anticoagulated.
- EDTA in the buffer and the low speed washing steps are important for removing platelets.

Leukapheresed Material

Wash cells once in PBS-0.5% BSA-5 mM EDTA, filter through 50 μm nylon mesh in order to remove clumps and resuspend in 300 μl PBS-0.5% BSA-5 mM EDTA per 10^8 white cells.

Frozen Material

Thaw very fast and wash two times with PBS-0.5% BSA-100 units DNAse per ml. Filter cells after each centrifugation step to remove clumps. Work quickly.

Magnetic Labeling and Separation

Cells should have a concentration of 10^8 white cells per 300 μl. For less than 10^8 cells use 300 μl.

Resuspend cells carefully by flushing 10 times up and down through an Eppendorf pipette.

Add 100 μl blocking reagent (Reagent A1) per 10^8 cells (not less than 100 μl), mix.

Add 100 μl antibody reagent (Reagent A2) per 10^8 cells (not less than 100 μl), mix well.

Incubate for 15 min at 4 to 8°C.

Wash cells in PBS-0.5% BSA-5 mM EDTA. Add 10 ml per 10^8 cells, spin for 10 minutes at 300 *g*, remove buffer *completely.*

Resuspend cell pellet carefully in 400 μl PBS-0.5% BSA-5 mM EDTA per 10^8 cells.

Add 100 μl reagent B per 10^8 cells (not less than 100 μl), mix gently.

Incubate for 15 minutes at 6 to 12°C (in refrigerator).

For flow cytometry analysis, add CD34-phycoerythrin (CD34-PE) conjugated antibody and incubate for 10 min (200 μl HPCA-2-PE [Becton Dickinson], or QBEND10-PE [Immunotech, France] per 10^8 cells, see below).

Add 5 ml PBS-0.5% BSA-5 mM EDTA per 10^8 cells. If any clumps are present, filter cells through 50 μm mesh. Always filter first if more than 10^8 cells are loaded per column. Spin for 10 min at 300 *g* and remove supernatant.

Prepare two separation columns (MiniMACS type MS or MACS type RS) per 2×10^8 total cells.

Place first column in MiniMACS or MACS cell separator.

Resuspend cells very carefully in 500 μl PBS-0.5% BSA-5 mM-EDTA per 10^8 cells. Flush cell suspension 15 times up and down through a 1 ml Eppendorf pipette.

Apply cells to prefilled column (maximum 5×10^8 total white cells per column), allow cells to pass through the column and wash with 4×500 μl PBS-0.5% BSA-5 mM EDTA.

Remove column from separator, place column on a suitable tube, pipette 1 ml buffer on top of column and elute retained cells using the plunger supplied with the column.

Repeat magnetic separation step: Apply the eluted cells to the second filled column, wash with 2×500 μl, and elute retained cells with 500 μl buffer using the plunger.

Take a sample for determination of cell numbers and purity.

NB:

- Bovine serum albumin (BSA) may be replaced by human serum albumin (HSA).
- Use degassed buffers for filling and running the separation columns.
- Other MACS separation column types may be used for larger cell numbers, however, several washing steps are necessary.
- 50 μm nylon mesh filters are available from different companies (e.g., Consul T. S., Bruimo, Italy).

Measurement of Purity and Recovery

The complete separation can be easily followed up by flow cytometry if all cells are stained with a fluorochromed CD34 prior to separation (see below).

Alternatively, only a sample of the original and final fraction may be stained.

NB:

- Miltenyi Biotec offers different MACS CD34 reagent kits using the HPCA-2 or the QBEND10 antibody for CD34 labeling. For fluorescent staining, HPCA-2-PE should be used in combination with the QBEND10 based separation system, whereas QBEND10-PE should be used in combination with the HPCA-2 based system. If the same antibody is used for separation and fluorochrome staining, cell discrimination may be insufficient.

- Staining of the primary CD34 antibody using a fluorochromed anti-mouse antibody often results in low intensity signal.

Flow Cytometry

Add to the sample 1 μl of 0.1 mg/ml propidium iodide for discrimination of dead cells. Acquire at least 10,000 cells of each fraction to minimize statistical error. See Figure 1.

Results

Figure 2 shows the magnetic labeling and separation process schematically. The typical enrichment factor for the first column is in the range of 200- to 1000-fold, e.g., resulting in an increase of CD34 from 0.1% to 33% or 1 to 80% (500-fold) depending on the frequency of CD34 cells in the starting sample and the quality of the preparation. For increasing the purity of the CD34 cells, the positive fraction recovered from the first column is separated a second time using a further column. This second separation (typically 10- to 100-fold enrichment) results in a total enrichment of 5,000- to 20,000-fold.

Enumeration of cell percentages can be done easily if the cells are stained before separation. In Figure 3 cells were stained with HPCA-2-PE allowing for quick enumeration of cell frequencies. The percentage of CD34 cells in the unseparated and first negative fraction is often overestimated due to the

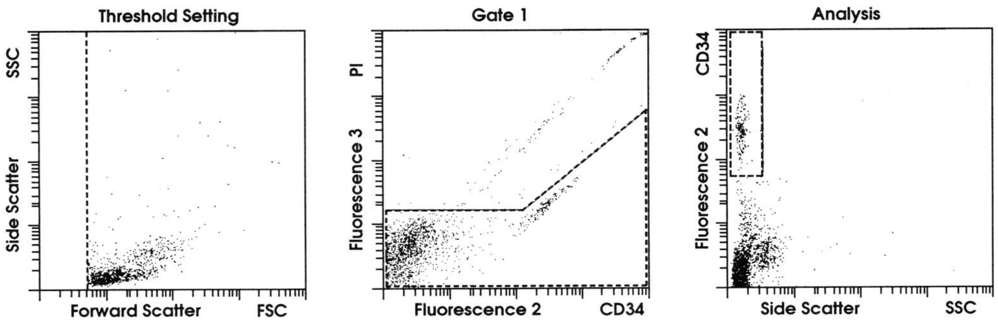

Fig. 1. Setting the gates for analysis. Typical gates on a FACScan flow cytometer for exclusion of debris and dead cells are shown. Debris and contaminating erythrocytes are excluded from analysis by adjusting the forward-scatter threshold level during collection to the lower end of the lymphocyte region. Dead cells are excluded by FL2-FL3 gating (gate 1). Enumeration is done in a FL2-side scatter dot plot excluding aggregates, nonspecifically stained and autofluorescent cells (high side scatter). Gates should be set using a pre-enriched sample (after first column). Data: isolation of CD34 cells from normal peripheral blood, first positive fraction.

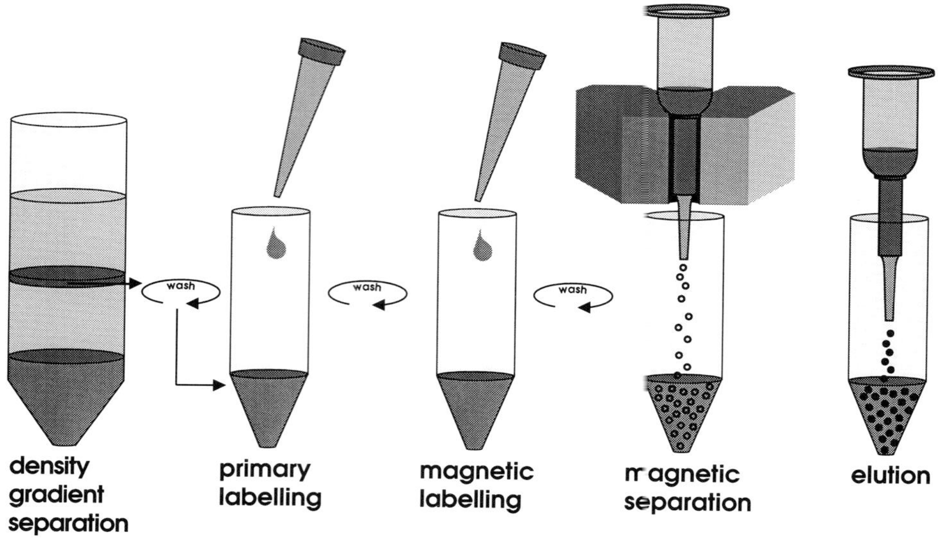

Fig. 2. Magnetic labeling and separation using the CD34-Isolation Kit and MiniMACS. Mononuclear cells are isolated by density gradient separation. The $CD34^+$ cells are labeled with a chemically modified CD34 antibody, which is magnetically stained with specific MACS microbeads. The cells are separated over a high-gradient magnetic separation column. Labeled cells are retained in the column. After washing the column, bound cells are eluted by removing the column from the magnetic separation unit and flushing the cells out.

background of the staining and the flow cytometry analysis. Measured percentages of less than 1% need careful interpretation. In the example given, the percentages of CD34 cells in the starting population are likely overestimated by a factor of two.

A small percentage (<10%) of the total CD34 cells is usually lost in the negative fraction of each separation. The negative fraction of the second separation may contain a high percentage of CD34 cells, however, the absolute cell number is low. Generally, absolute cell numbers have to be measured to calculate recovery.

As an alternative to staining with CD34-PE, other fluorochromed antibodies can be introduced in the process of magnetic labeling before separation. See Figure 4. Subpopulations of CD34 cells can be identified or sorted by staining with further antibodies e.g., by using flow cytometry. Figure 5 shows subtypes from peripheral blood.

The analysis of typical number $CD34^+$ cells recovered from peripheral blood in 23 experiments is summarized in Figure 6.

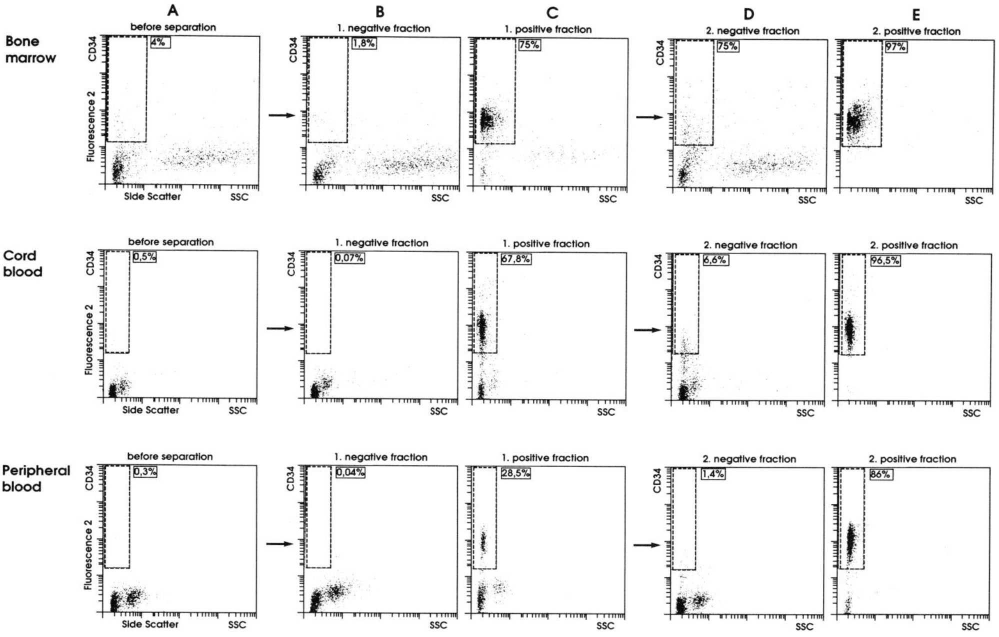

Fig. 3. Typical separation of CD34 expressing cells from bone marrow, cord blood and buffy coat. 1×10^8 bone marrow cells (after Ficoll) from hip joint surgery, 3×10^7 cord blood mononuclear cells and 1×10^8 PBMC were used as starting material. All samples were labeled magnetically using the QBEND10-CD34 Isolation Kit (Miltenyi Biotec), stained using CD34(HPCA-2)-PE and separated over two MiniMACS separation columns. Cell fractions were analyzed on a FACScan flow cytometer using FACScan research software and gating as shown in Figure 1. A) before separation, B) negative fraction of first column, C) positive fraction of first column, D) negative fraction of second column and E) final positive cells.

Discussion

The described CD34 cell isolation system shows extremely high enrichment rates with typically less than 1 in 10,000 nonspecifically retained cells. This high specificity is achieved by an optimized reagent combination of blocking and isolation reagents and enhancement steps. Therefore, CD34 cells can be isolated with high purity even from samples containing few CD34 expressing cells.

As dead cells are *not* nonspecifically labeled, even thawed cells can be successfully purified with the advantage of removing most debris and dead cells.

The separation process is compatible with flow cytometry since microbeads are too small to be detected by optical methods. This allows easy quality control of the separation, analysis of small CD34 subfractions or their separation in combination with fluorescent activated cell sorting.

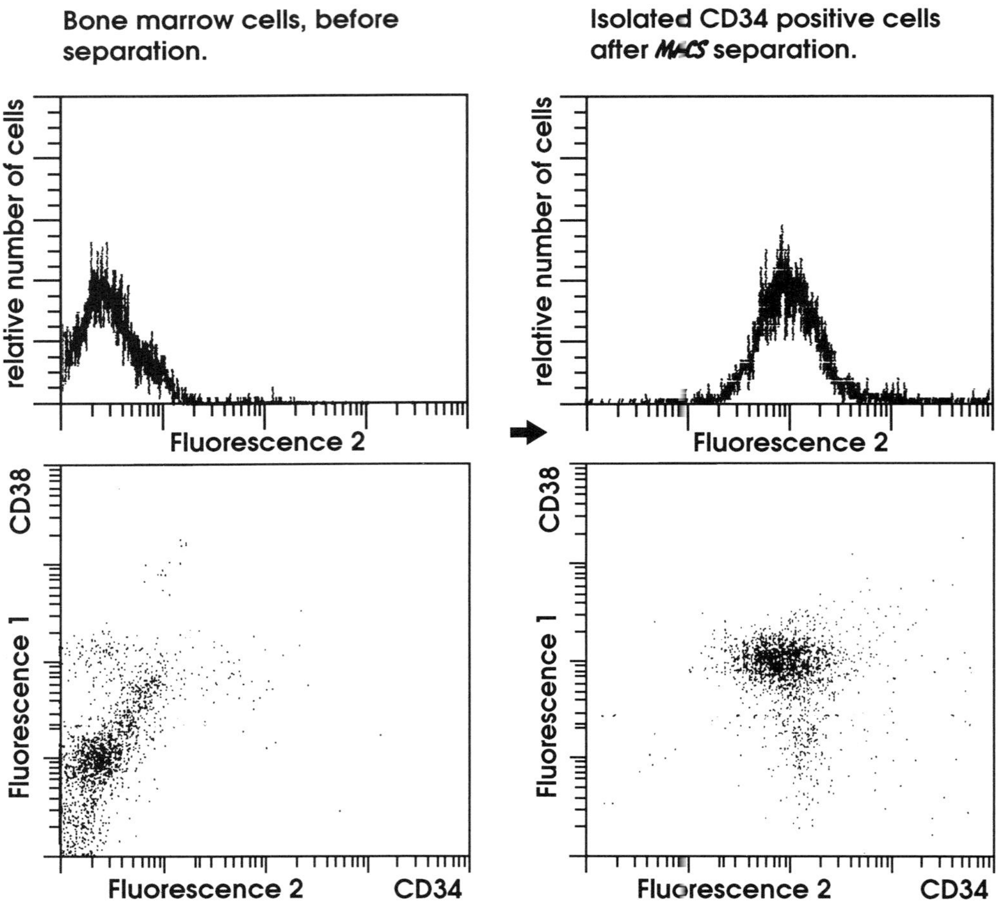

Fig. 4. Staining cells prior to magnetic separation. Bone marrow cells were stained with CD38-FITC (Becton Dickinson) and CD34-PE before separation and fractionated using MiniMACS. CD38 high and low expressing cells can be identified.

No effect on cell function due to bound antibodies or microbeads has been found so far. The microbeads seem to be released from the CD34 cells after one day culture as magnetic separations of cultured cells indicate. The enriched CD34 cells show normal hematopoietic colony formation in colony forming unit (CFU) assays [16].

This CD34 cell isolation technique is an interesting alternative to the currently available methods. Highly purified cells are of advantage if e.g., effects of cytokines or differentiation are explored whereby contaminating mature cells can modulate the effect on target cells, and this may result in wrong conclusions (see the chapter by *Wunder,* pp. 271-279).

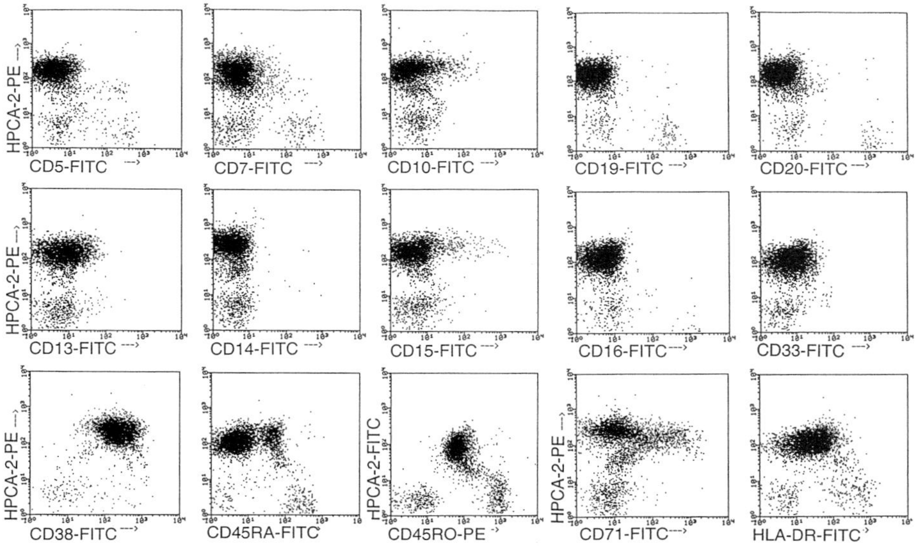

Fig. 5. Subtyping of isolated CD34 cells from peripheral blood. Cells were purified using a single run over the MiniMACS column, then stained with fluorochromed antibodies. In order to have CD34⁻ contaminating cells as a staining control present, only one round of separation was performed.

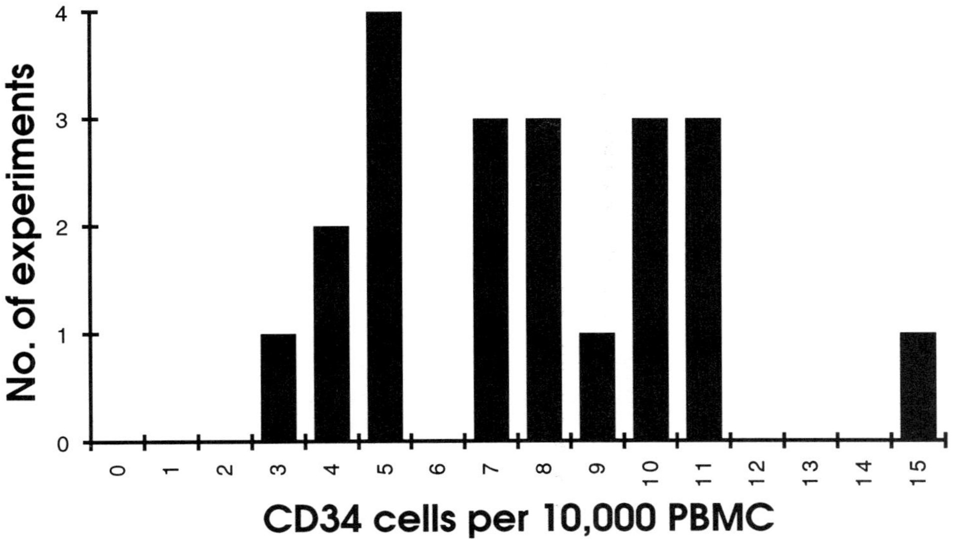

Fig. 6. Number of CD34 cells recovered from peripheral blood. An average of 7.8 CD34 cells per 10,000 PBMC could be isolated in 23 experiments (PBMC of normal donors after Ficoll isolation).

In combination with flow cytometry or fluorescence activated cell sorting, this technique makes the analysis and purification of CD34 subpopulations possible. Because of its high enrichment rates this technique will be useful in the future for clinical applications, e.g., purification of cells for gene therapy or transplantation when high purity is essential.

The combination of MACS with other bulk separation systems can be used for separation of subpopulation of CD34 cells or as a further step of CD34 purification. This opens the possibility of isolating cancer-cell-free CD34 cells for transplantation.

References

1 Civin CI, Strauss LC, Brovall C, Fackler MJ, Schwartz JF, Shaper JH. Antigenic analysis of hematopoiesis. III. A hematopoietic progenitor cell surface antigen defined by a monoclonal antibody raised against KG-1a cells. J Immunol 1984;133:157-165.

2 Katz FE, Tindle R, Sutherland DR, Greaves MF. Identification of a membrane glycoprotein associated with hematopoietic progenitor cells. Leuk Res 1985;9:191-198.

3 Tindle RW, Nichols RAB, Chan L, Campana D, Catovsky D, Birnie GD. A novel monoclonal antibody BI-3C5 recognizes myeloblasts and non-B non-T lymphoblasts in acute leukemias and CGL blast crisis, and reacts with immature cells in normal bone marrow. Leuk Res 1985;9:1-9.

4 Andrews RG, Singer JW, Bernstein ID. Monoclonal antibody 12.8 recognizes a 115 kD molecule present on both unipotent and multipotent hematopoietic colony-forming cells and their precursors. Blood 1986;67:842-845.

5 Watt SM, Karhi K, Gatter K, Furley AJW, Katz FE, Healy LE, Atlass LJ, Bradley NJ, Sutherland DR, Levinsky R, Greaves MF. Distribution and epitope analysis of the cell membrane glycoprotein (HPCA-1) associated with human hemopoietic progenitor cells. Leukemia 1987;1:417.

6 Simmons DL, Satterthwaite AB, Tenen DG, Seed B. Molecular cloning of a cDNA encoding CD34, a sialomucin of human hematopoietic stem cells. J Immunol 1992;148:267.

7 Beschorner WE, Civin CI, Strauss LC. Localization of hematopoietic progenitor cells in tissue with the anti-MY-10 monoclonal antibody. Am J Pathol 1985;119:1-4.

8 Simmons PJ, Torok-Storb B. CD34 expression by stromal precursors in normal human adult bone marrow. Blood 1991;78:2848.

9 Fina L, Molgaard HV, Robertson D, Bradley NJ, Monaghan P, Delia D, Sutherland DR, Baker MA, Greaves MF. Expression of the CD34 gene in vascular endothelial cells. Blood 1990;75:2417.

10 Silvestri FF, Banavali SD, Hulette BC, Civin CI, Preisler HD. Isolation and characterization of the CD34+ hematopoietic progenitor cells from the peripheral blood of patients with chronic myeloid leukemia. Int J Cell Cloning 1991;9:474-490.

11 Berenson RJ, Andrews RG, Bensinger WI, Kalamasz D, Knitter G, Buckner CD, Bernstein ID. Antigen CD34+ marrow cells engraft lethally irradiated baboons. J Clin Invest 1988;81:951-955.

12 Winslow JM, Liesveld JL, Ryan DH, Abboud CN. Enrichment of CD34+ progenitors: comparison of immunoadsorptive selection to flow cytometry. Blood 1991;68:300a.

13 Kirshenbaum AS, Kessler SW, Goff JP, Metcalfe DD. Demonstration of the origin of human mast cells from CD34+ bone marrow progenitor cells. J Immunol 1991;146:1410.

14 Landsdorp PM, Dougherty GJ, Humphries RK. CD34 epitopes. In: Knapp W, ed. Leucocyte Typing IV. Oxford: Oxford University Press. 1990.

15 Miltenyi S, Müller W, Weichel W, Radbruch A. High-gradient magnetic cell separation with MACS. Cytometry 1990;11:231-238.

16 Kato K, Radbruch A. Isolation and characterization of $CD34^+$ hematopoietic stem cells from human peripheral blood by high-gradient magnetic cell sorting. Cytometry 1993;14:384.

Isolation and Culture of Human CD34⁺ Hematopoietic Stem Cells Using AIS CELLectors™

Jane Lebkowski, Lisa Schain, Mark Harvey, Annemarie Moseley, Thomas B. Okarma
Applied Immune Sciences, Inc., Santa Clara, California, USA

Key Words. $CD34^+$ cell isolation • Stem cell expansion • Stem cells • Peripheral blood stem cells • Bone marrow • Transplantation • Cell separation

Introduction

The isolation and culture of large quantities of $CD34^+$ human hematopoietic stem cells have numerous applications in basic research and human therapy. For instance, isolated $CD34^+$ cells can be used as a purged graft in autologous bone marrow transplantation minimizing the reinfusion of tumor cells post-high-dose chemotherapy or irradiation. $CD34^+$ cells can also be used as a T cell depleted graft in allogeneic bone marrow transplantation, as a supportive care transfusion product post-chemotherapy, or as a target cell in gene therapy protocols. In this report we describe a simple system to isolate and culture human $CD34^+$ cells in large scale from a variety of sources using polystyrene devices containing covalently immobilized soybean agglutinin or the anti-CD34 monoclonal antibody, ICH3 [1]. The system can be used to process input samples as small as 1×10^7 cells to full size clinical bone marrow grafts. $CD34^+$ cells isolated using this procedure are 60-98% pure, have no detectable mouse immunoglobulin on their surfaces, and are functional in in vitro hematopoiesis assays. Since the devices are sterile culture vessels, isolated $CD34^+$ cells can also be directly cultured in the AIS CELLectors® yielding large expansions of progenitors.

Materials and Methodology

Isolation of $CD34^+$ Cells

Basic Scheme

Isolation of $CD34^+$ cells from any human cell source using AIS CELLectors involves three steps. In the first step, the sample is depleted of red blood cells (RBC) using either Ficoll/Hypaque density gradients or gelatin sedimentation. After RBC depletion, the majority of differentiated cells are depleted using the AIS CELLector SBA which contains the lectin, soybean agglutinin. The nonadherent, SBA^- cells, which are enriched in $CD34^+$ cells, are then loaded into the AIS CELLector CD34 for the purification of $CD34^+$ cells. The nonadherent, $CD34^-$ cells are washed from the device, and the adherent $CD34^+$ cells are collected by physical agitation.

Correspondence: Dr. Jane S. Lebkowski, Senior Director of Research, Applied Immune Sciences, Inc., 5301 Patrick Henry Drive, Santa Clara, CA 95054-1114, USA.

Cell Sources

Bone marrow was collected from the iliac crests of consenting volunteers. Normal peripheral blood was collected as a leukapheresis product from consenting volunteers. Aliquots of cytokine stimulated peripheral blood were collected either from normal volunteers who were stimulated six days with granulocyte-colony stimulating factor (G-CSF) or from myeloma patients undergoing peripheral blood stem cell collections after chemotherapy and G-CSF treatment as a part of their normal course of therapy.

Preparation of Bone Marrow or Peripheral Blood Mononuclear Cells

To prepare cells for $CD34^+$ cell isolation, mononuclear cells were isolated from bone marrow, growth factor stimulated peripheral blood stem cell preparations, or normal peripheral blood cells using Ficoll-Hypaque density gradients. Briefly, the cell sample was diluted 1:5–1:10 using Dulbecco's Phosphate Buffered Saline (Ca/Mg free) containing 1 mM ethylenediaminetetraacetate (EDTA) (DPBSE). Forty ml of this suspension were underlayered with 10 ml of Histopaque (Sigma, 1.077 g/ml) and centrifuged for 20 minutes at 900 *g* (no brake). The mononuclear cell layer was collected, diluted five fold with DPBSE, and the cells were collected at 900 *g* for 20 minutes. To eliminate platelets, the cells were subsequently diluted with DPBSE and centrifuged at 450 *g* for 10 minutes. The cells were resuspended in DPBSE, counted, and used in later separation procedures.

As an alternative procedure to eliminate red blood cells from the input samples, gelatin sedimentation was used. For this procedure, the bone marrow or peripheral blood was directly mixed 1:1 (v:v) with 3% gelatin in DPBSE. After a 20-40 minute incubation at room temperature, the white cell supernatant was extracted and diluted 3-5 fold with DPBSE. The white cells were collected at 900 *g* for 20 minutes and were ready to use in the AIS CELLector process.

Preparation of the AIS CELLectors

The AIS CELLectors are polystyrene vessels containing covalently immobilized protein. The AIS CELLector devices containing SBA have a variety of capacities; the 25 cm^2 and 150 cm^2 MicroCELLectors® SBA will separate up to 2×10^7 and 1.2×10^8 input cells, respectively. The large scale AIS CELLector SBA will process up to 4×10^9 cells. The AIS CELLectors CD34 also are designed to process a variety of cell loads. The AIS MicroCELLector CD34 (25 cm^2) will accommodate 2×10^7 cells, whereas the large scale device will process up to 5×10^8 cells. The devices collectively are referred to as the AIS CELLectors, and their instructions for use are, in general, identical. However, any differences in the specific operation of the individual devices is noted below.

The AIS CELLectors were prepared by rehydrating the surface with four consecutive washes with DPBSE. The device was shaken vigorously at each wash to remove the protective coating of the surface. The last wash was left on the device until use to protect the immobilized lectin or antibody.

Depletion of Mature Cells Using the AIS CELLector SBA

To remove most mature, differentiated elements, the RBC depleted cells were loaded into the AIS CELLector SBA. For this separation, the cells were incubated at 5×10^6 cells/ml in 0.5% human immunoglobulin (Ig)G (Gamimune N, Cutter Labs) in DPBSE for 15-20 minutes at room temperature. The 25 and 150 cm^2 AIS MicroCELLectors SBA were then loaded with 4 and 25 ml of cells, respectively, containing at maximum 2×10^7 and 1.2×10^8 cells. For the large scale 3000 cm^2 AIS CELLector SBA, up to 4×10^9 cells were incubated in 50 ml of 0.5% human IgG in DPBSE for 15-20 minutes at room temperature. After incubation, the cells were diluted to 265 ml with DPBSE and loaded directly into a primed 3000 cm^2 device. After loading, the AIS MicroCELLectors SBA were incubated at room temperature for one hour. The large scale 3000 cm^2 devices were incubated 30 min at room temperature on each of the two broad sides of the device. To remove the nonadherent SBA^- cells, the devices were rocked gently, and the nonadherent cell suspension was collected. The 25 and 150 cm^2 devices were then washed two times with DPBSE and the washes were pooled with the first nonadherent fraction. For the 3000 cm^2 AIS CELLector SBA, the device was rocked steadily during the collection of the nonadherent cells. If this procedure was followed, subsequent washes of the device were not necessary. The nonadherent cells from all devices were centrifuged at 900 *g* for 20 min, and subsequently resuspended at 5×10^6 cells/ml in 0.5% human Ig in DPBSE for processing on the AIS CELLector CD34 devices.

$CD34^+$ Cell Selection on the AIS CELLector CD34

After resuspension of the SBA^- cells in the human IgG solution, the 25 cm^2 and 624 cm^2 CD34 devices were loaded with a maximum of 2×10^7 and 5×10^8 SBA^- cells, respectively. The devices were then incubated at room temperature for 60 minutes. To remove the $CD34^-$ nonadherent cells, the devices were gently rocked and the fluid was drained. The devices were then washed 2-4 times using DPBSE containing 0.5% human serum albumin (HSA). After these washes, the 25 and 624 cm^2 CELLectors were filled with 4 and 50 ml of DPBSE containing 0.5% HSA, respectively, and the devices were agitated vigorously in the plane of the binding surface. The dislodged $CD34^+$ cells were drained into centrifuge tubes pre-coated with HSA, and the devices were rinsed twice with DPBSE. These washes were pooled with the dislodged $CD34^+$ cells in the HSA coated tubes, and the $CD34^+$ cell fraction was collected at 900 *g* for 20 minutes.

Culture of CD34+ Cells in the AIS CELLector CD34

To culture and expand CD34+ cells, the adherent cells from the AIS CELLector CD34 were not removed from the device. Instead, Dulbecco's Modified Eagles Medium (DMEM) containing 10% fetal calf serum and a variety of cytokines or growth factor combinations was simply added to the AIS CELLector. The device was incubated at 37°C at 5% CO_2. Half media changes were made twice weekly until the termination of the culture. For the experiments described in this report, IL-1, IL-3, IL-6, GM-CSF, G-CSF (all at 10 ng/ml), erythropoietin (0.5 U/ml) and stem cell factor (SCF) (50 ng/ml) were used to stimulate hematopoietic stem cell growth.

Assays and Determinations

Flow Cytometry

After purification, the CD34+ cells were held overnight at 4°C in DPBS containing 0.5% HSA. To assess final purity, the cells were stained using the fluorescein isothiocyanate (FITC) or phycoerythrin (PE) conjugated HPCA-2 (Becton Dickinson) anti CD34 monoclonal antibody. These FITC and PE conjugated antibodies were used for evaluation: control mouse Ig, anti-CD3, clone SK7; anti-CD19, clone 467; anti-CD33, clone P676; anti-CD38, clone HB-7; anti-HLA-DR, clone L243; goat anti-mouse IgG (heavy and light chain). These samples were analyzed on a FACScan flow cytometer (Becton Dickinson).

Methylcellulose Progenitor Colony Assay

Defined numbers of the different cell populations were plated in 1.5 ml of Terry Fox methylcellulose containing phytohemagglutinin (PHA)-stimulated leukocyte conditioned media. More recently, we have supplemented this media with 50 ng/ml SCF, which produces higher cloning efficiencies in the CD34+ cell fraction. The cells were plated in humidified 6-well culture dishes and incubated at 37°C in 5% CO_2. After 14 days, colony forming units-granulocyte-macrophage (CFU-GM), burst forming units-erythroid (BFU-E) and CFU-granulocyte-erythroid-macrophage-megakaryocyte (CFU-GEMM) were counted on an inverted microscope.

Long Term Bone Marrow Culture

Long term bone marrow cultures were initiated on well-established human stromal cultures that were irradiated with 25 Gy according to the methods of *Kaplan et al.* [2]. Within seven days after irradiation, 2-10 × 10^5 cells were seeded into each irradiated stromal culture flask. The cultures were grown at 37°C in a 5-7% CO_2 atmosphere. Equal numbers of each different cell population were used to seed the stromal layers. Once a week for the following six weeks, nonadherent cells from each cell culture were collected, and an aliquot was plated in methylcellulose assay. The remaining cells from each population were distributed to the original flasks.

Results

Human CD34⁺ cells can be isolated from a variety of sources using the AIS CELLector system which consists of polystyrene devices containing either covalently immobilized soybean agglutinin or the monoclonal antibody, ICH3. The process for utilizing these devices is outlined in Figure 1. Bone marrow or peripheral blood CD34⁺ cells are depleted of red cells using Ficoll/Hypaque density gradients or gelatin sedimentation. The mononuclear cell preparation is then loaded into an AIS CELLector SBA device to bind many differentiated cells such as red cells, B cells, fat cells, fibroblasts, endothelial cells, certain T cells and tumor cells which normally bind to the soybean lectin. The nonadherent SBA⁻ fraction, which is enriched in CD34⁺ cells, is collected; the adherent SBA⁺ cells can be eluted from the devices by incubation at 37°C with 200 mM N-acetylgalactosamine in RPMI for 0.5-3 hours. After concentration, the SBA⁻ population is subsequently loaded into an AIS CELLector CD34 for CD34⁺ cell isolation. Finally, the nonadherent, CD34⁻, cells are removed and the CD34⁺ cells are harvested after physical agitation of the device.

Table I shows the recovery of cells in the various SBA⁻ and CD34⁺ populations from bone marrow, cytokine stimulated peripheral blood stem cells

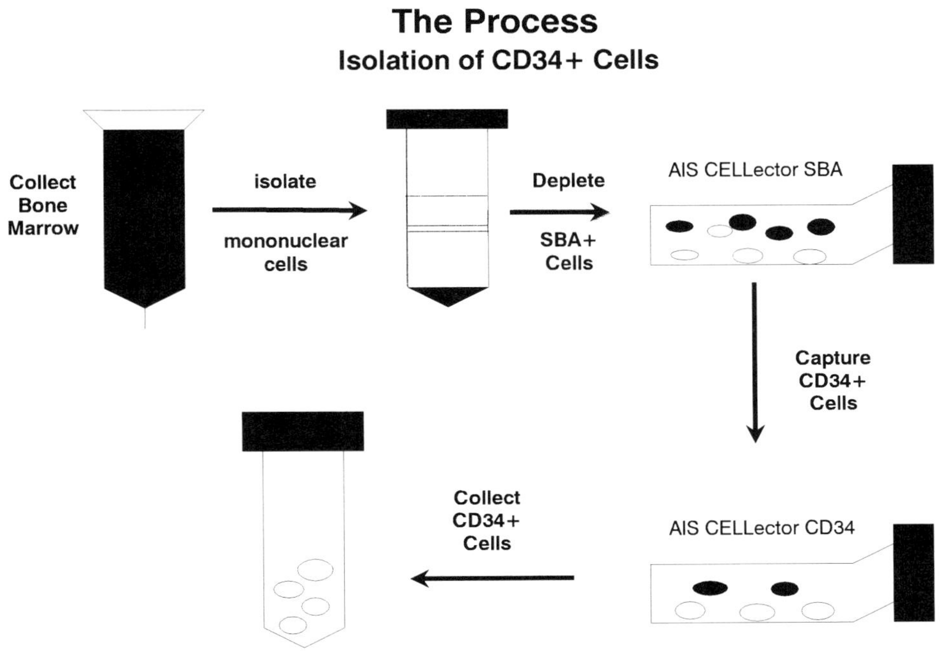

Fig. 1. Purification Scheme for CD34⁺ Cells. The procedures for isolation of CD34⁺ cells are detailed in Materials and Methodology.

Table I. Cell Recoveries

	% Recovery of Mononuclear Cells	
	SBA⁻ Fraction	CD34⁺ Fraction
Bone Marrow (n = 26)	20.4 ± 12.0	0.9 ± 0.6
Cytokine Stimulated Peripheral Blood (n = 5)	22.0 ± 6.6	0.8 ± 0.7
Nonmobilized Normal Peripheral Blood (n = 3)	15.0 ± 8.0	0.2 ± 0.1

The % recovery of mononuclear cells was determined from individual cell counts and was calculated as: # cells in output populations/# mononuclear cells × 100%. The results are expressed as the mean ± standard deviation.

and normal peripheral blood. On average, 15.0, 22.0 and 20.4% of the mononuclear cells were recovered after depletion of SBA binding cells from normal peripheral blood, cytokine stimulated peripheral blood or bone marrow, respectively. These recoveries are equivalent to those observed in the SBA⁻ fraction after soluble soybean agglutination (manuscript submitted). After purification of CD34⁺ cells, on average, 0.9% of the bone marrow mononuclear cells were found in the final stem cell fraction. This recovery is expected, as CD34⁺ cells comprise approximately 0.5-3.0% of normal bone marrow. From cytokine stimulated peripheral blood, on average, 0.8% of the mononuclear cells were collected in the CD34⁺ cell fraction, whereas normal unstimulated peripheral blood, which usually has CD34⁺ cell levels below the detection limits of flow cytometry, produced only 0.2% recoveries.

The CD34⁺ purities of the different cell fractions produced during the purification procedure were evaluated (Table II). For bone marrow, the mononuclear cell preparation was, on average, 2.4% CD34⁺. Upon depletion of the SBA⁺ population, there was a net enrichment of CD34⁺ cells to 8.1%. On average, 67.5% of the CD34⁺ cells were recovered in the SBA⁻ fraction. The majority of those CD34⁺ cells not recovered in the SBA⁻ fraction were CD34⁺CD19⁺ pre-B cells which normally bind SBA. After purification, the final CD34⁺ cell fraction from bone marrow was on average 74.2% pure, with a 30% overall recovery of CD34⁺ cells.

Similar purities were observed when CD34⁺ cells were isolated from G-CSF stimulated peripheral blood. The input mononuclear cell fraction had a mean 3.1% frequency of CD34⁺ cells, which upon depletion of SBA binding cells was enriched to 10.9% with greater than 90% recovery of CD34⁺ cells. The final CD34⁺ cell fraction was highly purified, being 81.5% pure with a 22% overall recovery of the CD34⁺ cells.

Table II. CD34$^+$ Cell Purity

	%CD34$^+$		
	Input Mononuclear Cells	SBA$^-$ Cells	CD34$^+$ Cells
Bone Marrow	2.4 ± 1.8	8.1 ± 4.2	74.2 ± 11.6
Cytokine Stimulated Peripheral Blood Mononuclear Cells	3.1 ± 2.0	10.9 ± 8.6	81.5 ± 8.9
Normal Peripheral Blood	< 0.2%	0.4 ± 0.4	43.4 ± 16.8

The CD34$^+$ purity of the above three cell fractions was determined using the PE conjugated HPCA-2 anti-CD34 MAb as described in Materials and Methodology. The purity was determined using a gate which excluded only debris. These data were collected from the same experiments described in Table I.

The covalently immobilized antibody surface provides high specificity binding for even extremely rare cell populations. For instance, CD34$^+$ cells from normal peripheral blood, which were essentially nondetectable (<0.2%) in the input mononuclear cell fraction, were isolated to 43.4% purity on the AIS CELLector devices, representing a greater than 200 fold purification of these CD34$^+$ cells (Table II).

To more fully characterize the cells at each step of the purification, two color flow cytometric analysis was performed. Figure 2 shows representative two color plots from the mononuclear cell, SBA$^-$ and CD34$^+$ cell fractions from bone marrow. CD3$^+$ T cells which were present in the input cell fraction were eliminated from the final CD34$^+$ fraction. Likewise, CD19$^+$ B cells were almost totally eliminated after SBA depletion and were less than 2% of the final CD34$^+$ cell fraction. Particularly evident in the figure is the enrichment of CD34$^+$ cells at both the SBA and final step of the purification process. In the final cell population, approximately 50% and 95% of the CD34$^+$ cells expressed the CD33 and CD38 antigens respectively, suggesting that the purified population contained a mixture of committed and uncommitted CD34$^+$ cells representative of those found in unfractionated bone marrow.

The final CD34$^+$ cell population does not have residual mouse immunoglobulin on its surface. In over 50 experiments, the CD34$^+$ cell population, after isolation on the AIS CELLectors, was phenotyped with many different anti-mouse immunoglobin antibodies directed against the heavy, light, Fab and Fc portions of the immunoglobulin molecule. In every test, no mouse immunoglobulin was found on the surface of the CD34$^+$ cells. Similar results were observed

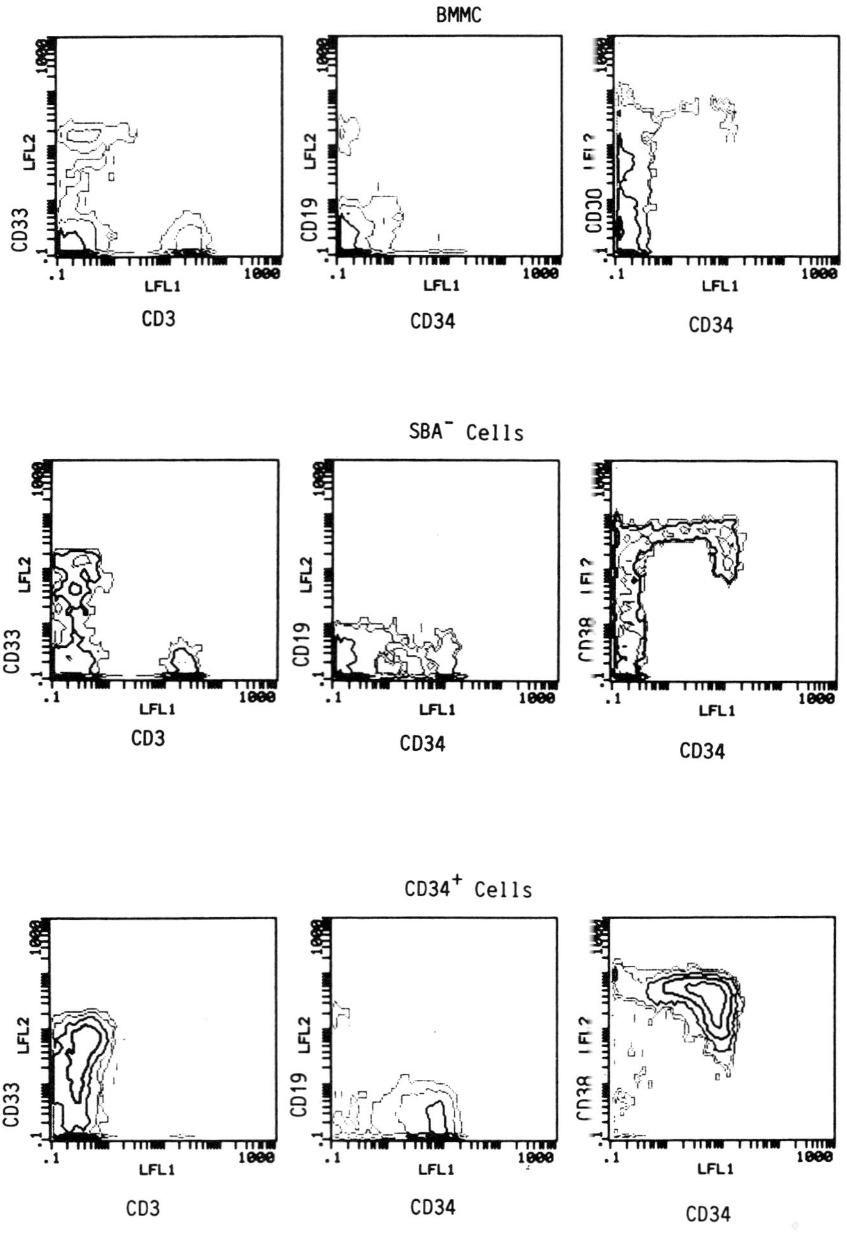

Fig. 2. Two Color Flow Cytometric Analysis. Two color analysis was performed as described in Materials and Methodology. A lymphoblastoid gate was used for the bone marrow mononuclear (BMMC) and SBA⁻ cell fractions to eliminate the autofluorescence of high side scatter cells. A total cell gate was used for the CD34⁺ cell fraction.

with the SBA⁻ fraction which was phenotyped with an anti-SBA polyclonal antibody. Therefore, the immobilized protein is an integral component of the AIS CELLector, which is not released upon use.

The isolated $CD34^+$ cells not only have high purity, but retain functional hematopoietic activity. Figure 3 shows the enrichment of CFU-GM, BFU-E and CFU-GEMM activity in the SBA^- and $CD34^+$ cell fractions from bone marrow (3A), cytokine stimulated peripheral blood (3B), and normal unstimulated peripheral blood (3C). On average, each of the three progenitor types are enriched approximately three fold after SBA^+ cell depletion. In addition, the $CD34^+$ cells from bone marrow and G-CSF stimulated peripheral blood are, on average, 25-30 fold enriched in CFU-GM and BFU-E progenitors. In general, 15-20 fold enrichments in CFU-GEMM were observed. It is important to note that in the assays reported here, SCF was not added to the methylcellulose progenitor cultures. If SCF is added, higher cloning efficiencies, especially of the $CD34^+$ cell fraction are observed, resulting in even higher progenitor enrichments (data not shown).

Substantial hematopoietic activity is also found in the $CD34^+$ cells isolated from nonmobilized normal peripheral blood. In these experiments, even higher enrichments of CFU-GM, BFU-E and CFU-GEMM are observed due to the very low level of these progenitors in the starting population. On average, 50, 90 and 38 fold enrichments of CFU-GM, BFU-E and CFU-GEMM, respectively, were observed after the AIS CELLector process.

The isolated $CD34^+$ cells also show enhanced activity in long term bone marrow culture. In these experiments, equal numbers of bone marrow mononuclear cells, SBA^- cells or $CD34^+$ cells were seeded on irradiated allogeneic stroma and the nonadherent cells were assayed weekly for cell number and progenitor activity. Figure 4 shows the results from one representative experiment. At each time point, cultures seeded with $CD34^+$ cells showed 2-50 fold more cells in the culture than did those cultures seeded with the unseparated mononuclear cells. Moreover, those cultures seeded with $CD34^+$ cells in general, proliferated 2-5 weeks longer than did those cultures seeded with the bone marrow mononuclear cell (BMMC) population. Similarly, CFU-GM production was much higher in those cultures seeded with $CD34^+$ cells, while the SBA^- fraction showed intermediate levels of activity. At every time point, 10-1000 fold more colonies were produced by the $CD34^+$ cells (Fig. 4B), yielding an overall 20-50 fold greater accumulation of CFU-GM. These results are consistent with the relative purity of the $CD34^+$ cells in each cell population, and indicate that the purified $CD34^+$ cells not only are viable but retain complete functionality as measured by both short and long term in vitro hematopoietic assays.

The AIS CELLector CD34 is a sterile culture vessel and will support the propagation of cells. To study the proliferation of stem cells, the purified $CD34^+$ cells were not dislodged from the device. Instead, culture media containing IL-1, IL-3, IL-6, GM-CSF, stem cell factor and erythropoietin was

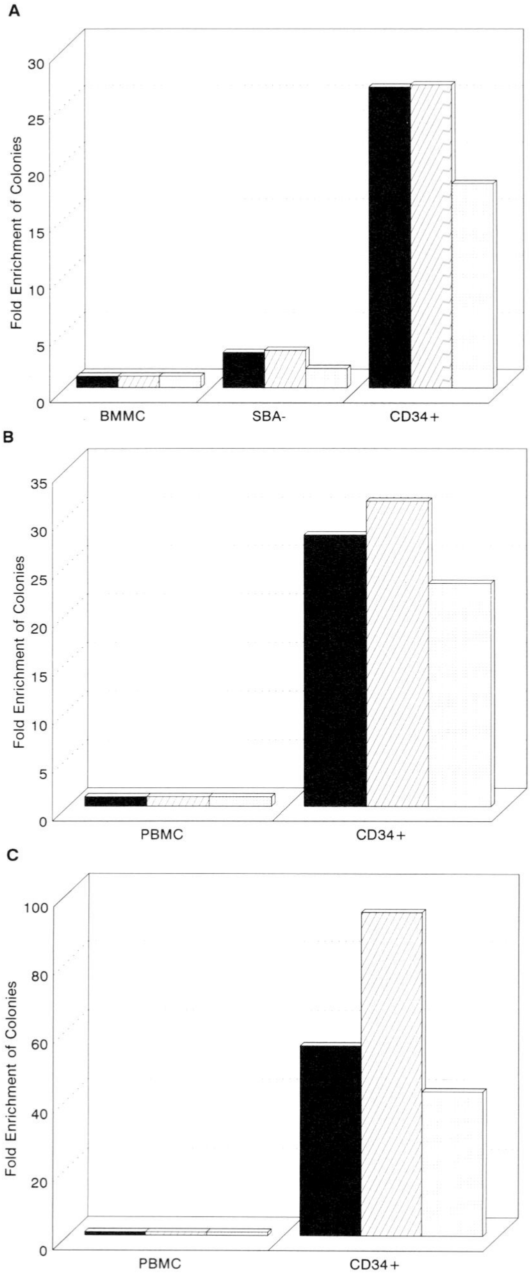

Fig. 3. Enrichment of Human Hematopoietic Progenitors. Aliquots of the indicated populations from bone marrow (A), cytokine stimulated peripheral blood (B), and unstimulated peripheral blood (C) were placed in methylcellulose culture as described in Materials and Methodology. The frequency of CFU-GM, BFU-E and CFU-GEMM were calculated in each population of cells. The fold enrichment of CFU-GM (solid bars), BFU-E (hatched bars) and CFU-GEMM (dotted bars) in the SBA^- and $CD34^+$ cell populations was then calculated in reference to the mononuclear cell fraction. The fold enrichment in the mononuclear cell fraction was defined as 1. The results shown in these figures are from the same experiments detailed in Table I.

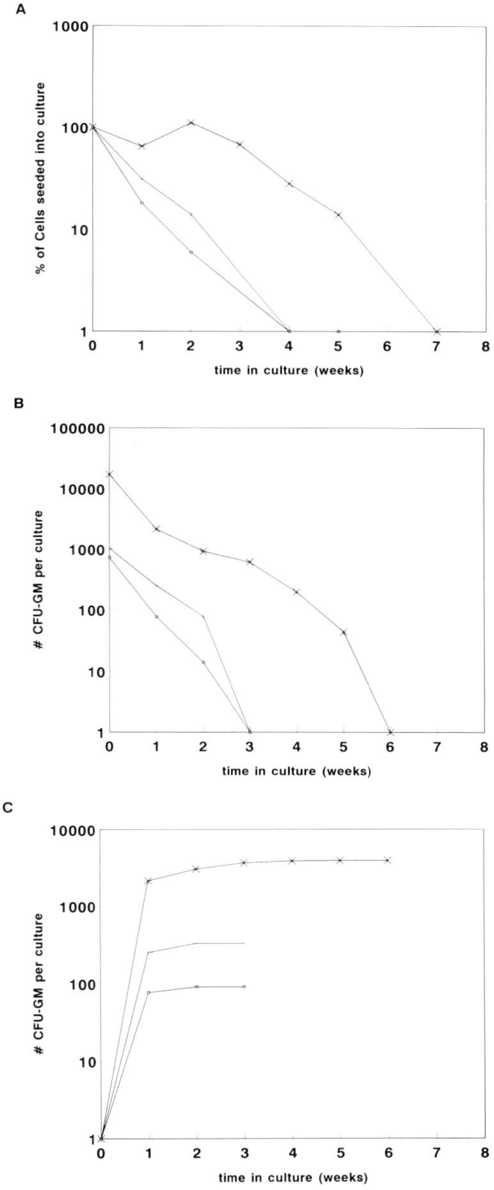

Fig. 4. Long Term Bone Marrow Culture of CD34+ Cells. Bone marrow mononuclear (■), SBA− (+) and CD34+ (*) cells were cultured in long term bone marrow culture as stated in Materials and Methodology. Two hundred thousand cells from each population were loaded into stromal layers and each population was tested in triplicate. Large scale (624 cm²) AIS CELLectors CD34 were used to isolate the cells for this experiment. Panel A), The number of cells in the nonadherent layer was counted at each time point and the % of the original number of seeded cells is plotted as a function of time. Panel B), The total number of CFU-GM produced at each time point during culture is plotted as a function of culture time. Panel C), The cumulative production of CFU-GM during long term bone marrow culture is plotted as a function of time. To plot accumulation, the number of CFU-GM at the start of the culture was defined as zero.

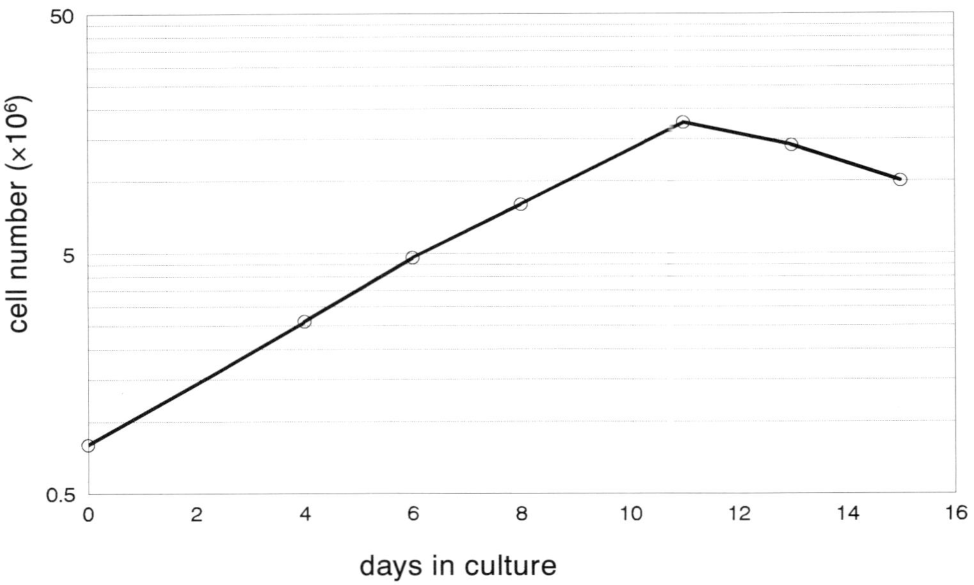

Fig. 5. Cell Number in CD34+ Cell Cultures. Viable cell number was determined by hemacytometer counts at various times during culture. AIS MicroCELLectors CD34 were used in this experiment.

simply added to the device and the AIS CELLector was incubated at 37°C in a 5% CO_2 incubator. At various time points during culture the cells were counted. Figure 5 shows the results from a representative culture. During the first week of culture, log phase expansion of cells occurred which eventually plateaued during the second and third weeks of incubation. By day 14 of culture, the total number of cells expanded up to 100 fold.

Flow cytometry was performed at various points to determine the phenotype of the propagating cells. At the initiation of culture, the cells were 85% CD34+ with approximately half of those cells carrying CD33 antigen. Moreover, the starting population was 90% CD38+, 70% HLA-DR+, 10% CD19+, and 5% CD3+. Upon culture, the cell population rapidly differentiated to the myeloid lineage with greater than 95% of the cells expressing the CD38, CD33 and HLA-DR antigens. CD3+ and CD19+ lymphoid cells were not detectable. The absolute number of CD34+ cells present in the cultures was calculated and is shown in Figure 6. During the initial week of the culture, the number of CD34+ cells was maintained at starting levels despite the logarithmic expansion of cells. At later time points, the number of CD34+ cells steadily declined as the majority of cells differentiated to a more mature phenotype.

The expansion of hematopoietic progenitors during CD34+ cell culture was also measured. Figure 7 shows a representative progenitor growth curve. Maximal

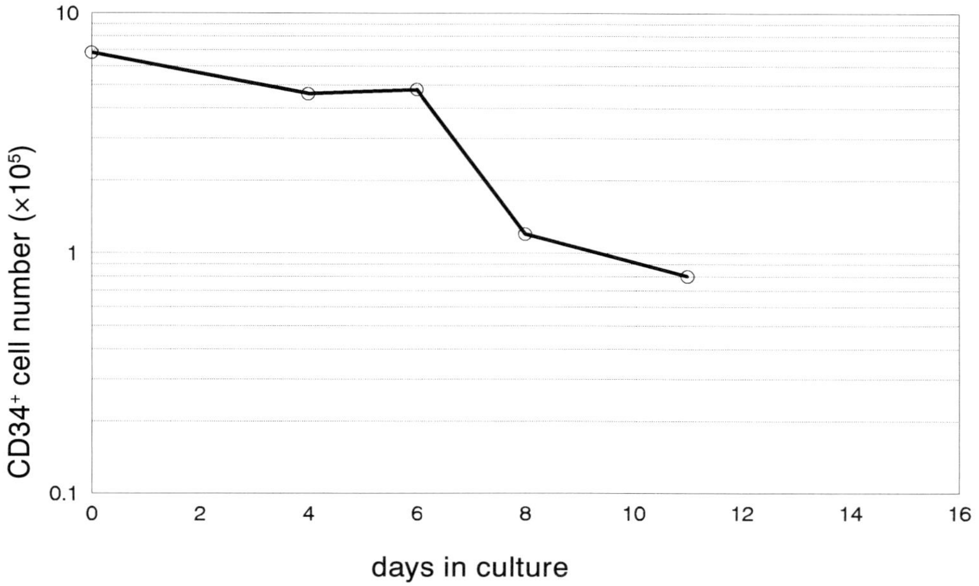

Fig. 6. CD34+ Cell Number in Cultures. The number of CD34+ cells present in the culture was calculated as the (# of cells in the culture) × (frequency of CD34+ cells in the culture as determined by flow cytometry). The results are from the culture described in Figure 5.

increase in both myeloid and erythroid progenitors occurred approximately one week after the initiation of the culture, at the point when CD34+ cell numbers remained high. On average, at peak levels, CFU-GM and BFU-E expanded 20 (range 4.5-40) and 3 (range 1.5-4.0) fold respectively, yielding a 12 fold overall increase in progenitor number.

Discussion

The results from these studies show that the AIS CELLector system can be used to isolate human CD34+ cells in large scale. The covalent attachment chemistry provides surfaces densely coated with the lectin or monoclonal antibody, allowing more efficient capture of target cells as compared to traditional "panning" [3] techniques. The isolated CD34+ cells have high purity and retain both short and long term culture hematopoietic activity. In previous studies we have also demonstrated that the system can readily be utilized for tumor purging [4]. The SBA device alone can produce a one log depletion in tumor cells with the whole purification procedure yielding a greater than 3 log reduction in tumor burden.

The CD34+ cell purification system takes advantage of the binding properties of the soybean agglutinin lectin. Soluble SBA has been utilized

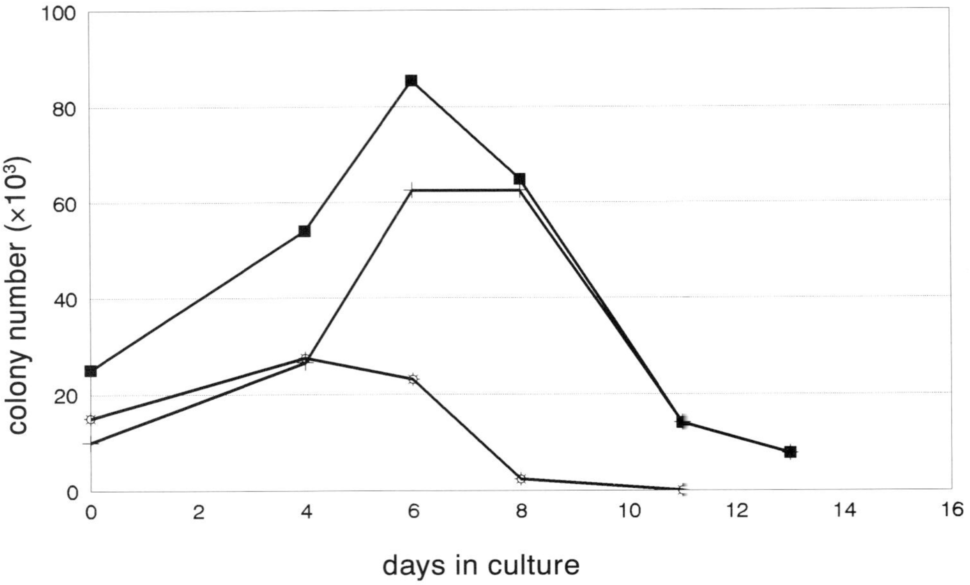

Fig. 7. Progenitor Number in $CD34^+$ Cell Cultures. Progenitor frequency was determined by culturing known numbers of cells in methylcellulose (Materials and Methodology). Progenitor number was calculated as (progenitor frequency) × (the cell number). (□), total progenitors (CFU-C); (+), CFU-GM; (*), BFU-E.

successfully in over 400 cell processing procedures to deplete T cells from bone marrow allografts [5]. SBA binds many differentiated cell types, yet $CD34^+$ cells almost quantitatively remain in the unbound fraction. Only $CD34^+CD19^+$ pre B cells are bound by the immobilized lectin. Use of the AIS CELLector SBA improves the purity of the final $CD34^+$ cell fraction 2-3 fold.

During the use of the AIS CELLector CD34, the device is vigorously agitated to remove the adherent $CD34^+$ cells. Other methods can also be employed to remove the purified $CD34^+$ cells. For the small 25 cm^2 devices, small magnetic propeller scrapers (post XCellerate™) can be easily used to recover the adherent fraction. In addition, the $CD34^+$ cells can be removed by incubation of the devices with media without growth factors for 3 hours at 37°C in a 5% CO_2 incubator. The adherent $CD34^+$ cells detach and can be collected by centrifugation.

An important feature of the AIS CELLector is that the immobilized protein is an integral component of the device and is not removed upon the binding or release of the specific target cell population. This feature is particularly important when the clinical application of these purified cells is considered.

Because of the antibody-free nature of these cells, repeated infusions of these cells into patients undergoing multiple rounds of chemotherapy should be possible without the risk of inducing a human anti-mouse immunoglobulin antibody response.

The AIS CELLector CD34 is also a sterile culture device and we have successfully used it to propagate CD34+ progenitors ex vivo. The expansions observed with this system are very similar to those observed by *Haylock et al.* using peripheral blood CD34+ cells [6]. In our studies, various combinations of IL-1, IL-3, IL-6, GM-CSF, G-CSF, erythropoietin and stem cell factor were used. The results indicate that maximal stimulation of cell and progenitor proliferation occurs when all of the growth factors are included. However, by eliminating some of the growth factors, especially G-CSF and GM-CSF, CD34+ cell frequency can be maintained at higher levels with reduced cell proliferation. It will be important to examine the effects of other growth factors such as IL-11 [7] and stem cell proliferation factor [8] on this system. Also important to examine is the media used for expansion. Our recent results indicate that certain serum free media formulations actually produce much greater expansion of progenitors, especially BFU-E, than do serum based media, and provide a suitable and reproducible system for clinical application.

The objective of these stem cell expansions is to culture to a time point when maximal progenitor and CD34+ cell activity can be returned to the patient. Under these circumstances, such cultured cells would not be expected to induce long term engraftment, but would provide a bolus of progenitors that could minimize or alleviate cytopenic periods due to repeated or intensive suppressive drug therapies. A system could also be devised where a single set of peripheral blood stem cell collections could conceivably provide enough CD34+ cells and progenitors to yield infusion products for multiple rounds of chemotherapy. This application could be especially important for later rounds of treatment when hematopoietic rebound can be delayed. We are currently scaling up this system for such clinical application.

Acknowledgments

We thank *Jacques Hatzfeld* and *Phil McCarthy* for sharing unpublished data.

References

1 Watt S, Karhi K, Gatter K, et al. Distribution and epitope analysis of the cell membrane glycoprotein (HPCA-1) associated with human hematopoietic progenitor cells. Leukemia 1987;1:417-430.

2 Gartner S, Kaplan HS. Long-term culture of human bone marrow cells. Proc Natl Acad Sci USA 1980;77:4756-4761.

3 Wysocki LJ, Sato VL. "Panning" for lymphocytes: a method for cell separation. Proc Natl Acad Sci USA 1978;75:2844-2849.

4 Lebkowski JS, Schain LR, Okrongly D, Levinsky R, Harvey M., Okarma TB. Rapid isolation of human CD34 hematopoietic stem cells—purging of human tumor cells. Transplant 1992;53:1011-1019.

5 Reisner Y, Kapoor N, Kirkpatrick D, et al. Transplantation for acute leukemia with HLA A and B nonidentical parental marrow cells. Lancet 1981;2:327-340.

6 Haylock DN, To LB, Dowse TL, Juttner CA, Simmons PJ. Ex vivo expansion and maturation of peripheral blood CD34+ cells into the myeloid lineage. Blood 1992;80:1405-1413.

7 Schibler KR, Yang YC, Christensen RD. Effect of interleukin-11 on cycling status and clonogenic maturation of fetal and adult hematopoietic progenitors. Blood 1992;80(suppl 4):900-909.

8 Lawman MJP, Wathana S, Donahue RE, Kessler SW, Lawman PD, Bagwell C. Identification, isolation and characterization of a novel cytokine which acts as a proliferative factor on human CD34+ cells. Blood 1992;80:149a.

Clinical Transplantation of CD34⁺ Hematopoietic Progenitor Cells: Positive Selection Using a Closed, Automated Avidin-Biotin Immunoadsorption System

Shelly Heimfeld, Ronald J. Berenson
CellPro, Inc., Bothell, Washington, USA.

Key Words. Stem cells • $CD34^+$ stem cell selection • Bone marrow transplantation • Stem cell expansion • Tumor cell purging

Introduction

CD34 antigen expression is limited to hematopoietic progenitor and stem cells, and is found neither on mature blood cells nor on most types of malignant cells. CellPro has designed a unique avidin-biotin immunoadsorption system (CEPRATE™ SC) for clinical scale purification of $CD34^+$ cells. This system has now been used in a wide variety of clinical settings. A Phase II study evaluated the ability of $CD34^+$ cells isolated from bone marrow or granulocyte-colony stimulating factor (G-CSF) mobilized peripheral blood progenitor cells (PBPC) to reconstitute hematopoiesis in breast cancer patients undergoing high-dose chemotherapy. Four cohorts were treated, receiving $CD34^+$ selected marrow and/or PBPC + G-CSF post-transplant as indicated below:

Patient Cohort	N	$CD34^+$ Marrow	$CD34^+$ PBPC	Growth Factor	Days to ANC>500	Days to Plat. Ind.
1	7	+++		None	23	23
2	10	+++		G-CSF	13	16
3	12	+++	+++	G-CSF	9	9
4	11		+++	G-CSF	9	13

These results indicate that $CD34^+$ bone marrow cells can engraft, that G-CSF given post-transplant accelerates neutrophil recovery, and that $CD34^+$ PBPC give even more rapid recovery of both absolute neutrophil count (ANC) and platelets. A sensitive immunohistochemical technique has shown that $CD34^+$ selection results in 2-5 logs depletion of contaminating breast cancer cells. Additional clinical trials utilizing the CellPro system of CD34 selection for autologous transplantation in breast cancer, lymphoma, myeloma, for allogeneic transplantation as an alternative to other T cell depletion methods to reduce graft versus host disease (GVHD), and for gene therapy are currently underway.

Correspondence: Dr. Shelly Heimfeld, CellPro, Inc., Suite 100, 22322 20th Ave. SE, Bothell, WA 98021, USA.

©AlphaMed Press ISBN 1-880854 17-1

The ability to expand progenitor cells ex vivo has broad potential for therapeutic benefit. We have focused on defining conditions to make expansion clinically practical. The CEPRATE system has been used to isolate large numbers of $CD34^+$ progenitor cells from bone marrow or cord blood, and then those cells were grown in suspension culture with recombinant cytokines. The cultured cells were analyzed for overall expansion (defined as fold-increase over the starting value) in total cell numbers, total $CD34^+$ cells, and colony-forming activity (colony forming units-granulocyte macrophage (CFU-GM), high proliferative potential-colony forming cells (HPP-CFC), and long-term culture-initiating cells (LTC-IC)). Our results indicate that CD34 purification enhances expansion >10-fold as compared with unseparated marrow. The addition of 5% human plasma augments growth 5-20 fold. Optimal expansion requires combinations of at least four cytokines. Using stem cell factor (SCF) + interleukin (IL)-1 + IL-3 + IL-6 results in a 30-50 fold-increase in CFU-GM and HPP-CFC progenitor cells by 7-14 days of culture. With no media exchange, optimal expansion occurs at starting cell densities of $<1 \times 10^5$ cells/ml. Frequent refeeding allows >10-fold expansion at plating densities of $1\text{-}4 \times 10^6$ $CD34^+$ cells/ml. These results indicate that large quantities of $CD34^+$ progenitor cells can be isolated and expanded in a clinically practical fashion ex vivo for subsequent transplantation.

Materials and Methodology

The CEPRATE system is currently being supplied in two different size formats, a research system for processing smaller numbers of cells, and a clinical system for large scale therapeutic applications. The basic components of both systems are similar, in which biotin-conjugated CD34 antibodies are used to specifically target the rare stem cells in bone marrow or peripheral blood. The antibody-labeled cell suspension is then put onto a column which contains avidin-coated beads. The strong affinity between biotin and avidin results in specific capture of the target cells, while the unwanted cells flow through the system. Because the cells are continuously flowing through the column, non-specific binding is kept to an absolute minimum. The purified stem cells are then released from the column by gentle agitation and washing, and collected for further processing or cryopreservation.

The CEPRATE system, in both the research and clinical setting, has been used to isolate and purify $CD34^+$ cells from a variety of sources, including bone marrow, peripheral blood and cord blood samples. The research kits include all the necessary reagents for processing and contain sufficient reagents and materials to process up to 10^9 starting cells and capture up to 40×10^6 target cells, while the clinical system has been used to process in excess of 100×10^9 cells and has a capture capacity of 5×10^9 cells. Total processing time is approximately 90 minutes for both systems, with the actual column separation procedure requiring 20-30 minutes. Details on the specifics of the methodology employed in the processing are given in a package insert supplied with each research kit or are included in the operators manual for the clinical system.

Listed below are overview descriptions of the operating procedures used for the research (CEPRATE LC) and the clinical (CEPRATE SC) systems, along with some warnings, observations and suggestions for improving and maintaining optimal performance.

CEPRATE LC

The CEPRATE LC CD34 kit is a disposable cell separation system for isolating $CD34^+$ cell populations from blood or tissue samples. The kit contains a complete set of quality controlled materials and reagents. The components are processed using standard sterilization techniques to minimize bioburden. All reagents have been filled using aseptic procedures to minimize risk of contamination. To maintain aseptic conditions, CellPro recommends performing all cell processing and separations under a laminar flow hood using sterile techniques. The following components are supplied with each kit:

- Sample/Wash chamber
- Avidin column
- Phosphate buffered saline; Ca, Mg free (PBS)
- 5% Bovine serum albumin (BSA) in PBS
- Pregel
- Anti-CD34 primary antibody-biotin (clone 12.8, mouse IgM)

Operating Procedures

A. Reagent preparation

1 Thaw antibody and store in refrigerator until use.

Warning: The CD34 antibody is shipped frozen to maintain stability. Once received, it is best kept frozen in a frost-free freezer for maximum shelf-life. The antibody may be thawed and kept at 2-8° C for a short period of time. Repeated freeze/thawing of the antibody is not recommended as it may result in precipitation. When thawing, avoid shaking or mixing of the vial as this may also lead to precipitation and loss of immunoreactivity.

2 Bring Sample/Wash chamber, Avidin column, and buffers to room temperature. (*Observation:* The temperature for antibody incubation and column separation does not appear to have a major influence on performance. Equivalent separation results have been found at room temperature and on ice.)

3 Prepare 60 ml of 1% BSA (12 ml of 5% BSA + 48 ml PBS).

Warning: It is important to not substitute other media for the PBS and 5% BSA. The use of other media which contain Ca and Mg will generally lead to lower purities and more non-specific binding to the column. Similarly, the particular BSA lot supplied in the kit has been screened to enhance the CD34 selection process and the use of substitute materials may decrease purity and yield results.

B. Sample Preparation and Antibody Incubation.

1 Samples may be prepared by red cell lysis, buffy coat centrifugation, or density gradient techniques. (*Suggestion:* It is usually beneficial to first deplete red cells from the sample prior to antibody incubation, although this is not an absolute requirement and samples of bone marrow and cord blood can be run without any prior processing. Density gradient preparation will improve final CD34 purities, although some loss of progenitor cells has been reported with this procedure.)

2 Wash samples with 1% BSA and resuspend to 100-200 × 10^6 cells/ml. There is enough primary antibody supplied to process 2.5 ml.

3 Add 80 μl of CD34 antibody per ml of cell suspension. (*Suggestion:* The cell concentration is not critical; from 10-500 × 10^6 cells/ml can be used for the antibody incubation. However, it is most critical that the correct dilution of antibody per ml be used.)

4 Incubate for 25 min with gentle mixing. (*Suggestion:* To minimize total processing time, priming of the avidin column should be done at this time.)

5 Dilute sample with 1% BSA, centrifuge once to pellet cells, and resuspend to 100-200 × 10^6 cells/ml in 5% BSA. (*Suggestion:* Again, the cell concentration is not critical, but optimal performance is obtained using the 5% BSA in PBS solution supplied in the kit.)

C. Priming CEPRATE system.

1 Assemble the system by attaching the Sample/Wash chamber to the operating platform, removing the Luer lock cap at the bottom of the three-way valve, and attaching the avidin column.

2 Remove air bubbles from the system by moving the three-way valve to 9 o'clock, squeezing the avidin column to displace media up into the sample chamber, and then adding in 5 ml of PBS to the sample chamber. Then turn the 3-way valve to 6 o'clock to allow PBS flow from sample chamber to wash chamber to remove air in connector. Turn valve back to 9 o'clock, add additional PBS to sample and wash chambers, and then add Pregel to sample chamber and allow to settle onto filter at bottom of sample chamber. Open outlet clamp and allow 5 ml of PBS to pass through avidin column; stop flow by closing outlet clamp when PBS reaches top of Pregel, and load 5 ml of 5% BSA into sample chamber. Open outlet clamp and let 5% BSA drain into avidin column until level reaches top of Pregel. Stop flow by closing clamp. The system is now ready for use. (*Observation:* It is important to remove large air bubbles from the avidin column and Sample/Wash chambers. Tiny air bubbles may remain in system and should not affect performance.)

D. Cell Separation. (*Note:* Described below is the procedure for operating the CEPRATE LC system using gravity feed to control flow rate. This system can also be used with a peristaltic pump. If using a pump, it should be calibrated to flow at approximately 1 ml per minute. Some improvements in yield can be obtained by slowing the flow rate to 0.5 ml/min during the cell loading phase, then switching to 1 ml/min for washing and elution.)

1 Load antibody-incubated cells in 5% BSA into sample chamber. (*Suggestion:* Try to layer cells so as not to disturb Pregel, and do not exceed 4 ml total volume. If sample volume exceeds 4 ml, add remaining sample after sufficient volume has been drained into avidin column.)

2 Release outlet clamp to flow cells through avidin column.

3 After sample reaches top of Pregel, add 1-2 ml of 5% BSA to flush remaining cells into column, then turn the 3-way valve to 12 o'clock to begin flow of PBS into column.

Warning: Do not completely drain sample chamber as this may introduce air bubbles into the column.

4 After 4 ml of PBS have drained through column, close outlet clamp for 60 seconds to stop flow. (*Observation:* This stop flow allows the gel bed to relax slightly, improving the washout procedure and resulting in some enhancement in purity.)

5 Resume flow and wash with an additional 2 ml of PBS.

6 Stop flow, add an additional 5 ml of PBS to wash chamber, and replace collection tube.

7 Resume flow, and squeeze avidin column vigorously 5-10 times along its length. Collect at least 4 ml of solution. The $CD34^+$ selected cells will drain into the collection tube.

CEPRATE SC

The CEPRATE SC system has been engineered to totally automate the process of stem cell concentration, making the procedure quick, easy and reliable. With this system, a trained operator can separate and concentrate $CD34^+$ cells from a clinical bone marrow or peripheral blood harvest within three hours, then cryopreserve the cells for later infusion into the patient. The basic principles of this clinical system are similar to the research columns described above. CellPro provides extensive operator training in the proper use of the CEPRATE SC system, as well as a complete operators manual detailing instrument operation.

The CEPRATE SC system consists of an instrument and a computer with monitor and keyboard, and disposables which include the biotin CD34 antibody, precolumn and avidin column, solutions, tubing sets and collection bags. The instrument controls the flow of antibody-treated samples through the column, the washing that removes residual unbound cells, the gentle agitation of the beads to release the target stem cells, and the final collection of the stem cells into a bag for cryopreservation. The computer's microprocessor controls all electromechanical components, and software directs the system to perform procedures in a standard sequence. The keyboard and video display allow the operator to monitor automatic system operation and to control instrument operation in manual mode.

The following components are supplied with each clinical kit. Each component meets the requirements of GMP production and uses clinically approved materials:

- Avidin column and precolumn assembly
- Reagent tubing set
- Collection tubing set
- Phosphate buffered saline; Ca, Mg free (PBS)
- 25% Human serum albumin (HSA)
- Anti-CD34 primary antibody-biotin (clone 12.8, mouse IgM)

Operation

Setup and priming: The clinical procedure has an initial priming step which involves installing the columns, tubing sets, and solution bags on the instrument, and then using the computer software to automatically purge the system of air trapped in the lines, wash out the columns with PBS + HSA, and then prepare the system for loading of the antibody-treated cells. Instructions on the computer screen will guide the operator during this priming step.

Sample Preparation:

1. Bone marrow samples from the operating room are usually first processed by standard blood washing procedures to produce a buffy coat preparation. Samples have also been used which have had no prior processing or different types of preprocessing, including mobilized peripheral blood as an apheresis product, elutriation samples, cord blood samples, and density separated samples. The clinical system is compatible with any of these types of starting materials, although it should be noted that final purities and yields may be affected by the type of preprocessing used.
2. Samples usually undergo one additional wash step and resuspension in 150 ml of PBS + HSA. One vial of biotin-CD34 antibody is added to the sample,

incubated at room temperature for 25 minutes, then the sample is washed and resuspended in 300 ml of PBS and loaded on the CEPRATE instrument.

Cell Separation:

1 After loading of the bag containing the antibody-treated sample, the operator simply chooses the Run command on the computer screen, and enters the volume of sample loaded. The automatic program will then complete the entire process of loading, washing and eluting the CD34 cells in approximately 25 minutes.

Analysis of Separation Performance

Two analytical methods are recommended for determining the degree of enrichment of target cells with the CEPRATE systems: 1) flow cytometry to measure the percent of $CD34^+$ cells in the starting, flow through, and selected fractions; and 2) colony formation in culture (CFC) to determine progenitor cell content. Optimal staining and analysis procedures and in vitro culture methods have been described in great detail in other chapters, and so will not be presented here other than to point out specific observations relative to the CEPRATE system.

Suggestion: For flow cytometric analysis, during the avidin column separation, the vast majority of the CD34 antibody is stripped from the surface of the target cells. Thus, immediate restaining with a fluorescent conjugated anti-mouse reagent results in a relatively poor fluorescence intensity and poor distinction between the $CD34^+$ and $CD34^-$ cells. Instead, use a directly conjugated anti-CD34 antibody, preferably one which recognizes a different epitope than the 12.8 antibody used in the CEPRATE selection.

Duplicate CEPRATE LC research separations were performed on bone marrow obtained from healthy or cadaver donors. Results are shown in Table I. In this series of experiments, purities averaged 83% and yields were 32%. The enrichment factor ranged from 20-123 × with an average of 60-fold enrichment. Note that while there was sample to sample variability, the CEPRATE kits gave consistently reproducible performance within the same set of samples.

Suggestion: For CFC analysis, to obtain a more accurate representation of the CFC content in the different fractions, a rich source of media and growth factors should be used to maximize progenitor cell growth. This is especially critical when analyzing the CD34 selected fraction, since these cells are depleted of accessory cells that can provide endogenous growth factor support. We recommend supplementing the methylcellulose cultures with various recombinant cytokines including IL-3 and SCF. Due to the high degree of variability in progenitor cell content from different tissue samples, several dilutions of cells should be plated per sample. We recommend 3×10^4, 1×10^5,

Table I. Results of LC Research Separations

	Starting Cell Population		Cells collected from CEPRATE Column			
Exp.	BM-MNC per Column (× 10⁶)	Percent CD34+ (%)	BM-MNC collected (× 10⁶)	Percent CD34+ (%)	Percent Yield[1] (%)	Enrichment Factor[2]
1	132.8	1.8	1.2	85.3	46.4	47.4×
			1.0	83.6	35.0	46.4×
2	150.4	1.3	0.6	83.8	25.7	64.5×
			0.6	75.2	23.1	57.8×
3	304.4	3.7	3.9	78.2	27.1	21.1×
			3.8	73.9	24.9	20.0×
4	304.4	3.7	3.8	79.8	26.9	21.6×
			3.9	79.5	27.5	21.5×
5	111.7	1.1	0.5	91.6	37.3	83.3×
			0.5	89.7	36.5	81.5×
6	180.8	0.6	0.6	68.7	38.0	114.5×
			0.6	74.0	40.9	123.3×
7	148.4	1.1	0.6	85.0	31.2	77.3×
			0.5	88.3	27.0	80.3×
8	148.4	1.1	0.6	86.8	31.9	78.9×
			0.5	85.9	26.3	78.1×
9	216.8	2.2	1.9	93.7	37.3	42.6×
			1.7	91.5	32.6	41.6×
Average	188.7	1.8	1.5	83.0	32.0	61.2×
SD	71.9	1.1	1.4	7.0	6.4	

[1]Yield is defined as the total number of CD34+ cells collected divided by the total number of CD34+ cells in the starting population. For example, in Experiment #1:

$$\text{Yield} = \frac{(1.3 \times 10^6 \text{ cells}) \times (85.3\% \text{ CD34}^+)}{(132.8 \times 10^6 \text{ cells}) \times (1.8\% \text{ CD34}^+)} \times 100\% = 46.4\%$$

[2]Enrichment factor is defined as the percentage of CD34+ cells in the enriched fraction divided by the percentage of CD34+ cells in the starting cell population. For example, in Experiment #1 again:

$$\text{Enrichment} = \frac{85.3\% \text{ CD34}^+}{1.8\% \text{ CD34}^+} = 47\times$$

3×10^5 cells per plate for the start and flow-through samples, 1×10^3, 3×10^3, 1×10^4 cells for the selected fraction.

Acknowledgments

We would like to acknowledge all the employees at CellPro whose efforts have resulted in the CEPRATE research and clinical systems, and all the investigators who were kind enough to provide their summary data.

Selected Readings

1 Berenson RJ, Levitt LJ, Levy R, Miller RA. Cellular immunoadsorption using monoclonal antibodies: selective removal of T cells from peripheral blood and bone marrow. Transplantation 1984;38:136-142.

2 Berenson RJ, Bensinger WI, Kalamasz DF. Positive selection of viable cell populations using avidin-biotin immunoadsorption. Journal of Immunological Methods 1986;91:11-19.

3 Berenson RJ, Bensinger WI, Kalamasz D, Martin P. Elimination of Daudi lymphoblasts from human bone marrow using avidin-biotin immunoadsorption. Blood 1986;67:509-515.

4 Berenson RJ, Besinger WI, Andrews RG, Kalamasz D, Hill R, Bernstein ID. Hematopoietic stem cell transplants. In: Gale RP, Golde DW eds. Recent Advances in Leukemia and Lymphoma. New York: Liss, 1987;527-533.

5 Berenson RJ, Bensinger WI, Kalamasz D, Schuening F, Deeg HJ, Storb R. Avidin-biotin immunoadsorption: a technique to purify cells and its potential applications. In: Progress in Bone Marrow Transplantation. New York: Liss, 1987;423-428.

6 Berenson RJ, Bensinger WI, Kalamasz D, Schuening F, Deeg HJ, Graham T, Storb R. Engraftment of dogs with Ia-positive marrow cells isolated by avidin-biotin immunoadsorption. Blood 1987;69:1363-1367.

7 Lemoli RM, Gobbi M, Tazzari PL, Grassi G, Dinota A, Gherlinzoni F, Mazza P, Tura S. Avidin-biotin immunoadsorption for ex vivo bone marrow purging: effect of percentage of target cells and flow rate. Haematologica 1988;73:183-185.

8 Brugger W, Möcklin W, Heimfeld S, Berenson RJ, Mertelsmann R, Kanz L. Albert-Ludwigs Univ. Med. Ctr. (Freiburg Germany) and CellPro, Incorporated (Bothell WA): Ex vivo expansion of enriched peripheral blood $CD34^+$ progenitor cells by stem cell factor, interleukin-1β(IL-1β), IL-6, IL-3, interferon-γ, and erythropoietin. Blood 1993;81:2579-2584.

9 Berenson RJ, Bensinger WI, Kalamasz DF, Heimfeld S, Goffe RA, Berninger RW, Peterson DR, Thompson P, Strong DM; CellPro, Incorporated (Bothell WA), Fred Hutchinson Cancer Research Center (Seattle, WA), and Northwest Tissue Center (Seattle, WA). Transplantation of stem cells enriched by immunoadsorption. In: Gross S, Gee AP, Worthington-White DA eds. Advances In Bone Marrow Purging and Processing. NewYork:Wiley-Liss, 1992;277:449-459.

10 Shpall EJ, Stemmer SM, Johnston CF, Hami L, Bearman SI, Berenson RJ, Jones RB; Univ. Colorado BMT Program & Cancer Center (Denver, CO) and CellPro, Inc. (Bothell, WA). Purging of autologous bone marrow for transplantation: the protection and selection of the hematopoietic progenitor cell. Journal of Hematotherapy 1992;1:45-54.

11 Heimfeld S, Fogarty B, McGuire K, Williams S, Berenson RJ; CellPro, Incorporated (Bothell, WA). Peripheral blood stem cell mobilization after stem cell factor of G-CSF treatment: rapid enrichment for stem and progenitor cells using the CEPRATE/immunoaffinity separation system. Transplantation Proceedings 1992;24:2828.

12 Berenson RJ; CellPro, Incorporated (Bothell, WA). Transplantation of $CD34^+$ hematopoietic precursors: clinical rationale. Transplantation Proceedings 1992;24:3032-3034.

Purification of Peripheral Blood CD34+ Cells by Immunoadsorption: Laboratory and Clinical Experience with the CellPro System

W. Brugger,[a] *R. Henschler,*[a] *R. J. Berenson,*[b] *S. Heimfeld,*[b] *R. Mertelsmann,*[a] *L. Kanz*[a]

[a]Albert-Ludwigs-University Medical Center, Department of Hematology and Oncology, Freiburg, Germany; [b]CellPro, Inc., Bothell, Washington, USA.

Key Words. CD34+ • Peripheral blood stem cells • Immunoadsorption • Ex vivo expansion • High-dose chemotherapy • Tumor cells

Introduction

Peripheral blood progenitor cells (PBPC) are increasingly used as an alternative to bone marrow stem cells for autografting following high-dose chemotherapy in patients with both hematological malignancies as well as solid tumors [1-4]. The hematopoietic reconstitution following autotransplantation has been demonstrated to be mediated by CD34+ cells [5-7], which comprise the most primitive hematopoietic stem cells as well as all committed progenitor cells. These cells can be enriched by several methods as detailed in other chapters of this manual. In order to clinically apply enriched CD34+ cells, we selected these cells by the large scale CEPRATE™ immunoadsorption device, a method shown to be highly effective and suitable for clinical purposes [6, 7].

This report describes the enrichment of CD34+ cells from PBPC preparations collected after conventional-dose etoposide(VP16)-ifosfamide-cisplatin (VIP) chemotherapy and subsequent administration of granulocyte-colony stimulating factor (G-CSF, Neupogen®) [8, 9]. In addition, preliminary data on the clinical application of CD34+ cells for autotransplantation after high-dose chemotherapy without bone marrow support are reported. Moreover, it will be demonstrated that CD34+ cells represent ideal starting cells for the ex vivo expansion which we and others have shown to be feasible in the presence of a variety of hematopoietic growth factors [10, 11], (see also *Haylock et al.*, pp. 291-301). The rationale for CD34+ selection is underlined by the finding of significant tumor cell contamination in PBPC of apheresed patients with solid tumors [12].

Mobilization and collection of PBPC

Patients undergoing PBPC transplantation are treated as part of the induction chemotherapy with conventional-dose VIP—etoposide (500 mg/m^2), ifosfamide (4 g/m^2) and cisplatin (50 mg/m^2)—and subsequent administration of

Correspondence: Dr. W. Brugger, Albert-Ludwigs-University Medical Center, Department of Hematology and Oncology, Hugstetter Str. 55, 79106 Freiburg, Germany.

©AlphaMed Press ISBN 1-880854 17-1

recombinant human (rh)G-CSF (Amgen, Munich, Germany) at a dose of 5 μg/kg/d s.c. for 12 days [8].

PBPC are harvested during a two hour leukapheresis with a CS3000® blood cell separator and a small volume collection chamber (Baxter, Munich, Germany) at day 10-12 after VIP chemotherapy [13]. At the time of leukapheresis, patients generally have a white blood cell count of >10,000/μl and a platelet count >75,000/μl. The proportion of CD34+ cells at that time is in the range of 0.5-11% of mononuclear cells. The leukapheresis preparation (50 ml) contains 80 ± 20% mononuclear cells with a hematocrit of 7-15%. Due to the small volume collection chamber, platelet counts are low and there is generally no clumping of cells.

Positive selection of CD34+ cells by immunoaffinity adsorption columns

This clinical-scale device is a computer controlled, almost-closed system with a loading capacity of more than 10^{10} mononuclear cells. A detailed description of the CEPRATE™ system is presented by *S. Heimfeld et al.*, pp. 231-239.

At our institution, freshly harvested PBPC containing approximately 10^{10} mononuclear cells are incubated in the apheresis bag with the biotinylated immunoglobulin (Ig)M anti-CD34 monoclonal antibody (clone 12.8) without prior density gradient separation or any other centrifugation step. After incubation, cells are washed in PBS and loaded onto the large-scale avidin-immunoaffinity column device, as described and recommended by the manufacturer [see chapter by *S. Heimfeld et al.*]. Adsorbed CD34+ cells (= target cell population) are removed from the avidin-column and resuspended in PBS supplemented with human serum albumin in a volume of 80-100 ml. An aliquot of the CD34+ target cell fraction as well as the unbound cell fraction are analyzed to assess cell count, morphology, CD34-purity and colony formation as described below. Unbound cells (= non-target cell fraction) and cells recovered in the wash bag are subsequently removed. Cell counts including trypan blue dye exclusion from each cell fraction are done to determine the actual number of non-target as well as target cells and thus to determine the cellular yield. Cell recovery, as compared to the total number of cells loaded, is usually 70%. We did not observe cell clumping in any of the bags. More than 99% of red cells and platelets are recovered in the non-target cell fraction. Within the target cell fraction, granulocytic and monocytic cells are detected in a frequency of less than 10% each. Purity of CD34+ cells, as analyzed by flow cytometry, was 52-82%, with a mean value of 59% in the 12 separations studied so far.

Freezing of the target cell fraction is performed with a computer controlled freezer in 6% dimethyl sulfoxide (DMSO) and 20 U/ml heparin at a density of 10-15 × 10^6 $CD34^+$ cells/ml, either in 5 ml vials or in Baxter Cryocyte freezing containers (Baxter, Munich, Germany).

Immunocytology of selected $CD34^+$ cells.

Selected $CD34^+$ cells were attached to alcian blue coated slides (Bio-Rad, Munich, Germany) and pre-fixed in 0.05% glutaraldehyde at room temperature for 5 min. For the evaluation and characterization of $CD34^+$ mononuclear cells the following mouse monoclonal antibodies (mAb) were used: anti-CD34 (clone My10, HPCA-1, IgG1 from Dianova, Hamburg, Germany), anti-CD33 (My 9, Coulter, IgG, Krefeld), anti-HLA-DR (IgG2a) and anti-CD38 (Leu17, IgG1; all from Becton Dickinson, Rodermark, Germany). An irrelevant, isotype-matched (IgG1) anti-rota virus mAb (Dianova, Hamburg, Germany) was used as a control antibody for nonspecific binding of anti-CD34 mAb. A peroxidase-anti-peroxidase (PAP) technique was applied followed by post-fixation with OsO_4, as described [14]. The percentage of $CD34^+$ cells was determined by counting the brown stained cells.

Multi-color flow cytometry analysis

Unseparated PBPC or positively selected $CD34^+$ cells were incubated with an anti-CD34-phycoerythrin (PE)-conjugated mAb and/or anti-CD33-fluorescein isothiocyanate (FITC)-conjugated mAb, anti-CD38-FITC conjugated mAb or anti-HLA-DR-FITC conjugated mAb (all from Becton Dickinson, Rodermark, Germany) for 30 min at 4°C. Cells were analyzed by flow cytometry using a FACScan analyzer (Becton Dickinson), equipped with a filter set for FITC-PE dual-color fluorescence. Each measurement contained 20,000-40,000 cells; the frequency of cells expressing CD34 and/or CD33, CD38, HLA-DR antigens was calculated as a percentage of all cells analyzed.

Culture assays for hematopoietic progenitor cells

Unseparated PBPC were cultured at 1 × 10^5 in supplemented Iscove's modified Dulbecco's medium (IMDM) in 0.9% methyl-cellulose with 30% fetal calf serum (FCS; Paesel, Frankfurt, Germany). Cultures were stimulated with 100 U/ml rhGM-CSF and 100U/ml rh-interleukin (IL)-3 (both provided by Sandoz, Nurnberg, Germany), as well as rh-erythropoietin (rhEPO) (1 U/ml; Connaught, Willowdale, Ontario, Canada). Total volume per dish was adjusted to 1 ml. CD34-selected cells were cultured at 5 × 10^3, 15 × 10^3 and 50 × 10^3, respectively. These cells were additionally cultured in the presence of stem cell factor (SCF), IL-1, IL-3, IL-6, GM-CSF (all 100 ng/ml), and

EPO (1 U/ml), in order to optimally stimulate colony growth. Plates were cultured in humidified atmosphere and 5% CO_2. The colonies (CFU-GM, BFU-E, CFU-GEMM) were scored with an inverted microscope 12-14 days after initiation of culture.

Clinical application of positively selected CD34+ cells

Pilot patients with advanced malignancies are currently treated at our institution in an ongoing study with positively selected $CD34^+$ cells following high-dose chemotherapy with etoposide (1,500 mg/m^2), ifosfamide (12 g/m^2), carboplatin (750 mg/m^2) and epirubicin (150 mg/m^2) (VIC-E). Up to now, 11 patients have been reconstituted with CD34 selected cells, and all of them have shown an identical reconstitution pattern as compared to patients who were treated with the same number of unseparated PBPC after the same conditioning regimen. The median number of $CD34^+$ cells retransfused was in a range of 0.5-5.5 × 10^6 $CD34^+$ cells/kg.

Ex-vivo expansion of CD34-enriched PBPC

To provide sufficient numbers of PBPC for repetitive use in high-dose chemotherapy, or to possibly provide enough PBPC in patients with low progenitor cell output, we investigated the ability of hematopoietic growth factor combinations to expand PBPC ex vivo [10]. VIP chemotherapy plus G-CSF recruited $CD34^+$ cells from 18 patients were enriched with the avidin-biotin immunoadsorption column to a purity of more than 85% $CD34^+$ cells and cultured in suspension up to 28 days. A combination of five growth factors including SCF, EPO, IL-1β, IL-3, and IL-6 was identified as the optimal combination for the expansion of clonogenic progenitors. Proliferation peaked at day 12-14 with a mean 190-fold increase (range 46-930) of clonogenic cells (CFU-GM, BFU-E, CFU-GEMM). The number of CFU-GEMM increased 250 fold as compared to pre-expansion values. Moreover, $CD34^+Lin^-$($CD34^+$/HLA-DR^-; $CD34^+$/$CD38^-$) cells as well as mafosfamide-resistant $CD34^+$ cells (4-HC resistant cells) increased during ex vivo culture. Interferon-gamma synergized with the 5-factor combination (1.5 fold increase in clonogenic cells), whereas the addition of G-CSF or GM-CSF decreased the number of clonogenic cells. Large-scale expansion of $CD34^+$ cells in autologous plasma supplemented with the 5-factor combination resulted in an equivalent expansion. These data indicate that CD34-enriched PBPC from cancer patients can be successfully expanded ex vivo. Moreover, our data suggest the feasibility of large-scale expansion, starting from small numbers of $CD34^+$ cells. The number of cells generated ex vivo might be sufficient for use in high-dose chemotherapy, possibly obviating the need for aphereses procedures.

References

1 Brugger W, Bross KJ, Frisch J, Dern P, Weber B, Mertelsmann R, Kanz L. Mobilization of peripheral blood progenitor cells by sequential administration of IL-3 and GM-CSF following chemotherapy with etoposide, ifosfamide and cisplatin. Blood 1992;79:1193-1200.

2 Elias AD, Ayash L, Anderson KC, Hund M, Wheller C, Schwartz G, Telpler I, Mazanet R, Lynch C, Pap S, Pelaez J, Reich E, Critchlow J, Demetri G, Bibbo J, Schnipper L, Griffin JD, Frei E, Antman KH. Mobilization of peripheral blood progenitor cells by chemotherapy and granulocyte-macrophage colony-stimulating factor for hematologic support after high-dose intensification in breast cancer. Blood 1992;79:3036-3042.

3 Juttner CA, To LB, Haylock DN, Cyson PG, Thorp D, Dart GW, Ho JQK, Horvath N, Bardy P. Autologous blood stem cell transplantation. Transplant Proc 1989;21:2929.

4 Pettengell R, Demuynck H, Testa NG, Dexter TM. The engraftment capacity of peripheral blood progenitor cells mobilized with chemotherapy ± G-CSF. Int J Cell Cloning 1992;10:59-61.

5 Berenson RJ, Bensinger WI, Hill RS, Andrews RG, Garcia-Lopez J, Kalamasz DF, Still BJ, Spitzer G, Buckner CD, Bernstein ID, Thomas ED. Engraftment after infusion of $CD34^+$ marrow cells in patients with breast cancer or neuroblastoma. Blood 1991;77:1717.

6 Berenson RJ, Andrews RG, Bensinger WI, Kalamasz D, Knitter G, Buckner CD, Bernstein ID. Antigen $CD34^+$ marrow cells engraft lethally irradiated baboons. J Clin Invest 1988;81:951.

7 Shpall EJ, Jones RB, Johnston C, Hami L, Stemmer S, Affronti ML, Curiel T, Berenson RJ. Purified CD34-positive marrow progenitor cells provide effective reconstitution for breast cancer and non-Hodgkins lymphoma patients receiving high-dose chemotherapy with autologous bone marrow support: recombinant G-CSF accelerates hematopoietic recovery. Proc Am Assoc Clin Oncol 1992;11:59a.

8 Brugger W, Birken R, Bertz H, Hecht T, Pressler K, Frisch J, Schulz G, Mertelsmann R, Kanz L. Peripheral blood progenitor cells mobilized by chemotherapy plus G-CSF accelerate both neutrophil and platelet recovery after high-dose VP16, ifosfamide and cisplatin. Br J Hematol 1993;84:402-407.

9 Brugger W, Mertelsmann R, Kanz L. High-dose VIP chemotherapy with or without peripheral blood progenitor cell support. Proc Am Assoc Cancer Res 1992;33:241a.

10 Brugger W, Möcklin W, Heimfeld S, Berenson RJ, Mertelsmann R, Kanz L. Ex-vivo expansion of enriched peripheral blood CD34+ progenitor cells by stem cell factor, interleukin-1β, interleukin-6, interleukin-3, interferon-gamma, and erythropoietin. Blood 1993;81:2579-2584.

11 Haylock DN, To LB, Dose TL, Juttner CA, Simmons PJ. Ex-vivo expansion and maturation of peripheral blood $CD34^+$ cells into the myeloid lineage. Blood 1992;80:1405.

12 Brugger W, Glatt M, Georgi F, Bross KJ, Mertelsmann R, Kanz L. Recruitment of tumor cells into peripheral blood of patients concomitant to the mobilization of peripheral blood progenitor cells. Blood (in press, 1993).

13 Lasky LC, Ash RC, Kersey JH, Zanjani ED, McCullough J. Collection of pluripotential hematopoietic stem cells by cytapheresis. Blood 1982;59:822.

14 Bross KJ, Pangalis GA, Staatz CB, Blume KG. Demonstration of cell surface antigens and their antibodies by the peroxidase-anti-peroxidase method. Transplantation 1978;25:331.

Isolation of CD34+ Cells from Leukapheresis Products: Evaluation of Lymphoma Cell Purging

S. Fruehauf,[a] *M. Haberkorn,*[b] *R. Hoeft,*[b] *W.J. Zeller,*[b] *R. Haas,*[a] *W. Hunstein*[a]

[a]Department of Internal Medicine V, University of Heidelberg, Heidelberg, Germany; [b]German Cancer Research Center, Research Program Experimental Diagnostics and Therapy, Heidelberg, Germany

Key Words. CD34-selection • Peripheral blood stem cells • Lymphoma cell purging • Fluorescent dye PKH26

Introduction

Peripheral blood stem cells (PBSC) are used for autografting after high dose consolidation therapy in non-Hodgkin's lymphoma (NHL). However, leukapheresis products may be contaminated by malignant cells. Normal hematopoietic progenitors may be separated from lymphoma cells using the CD34-antigen for targeting. CD34-selection may be performed with immunomagnetic beads. CD34+ cells may be detached from the beads enzymatically [1, 2] or using competing Fab-antibodies [3]. Immunoadsorption of CD34+ cells to an avidin column [4] as well as panning [5] are alternative techniques for progenitor cell enrichment.

The aim of the present study was to compare immunomagnetic and biotin-avidin CD34-selection with respect to progenitor cell purity, recovery and lymphoma cell purging efficiency. A follicular lymphoma cell line was admixed to leukapheresis products and used as a model system for tumor cell contamination. Cells were labeled with the fluorescent dye PKH26 which binds to lipid residues of the cell membrane and which can be detected by argon-ion laser based flow cytometry. PKH26 does not alter the antigen expression or viability of cells [6].

Materials and Methodology

Lymphoma cell line

We used the cell line K422 which is positive for CD19 and CD37 and also bears the t[14;18] translocation. Cells were grown in RPMI 1640 medium (GIBCO BRL, Eggenstein, Germany) supplemented with 10% heat-inactivated fetal calf serum (Serva, Heidelberg, Germany) and 1% penicillin/streptomycin (Seromed, Berlin, Germany). Immediately prior to the CD34-enrichment, K422 cells were incubated with the fluorescent vital dye PKH26 (Zynaxis Cell Science, Malvern, PA, USA) at a concentration of 2×10^{-6} M for 5 minutes and then irradiated with 50 gy to prevent tumor cell growth in methylcellulose

Correspondence: Dr. S. Fruehauf, Department of Internal Medicine V, University of Heidelberg, Hospitalstr. 3, D-69115 Heidelberg, Germany.

 ISBN 1-880854 17-1

assays. Stained K422 cells were admixed to the leukapheresis sample to give a final proportion of 5%.

Mobilization and Harvesting of Blood Stem Cells

Circulating blood stem cells were collected from a heterogeneous group of patients (2 low grade NHL, 1 Hodgkin's disease, 1 multiple myeloma, 1 breast cancer). Treatment with granulocyte-colony stimulating factor (G-CSF) (5 μg/kg, s.c., filgrastim, Amgen, Thousand Oaks, CA, USA) was started 24 hours after chemotherapy. After reaching a white blood count (WBC) of >1 $\times 10^9$/l, leukaphereses were commenced. Mononuclear cells (MNC) were collected from peripheral blood using a Baxter CS3000 Blood Cell Separator. Collections were performed with a modified version of Fenwal procedure #1. Flow rates were 50-70 ml/min, the volume processed was 10 liters and 50 ml collection chambers were used. A 5 ml aliquot was taken for CD34-enrichment studies.

Isolation of CD34-positive cells

Immunomagnetic beads

Aliquots of mobilized peripheral blood MNC were subjected to red blood cell lysis in 0.15 M NH_4Cl. Cells were counted and viability determined by trypan blue dye exclusion. The 5% PKH26-stained and irradiated K422 cells were admixed. If an additional monocyte depletion step was included, cells were incubated in a cell culture flask for 30 minutes at 37°C and the non-adherent cell fraction was taken for the experiment. A total of 2×10^8 cells/ml in RPMI 1640 containing 1% human serum albumin (Sigma, Deisenhofen, Germany; RPMI/HSA) were incubated (4°C, 30 min, on a rocker rotator REAX3, Heidolph, Kelheim, Germany) with 10 μg/ml purified HPCA-1 (Becton Dickinson, Heidelberg, Germany) monoclonal antibody. The cells were then washed twice in RPMI/HSA and mixed gently and continuously (4°C, 30 min) with anti-mouse immunoglobulin IgG_1-coated magnetic microspheres (Dynal) in a screw-top tube, at a ratio of two cells per microsphere. After incubation, the cells were separated in a second tube, using a strong magnet to hold the microspheres and microsphere-bound cells to the wall of the tube while unbound cells were poured off. The microsphere/cell complexes were washed in this fashion once with RPMI/HSA and three times with RPMI without additives. To release $CD34^+$ cells from the microspheres, chymopapain (Chymodiactin, Kanoldt Arzneimittel GmbH, Hoechstaedt, Germany; 200 U/ml, 15 min, 37°C) was added [1]. Released $CD34^+$ cells were then poured off, while the microspheres were retained on the magnet; the microspheres were again resuspended and washed to recover as many $CD34^+$ cells as possible. Cell viability was assessed using the trypan blue dye exclusion assay.

From each fraction, cells were analyzed by flow cytometry for the expression of the progenitor antigen CD34, lymphoid antigens and the pan-leukocyte marker CD45. K422 cells were detected by their red fluorescence (PKH26).

Biotin-Avidin-Adsorption Columns

These assays used 2×10^8 leukapheresis cells containing 5% K422 follicular lymphoma cells. $CD34^+$ cells were separated according to the manufacturer's (CellPro, Bothell, Washington, USA) suggestions. In brief, cells were incubated with the 12.8 antibody and a secondary biotinylated anti-mouse antibody. Samples were then run through avidin columns primed with phosphate buffered saline (PBS) containing 5% bovine serum albumin. Labeled cells attached to the columns while unadsorbed cells were flushed through the system. Retained $CD34^+$ cells were removed from the columns by vigorous squeezing and additional flushing. In one experiment, cells were allowed to drain through the system by gravity. This led to very slow and discontinuous flow rates so that for the rest of the study a peristaltic pump was attached to the tubing.

Flow cytometry

Samples taken from the various steps of CD34-enrichment were incubated with saturating concentrations of directly conjugated fluorescein isothiocyanate (FITC) labeled monoclonal antibodies (MAbs) for 30 minutes at 4°C. MAbs used were HPCA2-FITC (CD34), CALLA-FITC (CD10), Leu12-FITC (CD19), CD37-FITC, HLE-1-FITC (CD45) and the respective isotype controls (CD37-FITC from Dianova, Hamburg, all others from Becton Dickinson, Heidelberg). Leukapheresis aliquots containing 5% K422 cells not stained with the dye PKH26 but with a phycoerythrin-labeled control antibody were used as negative controls for PKH26-fluorescence. In each test $5 \times 10^4 - 2 \times 10^5$ cells/100 μl were used. Following antibody incubation, cells were washed twice with PBS and fixed in 1% paraformaldehyde. Quantitative fluorescence analysis was performed using a five-parameter FACScan flow cytometer equipped with an argon-ion laser tuned at 488 nm and 0.3 W (Becton Dickinson). Emission from fluorescein was measured using a short band pass filter of 530 ± 15 nm and from PKH26 using a 575 ± 15 nm filter, respectively. Data were acquired using FACScan Research software. Each measurement contained 10^4 events. For analysis, windows were drawn so as to include positive events only, while negativity for control samples was confirmed by backgating.

Culture assay for hematopoietic progenitor cells

Leukapheresis cells taken from the various CD34-enrichment steps were grown in methylcellulose (0.8%) containing 30% fetal calf serum, 1% bovine serum albumin, 10^{-4} M 2-mercaptoethanol, 3 units/ml erythropoietin and 5% phytohemagglutinin-lymphocyte-conditioned medium (PHA-LCM) (all

Terry Fox Laboratory, British Columbia Cancer Research Centre, Vancouver, Canada). Cell concentrations seeded were 1×10^5 for unseparated bone marrow MNC, 1×10^5 for the $CD34^-$, and 1 and 2×10^3 for the $CD34^+$ cell fraction. Duplicate plates were incubated for 14 days at 37°C, ambient oxygen and 5% CO_2 in a humidified atmosphere. Colonies were scored as colony forming units-granulocyte-macrophage (CFU-GM), burst forming units-erythrocyte (BFU-E) and colony forming units-granulocyte-erythrocyte-megakaryocyte-macrophage (CFU-GEMM). For comparison, the colony count per 10^5 cells was calculated from these data.

Statistics

Mean values ± standard error (SE) are given.

Results and Discussion

Immunomagnetic bead CD34-selection (IMB) was compared to a biotin-avidin column (BAC) system. After red blood cell lysis and the addition of 5% K422 follicular lymphoma cells, the leukapheresis samples contained 2.7% ± 0.7% $CD34^+$ cells. In the enriched fraction, comparable CD34-purities were observed after bead selection (57.5% ± 14%) and immunadsorption (66.1% ± 11.1%). The variation of CD34-purity among patients was higher in the IMB group (range 10.5%-85.2% versus 57%-78.5% $CD34^+$ cells in the BAC group).

Recovery of hematopoietic progenitor cells was 15% ± 5% (IMB) and 18% ± 9% (BAC) of the initial $CD34^+$ cell number (Table I). A considerable number of $CD34^+$ cells was still detectable in the non-adherent "CD34-negative" cell fractions (IMB, 39% ± 9.6%; BAC 31% ± 9.9% of the starting $CD34^+$ population). Why such a high proportion of $CD34^+$ cells are not amenable to CD34-selection is not clear yet. Although a comparable loss of hematopoietic progenitors was observed with both CD34-selection methods,

Table I. Recovery of $CD34^+$ cells after CD34-enrichment. Immunomagnetic bead separation and biotin-avidin column separation are compared.

Patient	Unseparated		Immunomagnetic beads		Biotin-avidin column	
	$CD34^+$ cells	Recovery (%)	$CD34^+$ cells	Recovery (%)	$CD34^+$ cells	Recovery (%)
#1	9.32×10^6	100	0.97×10^6	10.4	0.72×10^6	7.7
#2	1.88×10^6	100	0.12×10^6	6.5	0.12×10^6	6.5
#3	6.74×10^6	100	1.51×10^6	20.6	1.11×10^6	15.1
#4	4.08×10^6	100	1.29×10^6	31.5	2.19×10^6	53.7
#5	3.86×10^6	100	0.31×10^5	8.1	0.27×10^6	7.1
Mean	**5.18×10^6**	**100**	**0.84×10^6**	**15.4**	**1.37×10^6**	**18.0**
SE	**1.29×10^6**		**0.27×10^6**	**4.7**	**0.47×10^6**	**9.1**

Table II. Hematopoietic colony growth of peripheral blood progenitor cells after CD34-selection with immunomagnetic beads or biotin-avidin columns (mean values ± SE). Colonies/10^5 cells.

	CFU-GM	BFU-E	CFU-GEMM
Unseparated	370 ± 132	240 ± 115	0.7 ± 0.3
Immunomagnetic Beads			
$CD34^-$ fraction	98 ± 62	151 ± 8	0.5 ± 0.5
$CD34^+$ fraction	6033 ± 1991	6633 ± 3175	160 ± 46
Biotin-Avidin Column			
$CD34^-$ fraction	98 ± 1	242 ± 170	0.5 ± 0.5
$CD34^+$ fraction	8300 ± 1200	9475 ± 6974	138 ± 37

the underlying etiology may be different. In the column system, an IgM CD34-antibody (clone 12.8) with low avidity to its antigen is used [7]. Therefore, cells flowing through the columns may have escaped antigen binding. In contrast, the My-10 (HPCA-1) antibody used for CD34 bead selection is known for its high avidity [7]. In the bead system, a higher bead to cell ratio will also lead to a higher $CD34^+$ cell recovery. However, as more monocytes bind nonspecifically to the beads, $CD34^+$ purity is going to decrease as well (*Dr. Ping Law,* personal communication).

The flow cytometry data are paralleled by the results of the colony assays (Table II). From a starting value of 370 ± 132 total colonies, a 34-fold increase was found after IMB selection versus a 48-fold increase after immunadsorption. There was no significant difference in colony growth after bead selection, suggesting that chymopapain is not more toxic to $CD34^+$ progenitor cells than non-enzymatic detachment of the cell-antibody complex using the column separation technique. The core separation time for both methods was comparable and ranged approximately 3 hours.

After incubation with the fluorescent dye PKH26, K422 cells were readily detectable by flow cytometry (Fig. 1). In the enriched fraction, 0.53% ± 0.1% (IMB) and 1.7% ± 0.47% (BAC) K422 cells were present. Considering the absolute tumor cell number in the starting and the enriched cell fractions, purging efficiencies of log 3.3 ± 0.17 (IMB) and log 3.02 ± 0.67 (BAC) were reached. This is comparable to negative selection of tumor cells where a purging efficiency of more than log 3 could only be achieved after two cycles of antibody and bead incubation [8]. Pilot experiments with monocyte depletion before CD34-enrichment showed that even a purging efficiency of log 4.8 and a CD34-purity of 90% can be achieved, but only at the expense of the CD34-recovery (6.5% of the initial $CD34^+$ cells recovered).

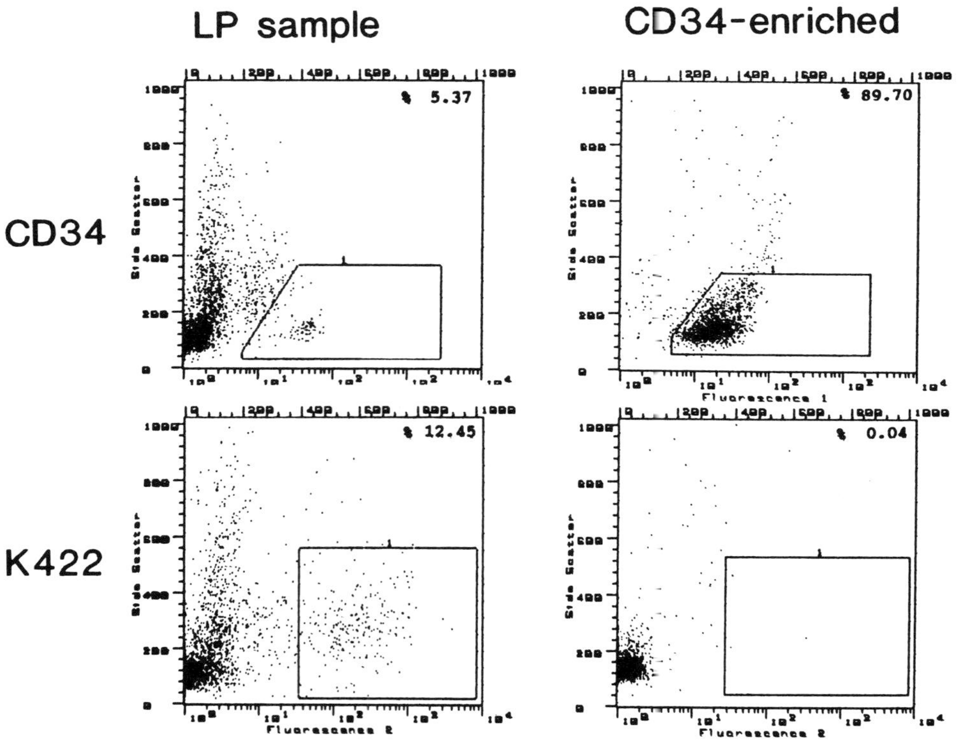

Fig 1. Representative flow cytometric profile of CD34+ cells (top row) in a leukapheresis sample before and after CD34-enrichment with immunomagnetic beads. K422 follicular lymphoma cells stained with the fluorescent dye PKH26 (bottom row) are depleted in the CD34-enriched cell fraction. Fluorescence intensity of cells is plotted versus orthogonal light scatter (SSC).

CD34-enrichment using immunomagnetic bead selection or biotin-avidin columns therefore is an effective approach for tumor cell depletion from leukapheresis products. However, due to the significant loss of progenitor cells only patients with a good hematopoietic reserve will be eligible for future clinical trials.

Acknowledgments

We are indebted to the expert technical assistance of *Mrs. Sigrid Heil.*

References

1 Civin CI, Strauss LC, Fackler MJ, Trischmann TM, Wiley JM, Loken MR. Positive stem cell selection—basic science. In: Gross S, Gee AP, Worthington-White DA eds. Bone marrow purging and processing. Progress in Clinical and Biological Research, Vol. 333. New York: Wiley-Liss, 1990:387-402.

2 Marsh JC, Sutherland DR, Davidson J, Mellors A, Keating A. Retention of progenitor cell function in CD34+ cells purified using a novel O-sialoglycoprotease. Leukemia 1992;6:926-934.

3 Smeland EB, Funderud S, Kvalheim G, Gaudernack G, Rasmussen AM, Rusten L, Wang MY, Tindle RW, Blomhoff, Egeland T. Isolation and characterization of human hematopoietic progenitor cells: an effective method for positive selection of CD34+ cells. Leukemia 1992;6:845-852.

4 Berenson RJ, Andrews RG, Bensinger WI, Kalamasz D, Knitter G, Bruckner CD, Bernstein ID. Antigen CD34+ marrow cells engraft lethally irradiated baboons. Journal of Clinical Investigation 1988;81:951-955.

5 Lebkowski JS, Schain LR, Okrongly D, Levinsky R, Harvey MJ, Okarma TB. Rapid isolation of human CD34 hematopoietic stem cells—purging of human tumor cells. Transplantation 1992;53:1011-1019.

6 Slezak SE, Horan PK. Fluorescent in vivo tracking of hematopoietic cells. Part I. Technical considerations. Blood 1989;74:2172-2177.

7 Civin CI, Trischmann TM, Fackler MJ, Bernstein ID, Bühring HJ, Campos L, Greaves MF, Kamoun M, Katz DR, Lansdorp PM, Look TL, Seed B, Sutherland DR, Tindle RW, Uchanska-Ziegler B. Report on the CD34 cluster workshop. In: Knapp W, Dörken B, Gilks WR, Rieber EP, Schmidt RE, Stein H, von dem Borne AEGK eds. Leucocyte Typing IV—white cell differentiation antigens. Oxford New York Tokyo: Oxford University Press, 1989:818-825.

8 Negrin RS, Kiem HP, Schmidt-Wolf IG, Blume KG, Cleary ML. Use of the polymerase chain reaction to monitor the effectiveness of ex vivo tumor cell purging. Blood 1991;77:654-660.

Large Scale Enrichment of CD34+ Cells by Percoll Density Gradients: A CML-Based Study Design

Francesco Lanza,[a,b] *Gianluigi Castoldi*[a]

[a]Institute of Hematology, University of Ferrara, Ferrara, Italy; [b]LRF Centre for Adult Leukaemia, Hammersmith Hospital, London, United Kingdom

Key Words. Percoll • CML • CD34+ cells • Calibration microbeads • Layering technique • Mixing of blood/BM with SIP • Large scale separation • Enrichment of progenitor cells • Phenotype of CD34+ cells

Introduction

CD34 expression in blood/BM CML cells

Chronic myeloid leukemia (CML) comprises 20% of all leukemias in the western countries and has an annual incidence of 1:100,000 of the population [1, 2]. The assessment of the stem and progenitor cell compartment in CML could be done with different procedures, i.e., colony assays (colony forming units-granulocyte-macrophage (CFU-GM) and burst forming units-erythroid (BFU-E) determination in solid agar- or semisolid methylcellulose medium), CD34 measurement by flow cytometry, etc. [3, 4]. In clinical practice, the enumeration of CD34+ cells in the peripheral blood (PB) or bone marrow (BM) has to be done in whole blood samples in order to avoid substantial cell losses which may occur during the separation procedures. The percentage of CD34+ cells evaluated by flow cytometry in the PB and BM varies significantly from patient to patient, depending on the clinical phase of the disease and the monoclonal antibody (MAb) used (Table I) [4]. Based on our findings, less than 5% of CML patients in blastic crisis show no reactivity with the CD34 MAbs, while the remaining cases are CD34+. Moreover, the number of epitopes so far recognized for the CD34 molecule is probably four, and therefore the type of MAb used for CD34 measurement is critical in

Table I. CD34 expression in PB and BM cells from CML patients at different phases of the disease.

	Chronic phase		Blast crisis[a]	
	PB (N = 82)	BM (N = 58)	PB (N = 37)	BM (N = 16)
Q-Bend 10 (%)	0.65(0.09-2.1)	0.76(0.18-2.2)	31(5-78)	36(9-81)
8G-12 (%)	0.78(0.12-2.9)	0.84(0.25-2.6)	33(3-81)	37(8-87)

Data are expressed as mean and range (in parenthesis). CD34 quantitation has been performed on whole PB/BM using a FACScan flow cytometer.
[a]% of blasts assessed morphologically: 38% ±15% (mean ± SD).

Correspondence: Dr. Francesco Lanza, Institute of Hematology, University of Ferrara, St. Anna Hospital, Via Giovecca N.203, I-44100 Ferrara, Italy.

©AlphaMed Press ISBN 1-880854 17-1

the evaluation of cell reactivity. In our experience, derived from more than 100 CML samples analyzed, the number of $CD34^+$ cells measured with a fluorescein isothiocyanate (FITC)-conjugated 8-G12 MAb (Becton Dickinson) was significantly higher than that detected by the FITC-conjugated Q-Bend 10 MAb (Immunotech). On the contrary, no significant differences in cell reactivity were observed between the two MAbs when analyzing BM/PB samples derived from healthy donors.

The flow cytometry method we used to detect the $CD34^+$ cell population in whole PB or BM samples was similar to that described by *Wunder* and coworkers [5]. The CD34 determination was performed on the entire nucleated cell population; fluorescence expression was evaluated on a cytogram generated by combining side scatter (SSC) and fluorescence 1 (FL1) or FL2 (as appropriate) parameters. A direct-staining technique was used in all cases.

Use of calibration microbeads. A reliable approach for fluorescence quantitation.

In order to obtain a reliable quantitation of the CD34 positivity, it is fundamental that the performance of the flow cytometer be optimal (i.e., power and alignment of the laser, fluidics system, etc.). Therefore, we suggest using FITC or phycoerythrin (PE) (as pertinent) quantitative microbead calibration standards (also called microbeads) as a reference standard to compare to the fluorescence intensity of cells stained for CD34 antibodies. The use of pre-mixed calibrated microbeads makes it possible to express the flow cytometry data in the form of Mean Equivalent Standard Fluorescence (MESF) values [6]. The calculation of MESF is based on the evaluation of the peak channel expressed by cells and different populations of microbeads (four or five, depending on the type and source of beads). The values for the slope, intercept and correlation coefficient allow the calculation of the regression line, which gives information on the linearity and stability of the instrument response, the noise level of the flow cytometer, the MESF values of the stained and unstained cells, the resolution indexes for fluorescence, and the coefficient of variation (CV) of microbead fluorescence [7, 8]. The "minimum detection threshold" (also called "calculated sensitivity" or "instrument fluorescence threshold") of the instrument corresponds to the MESF value for the blank beads, and provides information on the sensitivity of the flow cytometer in detecting fluorescence signals. The advantage of using microbeads also permits the possibility to compare the flow cytometry data over time and between one laboratory and another. Various types of pre-mixed calibration microbeads are available from different companies (Flow Cytometry Standards Corporation, Becton Dickinson, Polysciences, etc.).

The procedure that we follow for using microbeads is that recommended by the organizers of the Fifth International Workshop on Leukocyte Differentiation Antigens, Boston 1993 (*Prof. R. F. Todd*: Myeloid Section Chairman; *Dr. S. Shaw*: Chairman of the Data Management Section; *Dr. A. Schwartz*: Flow Cytometry Standards Corporation), and is intended for the quantitation of flow cytometry data. The microbeads used for data evaluation during the above-mentioned workshop were stained with the same fluorescent dyes as those used to stain cells with MAbs of the myeloid panel, and were released from the Flow Cytometry Standards Corporation. They are composed of five different calibrated fluorescence levels plus a blank. The preliminary fluorescence intensities assigned to this microsphere lot were the following: first level = 4,985; second = 15,667; third = 82,093; fourth = 291,669; fifth = 702,662 [9].

To conclude, labeling the microbeads with either a specific monoclonal antibody or a fluorescent dye enables the construction of a reference standard which can be utilized to calibrate the flow cytometer response to the chosen monoclonal antibody. This is a unique opportunity to assess cell positivity and fluorescence emission in a very standardized way using monoclonal antibodies of known origin in either direct or indirect technique.

Materials and Methodology

Guidelines for using microbeads with a flow cytometer

1 Prepare cell samples according to standard procedures.

2 Align and set up the instrument for cell analysis.

3 Dilute 3-4 drops of the pre-mixed FITC quantitative microbead calibration standards with 0.5 ml of the same solution in which you suspend the cell samples. The beads should be prepared a few minutes before their use.

4 Without changing any instrument setting, run the diluted microbeads and determine the peak channel (see below) of each of the six populations (%FITC labeled beads and a blank). If only five populations are on scale at your normal instrument settings, you may proceed so long as the unstained cell population is to the right of the blank microbeads and on scale. It is also possible to reset your instrument by increasing the FL1 PMT voltage such that the blank microbeads are on scale. Adjust the flow rate so that the count rate is optimal for your flow cytometer.

5 Without changing any instrument settings, run the cells and determine the peak channels of the labeled and unlabeled cell populations, and the percentage of positive staining.

6 The single histograms of each of the five populations of beads should be smoothed.

7 Locate the position for markers between the six populations and then determine the peak channel of each of these populations. The operator should make sure that a line has been drawn exactly at the peak of each population.

8 Plotting the calibration line: once the peak channel of each calibrated standard has been determined, a calibration curve can be constructed and data can be converted to MESF values. Along with the regression plot, a measure of "average residual percent" (ARP) can be performed. The ARP is an overall indicator of the agreement between assigned and observed values of the microbead populations. The residual values are calculated by comparing the assigned MESF value of the FITC or PE microbeads with the values of the regression line for the same channel numbers. Perfect agreement would be indicated by an ARP of 0.000. Software programs allowing a quick calculation of MESF are now available from Flow Cytometer Standards Corporation (QuickCal®).

9 After data acquisition, run the diluted microbeads again and determine their peak channel in order to see whether any significant changes in MESF values occurred. In that case the performance of your flow cytometer should probably be reviewed.

CD34 analysis in cell preparations enriched for hematopoietic progenitors: assessment of their engraftment potential

Background

Successful bone marrow transplantation (BMT) depends on engraftment of pluripotent hematopoietic stem cells in the marrow microenvironment. However, the speed of engraftment relies on the functional and phenotypic characteristics of the progenitor cells, which are associated with a varying capacity of repopulating the marrow and providing long term maintenance of engraftment. A subpopulation of progenitor cells (probably the lineage Lin^+CD34^+ cell subpopulation) is responsible for early engraftment, while the Lin^-CD34^+ cells more likely permit late engraftment [10]. Either PB or BM cells can be used as a source of autologous hematopoietic cells (AHSC), being able to provide a successful bone marrow reconstitution after supralethal myeloablative chemo-radiotherapy in patients suffering from different hematologic malignancies including CML [11, 12]. Autografting has the advantage of being available to all patients up to the age of 65 years [13]. In CML however, the situation is rather complex, since the vast majority of progenitor cells carry the Philadelphia (Ph) chromosome, and therefore belong to the neoplastic clone. In CML, autografting with AHSC may lead to sustained Ph negativity in about 10-20% of patients and probably prolongs life in a subgroup of CML patients [12, 13]. The phenomenon of Ph-reconstitution following autologous BMT (AuBMT) can be explained by the persistence of residual "normal" stem cells which under suitable conditions can re-establish Ph negativity. By 9-10 months after AuBMT, however, the percentage of Ph^+ cells increases up to 100% in most cases [11]. In the *Hammersmith* series two of the 14 patients autografted with autologous blood stem cells remained completely Ph^- 4 and 5 years respectively after autograft, suggesting the Ph^- cells could have (at least in some circumstances) a proliferative advantage over the Ph^+ clone [13].

For these reasons, a number of methodologies aimed at expanding the Ph^- clone in vitro or in vivo have been developed so far, and used, on some occasions, for improving the results of the AuBMT procedure [12]. By looking at the phenotype of $CD34^+$ CML cells, it seems now clear that only the $CD34^+HLA\text{-}DR^+$ population (which represents more than 90-95% of the total $CD34^+$ cells from CML patients in chronic phase) is Ph^+ and $BCR\text{-}ABL^+$, while the $CD34^+HLA\text{-}DR^-$ fraction is mainly Ph^- and $BCR\text{-}ABL^-$ [14, 15]. Thus, from a theoretical point of view, the selective removal of $CD34^+HLA\text{-}DR^+$ cells from BM/PB cells before autografting may permit a Ph^- marrow reconstitution and probably long-term disease-free survivals. In practice, however, this goal seems very difficult to reach at the present time, since the number of $CD34^+DR^-$ cells is very low, and the kinetic characteristics of this subpopulation does not allow (probably) an early engraftment due to its position in the G_0/G_1 phase of the cell cycle [16, 17]. It is possible that the use of a combination of growth factors might expand this fraction and push these cells into active phases of the cell cycle and therefore allow marrow reconstitution after AuBMT [17-19].

However, in order to make these purging techniques more efficient and reduce the amount of reagent to be used it is important to decrease the volume and the total cell number to be reinfused during AuBMT. Hematopoietic progenitors are of low density (1.055-1.065 g/ml) and can be separated from more mature myeloid cells and red blood cells of higher density by a number of methodologies including counter elutriation, centrifugation on a Percoll or Ficoll density gradient, etc. [20-22]. Moreover, based on the experience from different centers, hematopoietic progenitors obtained in this way have shown normal engraftment, with only sporadic evidence of delay in the speed of marrow reconstitution [23].

Layering of cells on Percoll of known density

Percoll is an inert, non-toxic polyvinylpyrrolidone-covered particle of silica which can be diluted with a calculated volume of isotonic solution or plasma to give a range of desired densities (Sigma-P 1644; Pharmacia, Upsala, Sweden) [20-22]. We have used Percoll at a variety of densities to separate low density cells from leukapheresis (PB) or BM harvest samples obtained from normal donors and patients with CML.

Whole blood or bone marrow samples (either diluted or undiluted) should be carefully layered over Percoll of known density in either tubes of different size or, alternatively, in a plastic bag in a cell washer. The tubes are spun at 800 *g* for 30 min without the brake on. After centrifugation the cells with a density lower than that of the starting Percoll are clearly visible as a cell layer (interface), and can be recognized as a cloudiness at the top of the Percoll. The cells should be removed along with some of the Percoll below using a sterile

Pasteur pipette (glass or plastic). It is mandatory to remove less than 15% of the total volume of Percoll, since removal of larger amounts can cause difficulties in spinning down the cells during cell washings, and therefore considerably increase cell losses. At the same time, separate the waste Percoll and deposit (cells situated between the red blood cell fraction and the Percoll) in order to evaluate the cell number and the CD34 count in each fraction. The volume and the leukocyte count of each fraction are thereby measured, and the total cell recovery present in each fraction is calculated. The percentage of cells present in each fraction is expressed as a percentage of the total cells recovered in all three fractions. An aliquot from the waste Percoll is used to check the density achieved after centrifugation.

Measurement of density on starting and final solutions

The density of solutions and of patient samples is measured on a densitometer (DMA 35, Pear Scientific Ltd., Paar, Austria). The machine is calibrated regularly using distilled water (density: 0.999 g/ml), Ficoll-Hypaque (density: 1.077 g/ml), and Hank's medium (1.006 g/ml). The density of all reagents should be measured at room temperature, as temperature may significantly affect the density values. The density of the calibrating agents is also checked using a hydrometer.

Preparation of standard isotonic Percoll (SIP)

1 One hundred ml of × 10 phosphate buffered saline (PBS) is added to 10 ml of 1M HCl and filtered.

2 One hundred-ten ml of PBS/HCl is added to one l of stock solution of Percoll (Sigma) to make the working solution of SIP. The pH, osmolarity and density of each batch of SIP is recorded.

It is fundamental that the osmolarity be in the physiological range, as too high an osmolarity will dehydrate the cells and make them less dense (more buoyant), and a low osmolarity will cause the cells to swell and become more dense.

Preparation of Percoll of required density

The volume of medium (Hank's or other types of isotonic buffer such as buffered saline) to be added to the Percoll solution can be calculated according to the following formula:

$$\text{Volume of medium (ml)} = \frac{220.5 \times 0.130 \text{ (density of the Percoll)}}{\text{desired density } (1.068) - 1} \times 220.5$$

Table II. Distribution of CD34⁺ cells in different fractions obtained after layering of BM cells on Percoll of various density (1.065-1.071 g/ml).

	1.065 g/ml	1.068 g/ml	1.071 g/ml
Cell layer	67	70	58
Percoll waste	30	26	32
Supernatant	0.01	0.02	0.01
Deposit	3	4	10

Data are expressed as a mean. The percentage of $CD34^+$ cells means % of total $CD34^+$ cells recovered in the different fractions. Similar results were observed after fractionation of BM or PB cells derived from CML patients in chronic phase.

Results

Table II shows the mean percentage and absolute counts of $CD34^+$ cells recovered from different fractions (cell layer, supernatant, waste Percoll and deposit) of three different Percoll density gradients (1.065, 1.068, 1.071 g/ml) obtained after fractionation of bone marrow cells from CML and normal subjects.

There was a significant number of $CD34^+$ cells (26-32% of the total $CD34^+$ population) in the waste Percoll, and, to a lesser degree, in the deposit (3-10%). In the cell layer, the enrichment of $CD34^+$ cells was 14 times for the 1.065, 15 times for the 1.068, and 11 times for the 1.071. The 1.071 gradient resulted in the loss of the largest number of $CD34^+$ cells. This phenomenon is probably due to a higher overloading of the gradient itself. In CML, the highest number of $CD34^+HLA\text{-}DR^-$ cells was observed in the cell layer using the 1.068 g/ml gradient.

On the basis of these findings we conclude that discarding the Percoll solution during cell separation procedures causes a considerable loss of $CD34^+$ cells irrespective of the Percoll density gradient used (1.065-1.071 g/ml). A careful analysis of data obtained through the application of layering techniques allowed us to speculate a poor reproducibility and reliability of this technique in terms of progenitor cell recovery. In fact, we observed that the final density achieved after centrifugation was frequently much lower (average 0.005 g/ml lower) than that expected, due to dilution of the Percoll after spinning.

A number of factors can affect the reliability of the results: 1) temperature; 2) type of centrifuge; 3) speed of centrifugation; 4) ratio of dilution of the sample (1:1, 1:2, undiluted); 5) medium used for diluting blood or BM; 6) density gradient aimed for; 7) number of cells present in the sample; 8) characteristics of the sample (hemoglobin concentration, hematocrit).

Table III. The effect of temperature on various Percoll and Ficoll solutions.

	4°C	21°C	37°C
Ficoll (1.077 g/ml)	1.083	1.077	1.073
Stock Percoll (1.130 g/ml)	1.133	1.130	1.127
Percoll (1.068 g/ml)	1.073	1.068	1.065
SIP (1.126 g/ml)	1.129	1.126	1.123

Data are expressed as a mean of five experiments.

In fact, a positive correlation between the hemoglobin concentration and the density of the sample was demonstrated. The effect of temperature on Percoll density gradients is shown in Table III. However, overloading of the gradient was observed in hyperleukocytotic samples using gradients of density higher than 1.070 g/ml. On the basis of our experience we therefore propose to use Percoll solutions according to these basic rules:

1 The Percoll solutions should be used at room temperature.

2 The cells should be spun at 1600 *g* for 30 min using a late-model centrifuge whose performance has been carefully checked.

3 Use undiluted or diluted in the ratio of 1:2 (medium:sample) BM or PB samples. It is mandatory to dilute the specimen if the leukocyte count is very high (leukapheresis product, hyperleukocytotic samples).

Mixing of blood or BM with SIP

Since the layering technique was unsatisfactory in terms of reproducibility and reliability of the results, we developed an alternative way for enriching progenitors using Percoll density cuts. This principle can be applied on a large scale in a closed system or on a small scale, and is based on the direct mixing of blood or BM with a calculated amount of SIP. In order to calculate the volume of SIP to be added, the volume and density of plasma, blood or BM, and suspending medium should be carefully evaluated on a densitometer.

Calculation of final density of Percoll

Before any samples are taken, 5,000 units of preservative-free heparin are added to the leukapheresis or bone marrow bag and mixed well. The hematocrit (HCT) of the sample should be measured in a microhematocrit. An aliquot of PB/BM is spun at 3000 rpm and the plasma is pipetted off. The density of the plasma (or diluting medium) is measured at room temperature in a densitometer. The volume of SIP to be added to a known volume of isotonic solution, blood or bone marrow has to be calculated according to the following formula:

$$V_p = \frac{V_m(D_r - D_m)}{(D_p - D_r)}$$

where V_p = volume of SIP; V_m = volume of medium or plasma (i.e., excluding packed cells); D_r = final density required; D_m = density of medium or plasma; D_p = density of SIP.

Example:
Volume of leukapheresis blood product = 260 ml.

Hct = 18%

therefore the volume of plasma $V_m = (1 - 0.18) \times 260 = 213$ ml

measured density of plasma $D_m = 1.023$ g/ml

measured density of SIP $D_p = 1.125$ g/ml

desired final density = 1.067 g/ml

$$\frac{213\ (1.067 - 1.023)}{(1.125 - 1.067)} = \frac{213 \times 0.044}{0.058} = 162 \text{ ml}$$

Therefore the volume of SIP (V_p) to be added is 162 ml, which means 182 g of SIP (162 × 1.125 g/ml-measured density = 182 g). The volume of PB/BM can also be calculated by dividing the weight (268 g in this example) by the density of the PB/BM (1.032 g/ml in this example).

In all samples we analyzed (more than fifty), the required Percoll density was achieved or was within 0.001 g/ml of the desired density. In some samples from CML leukapheresis, overloading of the density gradient resulted in a higher final density than that desired, probably due to the effect on the density of the suspended leukocytes in the waste Percoll. Also in these samples, however, the difference between final and desired density was within 0.001 g/ml.

When performing the procedure in the cell washer on a large scale, if any SIP or blood is left in the connecting tubes or bags (even as little as 5 ml) the final density will be modified. According to our example, if 5 ml were left in the connecting tubes, the expected final density would be 1.067 g/ml.

Separation procedure

The PB or BM sample was mixed thoroughly with the SIP and then centrifuged at 1000 *g* for 30 min on a Cobe 2991 cell washer for large scale separation or in 50 ml tubes for small scale separation. On the large scale system the cell layer (cells with a density lower than that of the Percoll aimed for) was collected into 50 ml of TC 199 medium and 5,000 units of heparin.

Recovery of cells after centrifugation (small and large scale)

On small scale systems the recovery of cells from the cell layer was performed visually, bearing in mind the general rule of not taking more than 15-20% of the total volume of Percoll. On large scale procedures (using a cell washer) the volume of cell layer to be removed was judged visually when the fluid in the collecting tubes became less cloudy. In a few experiments we collected the cell layer in 10 ml aliquots in order to check the cell count and the number of $CD34^+$ cells. We found that most of the cells were in the first 20 ml; and after approximately 60 ml, the count significantly decreased. The proportion of $CD34^+$ cells in each of the first five 10 ml aliquots from a separation performed at density 1.069 g/ml was consistently high (5-7%). In each of the following ten aliquots the percentage of $CD34^+$ cells significantly declined (0.5-1.3%). In the initial material from a few experiments, most of the counts were higher than $200 \times 10^6/\mu l$ and it was difficult to see a transition between the cell layer and the waste Percoll, due to the presence of trapped cells in the latter which produces a cloudiness. In these cases it was arbitrarily decided to collect the first 60 ml, measured on a spring balance.

The number of cells recovered in the cell layer was different in individual patients depending on the specimen (PB leukapheresis, BM) and the density cut. For some CML patients, the same sample was separated at different density cuts, and generally a lower density gradient produced a lower recovery of cells in the cell layer (and vice versa).

CD34 enumeration

An aliquot of cells from each fraction was washed three times in RPMI 1640 medium without phenol red (GIBCO). On cells from each fraction, a two-fluorescence staining with FITC-conjugated CD34 MAb (Q-Bend 10, Immunotech) and PE-conjugated HLA-DR MAb (Becton Dickinson) was performed. An isotype matched control (IgG1 FITC/IgG2 PE conjugated MAb) was performed. For each sample 1×10^6 cells were suspended in 100 μl of Hank's buffered salt solution and incubated for 15 min at 4°C with

20 μl of AB serum to block nonspecific binding. The cells were then washed × 3 and either 10 μl of CD34-FITC and 20 μl of HLA-DR-PE or isotypic control were added to the cells in 100 μl of Hank's. The cells were incubated for 30 min at 4°C then washed × 3 in Hank's and resuspended in 1 ml of Hank's. Red cells in the deposit were lysed using FACS lysing solution (Becton Dickinson) before washing. At least 10^4 cells were analyzed using a FACScan flow cytometer (Becton Dickinson). There was no gate during data acquisition.

Cell depletion by immunomagnetic beads

The method we use to isolate the CD34$^+$ progenitor cells from PB/BM is the following.

1 Separate equal volume of either PB or BM on 1.068 g/ml Percoll density gradient.

2 Block Fc receptors with 2% AB serum at room temperature for 15 min.

3 Incubate 2×10^8 cells with the required MAbs (see below) for 30 min at 4°C with agitation. Have cells suspended in about 1.5 ml.

The following MAbs were used: CD3 (15 μl), CD19 (15 μl), CD14 (30 μl), CD16 (15 μl), anti-glycophorin A (30 μl, to be used in BM samples only), CD41 (15 μl, to be used in BM samples only), CD15 (40 μl, to 120 μl in CML samples), CD11c (20 μl), L12-2 (which recognizes mature neutrophils: 40 μl, to be added in CML samples only).

4 Centrifuge cells (10 min at 1500 rpm) with fetal calf serum (FCS = 10%) to remove unbound MAbs.

5 Wash the cells once with a colorless medium.

6 Incubate for 30 min at 4°C with Dynabeads coated with sheep anti-mouse IgG (M-450, Dynal). Bead:cell ratio should be 5:1. Have cells and beads suspended in about 1 ml.

7 Dilute to 3 ml and remove beads with magnet for 2 minutes. Repeat × 2.

8 Wash cells × 2 and analyze their reactivity by flow cytometry using the required MAbs.

9 Repeat steps 3-8 (using a half amount of MAbs) if purity of CD34$^+$ cells is less than 60%. Values of purity higher than 90% are less likely to be obtained in CML samples than in normal samples.

Results

Recovery of CD34$^+$ cells

On a large scale procedure, using a density cut ranging from 1.065 to 1.068, the large majority of CD34$^+$ cells were recovered in the cell layer (66-97%), while 0-33% were in the waste Percoll and less than 10% in the deposit. Table IV gives details of the cell number, CD34 and CFU-GM counts, and percentage of blasts recovered in each fraction after large scale separation using a continuous-flow blood cell separator (Cobe Spectra). The morphological analysis showed that the majority of the blast cells (>90%) were found in the cell layer. Furthermore, the percentage of blasts in the cell layer was 3- 6-fold higher than the percentage of $CD34^+$ cells detected in that fraction.

In CML, the vast majority of $CD34^+$ cells (mean 95%) co-express the HLA-DR antigen. Furthermore, we found that the $CD34^+$HLA-DR^- cell population peaked at a density of 1.067 g/ml, while the $CD34^+DR^+$ cells showed a broader distribution (1.055–1.067) with the highest concentration at 1.062 g/ml. These findings were consistent either in normal or in CML BM samples.

Clinical findings

So far, three patients with CML have been autografted at Hammersmith Hospital (London) with cells derived from large scale separations on a closed system using Percoll density cuts. All patients engrafted successfully and showed no delay in marrow reconstitution. Similar results were observed by *Thomas* and coworkers, who demonstrated that patients receiving Percoll-separated marrow cells engrafted as quickly as patients receiving unmanipulated cells [23]. The procedure they used for large scale separation of BM cells was similar to that developed at Hammersmith.

Phenotypic profile of purified CML progenitor cells and comparison with their normal counterpart

The phenotypic profile of either CML or normal progenitor cells purified by negative depletion of non-$CD34^+$ cells is shown in Table V [24, 25]. Interestingly, in CML the $CD34^+$ cells expressed at least two antigenic markers CD35 (also called CR1-complement receptor 1 [26, 27]) and CD56 (also called N-CAM-neural cell adhesion molecule [25]), which were found to be mainly negative in their normal counterpart. Furthermore, both the mean fluorescence intensity and the percentage of positivity for the HLA-DR molecule was higher in the CML $CD34^+$ cells than in their normal counterpart [28].

Reagents

Becton Dickinson Immunocytometry Systems, 2350 Qume Drive, San José, California 95131-1807 USA, Tel: 1-800-223-8226, European HQ: Denderstraat 24, B-9320 Erembodegem-Aalst, Belgium, Tel: 32-53-720211, Fax: 32-53-720450.

Table IV. Recovery of $CD34^+$ cells, CFU-GM and blast-appearing cells after large scale separation using a Percoll density cut ranging from 1.066-1.068 g/ml. Data are obtained from 31 chronic phase CML samples.

	Initial WBC $\times 10^9$/l	% of nucleated cells	% of total $CD34^+$ cells	enrichment factor for $CD34^+$ cells	CFU-GM	% blasts
Cell layer	254 (32-413)	24 (8-31)	82 (71-94)	8 (5-12)	112	22
Percoll waste		17 (6-38)	15 (4-23)	< 1	21	2
Cell deposit		59 (33-86)	3 (0-8)	< 1	16	0.1

The mean % of total $CD34^+$ cells recovered in the cell layer after large scale separation of BM cells from eight normal donors was slightly higher (86%) than that from CML samples.

Table V. Immunophenotypic profile of $CD34^+$ cells isolated using a negative depletion technique.

	CML (Ph^+, CP) (N = 10)	Normal donors (N = 8)
CD33	64	45
HLA-DR	98[a]	82
CD38	93	90
CD56	0-40	<0.5
CD35	0-60	0-10
CD45RO	31	44

[a]increased mean fluorescence compared to that of donors.

Dynal International, PO Box 158, Skoyen, N-0212 Oslo, Norway, Tel: + 472-529450, Fax: + 472-507015, USA/Canada: 475 Northern Boulevard, Great Neck, NY 11021, Tel: 1-800-638-9416, Fax: 1-516-829-0045.

Flow Cytometry Standards Corporation, P.O. Box 12621, Research Triangle Park, NC 27709 USA, Tel: 1-800-227-8143, Fax: 1-919-967-7325.

Sigma Chemical Company, P.O. Box 14508, Saint Louis, Missouri 63178, USA, Tel: 1-800-325-3010, Fax: 1-800-325-5052.

Acknowledgments

Several coworkers (*Dr. Chris Hoyle, Dr. Christine McDonald,* and *Mr. John Davidson,* London, UK) have collaborated with me on this project and their contribution is acknowledged. I wish to express my gratitude to *Prof. John M. Goldman* (LRF Centre for Adult Leukemia, Hammersmith Hospital, London) for his support and discussions about the project. Without the co-operation of each of the scientists listed above, this work would not have been possible.

References

1 Goldman JM. Molecular biology and treatment of chronic myelogenous leukemia. Current Opinion in Oncology. 1990;2:49-54.

2 Hughes TP, Morgan GJ, Martiat P, Goldman JM. Detection of residual leukemia after bone marrow transplant for chronic myeloid leukemia: role of polymerase chain reaction in predicting relapse. Blood 1991;77:874-878.

3 Dowding CR, Gordon MY, Goldman JM. Primitive progenitor cells in the blood of patients with chronic granulocytic leukemia. Int J Cell Cloning 1986;4:331-340.

4 Banavali S, Silvestri F, Hulette B, Hurtubise P, Srivastava A, Civin C, Preisler H. Expression of hematopoietic progenitor cell associated antigen CD34 in chronic myeloid leukemia. Leuk Res 1991;15:603-608.

5 Wunder E, Sovalat H, Fritsch G, Silvestri F, Hénon P, Serke S. Report on the European workshop on peripheral blood stem cell determination and standardization—Mulhouse, France, February 6-8 and 14-15, 1992. J Hematol 1992;1:131-142.

6 Vogt RF, Cross GD, Henderson LO, Phillips DL. Model system evaluating fluorescein-labeled microbeads as internal standards to calibrate florescence intensity on flow cytometers. Cytometry, 1989;10:294-302.

7 Brando B, Sommaruga E. Nationwide quality control trial on lymphocyte immunophenotyping and flow cytometer performance in Italy. Cytometry 1993;14:294-306.

8 Vogt RF, Cross GD, Phillips DL, Henderson O, Hannon H. Interlaboratory study of cellular fluorescence intensity measurements with fluorescein labeled microbeads standards. Cytometry 1991;12:525-536.

9 Schwartz A. Fluorescent microbead standards (monograph). Flow Cytometry Standards Corporation, Research Triangle Park, NC, 1988.

10 Moore MAS. Clinical implications of positive and negative hematopoietic stem cell regulators. Blood 1991;78:1-19.

11 Brito-Babapulle F, Bowcock SJ, Marcus R, Apperley J, Th'ng KH, Dowding C, Rassol F, Catovsky D, Galton DSG, McCarthy D, Goldman JM. Autografting for patients with chronic myeloid leukaemia in chronic phase: peripheral blood stem cells may have a finite capacity for maintaining hemopoiesis. Br J Haematol 1989;73:76-81.

12 Barnett MJ, Eaves CJ, Phillips GL, Kalousek DK, Klingemann HG, Lansdorp PM, Reece DE, Shepherd JD, Shaw GJ, Eaves AC. Successful autografting in chronic myeloid leukemia after maintenance of marrow in culture. Bone Marrow Transplant 1989;4:345-351.

13 Goldman JM. Autografting for chronic myeloid leukaemia. Palliation, cure or nothing? Leuk Lymph 1992;7:51-54.

14 Verfaille CM, Miller WJ, Boylan K, McGlave PB. Selection of benign primitive hematopoietic progenitors in chronic myelogenous leukemia on the basis of HLA-DR antigen expression. Blood 1992;79:1003-1010.

15 Dunbar C, Stewart FM. Separating the wheat from the chaff: selection of benign hematopoietic cells in chronic myeloid leukemia. Blood 1992;79:1107-1110.

16 Srour EF, Brandt HE, Leemhuis T, Ballas CB, Hoffman R. Relationship between cytokine-dependent cell cycle progression and MHC class II antigen expression by human $CD34^+$ $HLA\text{-}DR^-$ bone marrow cells. J Immun 1992;148:815-820.

17 Hatzfeld JH. Control of G_0 phase of human bone marrow stem cells. Sem Hematol 1992;29:2-6.

18 Cashman JD, Eaves AC, Raines EW, Ross R, Eaves C. Mechanisms that regulate the cell cycle status of very primitive hematopoietic cells in long term human marrow cultures. I. Stimulatory role of a variety of mesenchymal cell activators and inhibitory role of TGF-β. Blood 1990;75:96-101.

19 Caux C, Favre C, Saeland S, Duvert V, Mannoni P, Durand I, Aubry JP, de Vries JE. Sequential loss of CD34 and class II MHC antigens on purified cord blood hematopoietic progenitors cultured with IL3: characterization of $CD34^-$, $HLA\text{-}DR^+$ cells. Blood 1989;74:1287-1294.

20 Olofsson T, Gartner I, Olsson I. Separation of human bone marrow cells in density gradients of polyvinylpyrrolidone coated silica gel (Percoll). Scand J Haematol 1980;24:254-262.

21 Ellis WM, Georgiou GM, Roberton DM, Johnson GR. The use of discontinuous Percoll gradients to separate populations of cells from human bone marrow and peripheral blood. J Immunol Meth 1984;66:9-16.

22 Anonymous. Percoll, methodology and applications, density marker beads for calibration of gradients of Percoll. Upsala:Pharmacia, 1986.

23 Thomas TE, Abraham S, Phillips G, Lansdorp P. A simple procedure for large scale density separation of bone marrow cells for transplantation. Transplantation 1992;53:1163-1165.

24 Lanza F, Bi S, Goldman JM. Similarity of p53 expression by CD34+ cells in chronic myeloid leukemia and normal progenitors detected by flow cytometry. Blood 1992;80:1857-1858.

25 Lanza F, Bi S, Castoldi GL, Goldman JM. Abnormal expression of N-CAM (CD56) adhesion molecule on myeloid and progenitor cells from chronic myeloid leukemia. Leukemia 1993 (in the press)

26 Lanza F, Fagioli F, Gavioli R, Spisani S, Malavasi F, Castoldi GL. Evaluation of CR1 expression in neutrophils from chronic myeloid leukemia: relationship between prognosis and cellular activity. Br J Haematol 1991;77:66-72.

27 Lanza F, Castoldi GL. Complement receptor 1 (CR1) expression in chronic myeloid leukemia. An overview. Leuk Lymph 1992;8:35-41.

28 Dowding CR, Gordon MY, Goldman JM. Increased DR antigen expression by committed hemopoietic progenitor cells but not primitive progenitor cells in chronic myeloid leukemia. Exp Hematol 1988;16:171-175.

Separation of Hematopoietic Cells of Different Maturity in Mononuclear Cell Subsets Generated by Elutriation

E. Wunder,[a] *G. Herbein,*[b] *H. Sovalat,*[a] *A. Kirn*[c]

[a]Institut de Recherche en Hématologie et Transfusion, Hôpital du Hasenrain, Mulhouse, France; [b]Sir William Dunn School of Pathology, Oxford, United Kingdom; [c]Institut de Virologie et Unité INSERM, Faculté de Médecine, Strasbourg, France

Key Words. Elutriation • CD34+ cells • Cell size • Buoyant density • CFC • Non-CFC • Bone marrow repopulation

Introduction

In the past elutriation was mainly used for removing T cells from grafting material in order to avoid graft-versus-host disease in allografts [1]; this strategy was abandoned, since it turned out that these grafts fail. However, the basic technology of elutriating cells prior to grafting has been developed in this context [2]; hematopoietic cells were monitored in the cell fractions by short-term colony growth after stimulation, which of course is limited to committed progenitors. Meanwhile more immature cells can be detected and measured by phenotyping and by long-term culture; in addition, these can be subject to ex vivo expansion by exposing them to stem cell factor and some other growth factors. Thus, exploration of the capacities of elutriation to separate early non-colony forming cells (pre-CFC) from advanced hematopoietic cells gains new interest. Isolation of CD34+ cell subsets of course is also possible by flow sorting or by immunoadsorption techniques; however, for preparing these extremely rare target cells in sufficient quantity for experiments, one has to start out with high numbers of total mononuclear cells (MNC), and therefore sorting time and costs increase tremendously for immunoadsorbing devices or fluorescent monoclonal antibodies (MAbs) being consumed. In this case, the combination of a preenrichment step, which already narrows down on a fraction of MNC containing the desired CD34+ cell subset, and the definitive isolation of the target cell by positive selection from this reduced cell mass can be a reasonable strategy. Elutriation of nonmobilized peripheral blood MNC, containing very few CD34+ cells, may serve as a guide for such applications, which of course can be extended to any other material containing CD34+ cells.

As opposed to positive selection techniques for CD34 hematopoietic cells being based on immunoadsorption, centrifugal counter flow elutriation (CCE) uses cell size and buoyant density as separation criteria. It is known from cytofluorimetric analysis that CD34+ cells are a very heterogeneous population with regard to light scatter, suggesting that all size classes are present that are

Correspondence: Dr. Eckart Wunder, Institut de Recherche en Hématologie et Transfusion, Hôpital du Hasenrain, 87 Avenue d'Altkirch, 68051 Mulhouse, France.

©AlphaMed Press ISBN 1-880854 17-1

also found in mature cells. Consequently it can be expected that they coelutriate with mature cells and simultaneously are subdivided into different fractions corresponding to elutriation parameters. Of course CD34$^+$ cell subsets are not necessarily related to coelutriating mature cells with regard to their line of differentiation, but their size classes correspond to degrees of maturation and lineage commitment. By analysis of CD34$^+$ cell subsets in elutriated fractions for their immune phenotype, and also by assessing their clonogenicity in vitro after stimulation, their commitment and maturity can be evaluated.

Materials and Methodology

Preparation of MNC from Peripheral Blood

As starting material, buffy coats from healthy adults are used, which are recovered from 400 ml fresh heparinized blood in transfusion bags after centrifugation. This suspension (70-100 ml) is diluted 1:1 (v/v) with phosphate buffered saline (PBS) and transferred onto a 80 ml Ficoll-Hypaque underlayer (Pharmacia, Upsala, Sweden) in sterile 250 ml conical-bottom tubes with screwcap (Corning, Avon, France). After centrifugation at 2,500 rpm on a Beckman TJ6 centrifuge for 30 min at 20°C, the opaque ring of MNC is removed by careful pipetting from the interphase of the density gradient. Occasionally this cell suspension has a slight pink color indicating the presence of erythroid cells, which can be ignored. Cells are counted and centrifuged in 50 ml Falcon tubes at 4°C for 10 min and resuspended in 10 ml of Gray's solution (or Ca^{++}/Mg^{++}-free PBS) containing 0.5% bovine serum albumin (BSA). Usually 4-8 × 10^8 MNC will be recovered.

CCE

For elutriation, a cooled centrifuge is used (Beckman JI6-MC, Beckman Instruments Inc., Palo Alto CA; Gagny, France) equipped with a JE6.0 rotor; this rotor houses one or two separation chambers (content 4 ml each) made of transparent plastic material. The central part of the rotor does not move and is connected with the separation chamber(s) in the rotating part by a waterproof bearing; it contains space for the incoming MNC suspension, from which cells are gated to the periphery of the rotor and flow back towards the center into the conical shaped separation chamber. Since the rotor is spinning during separation, a centrifugal force acts on the cells, which is counteracted by the flow of the cell suspension being generated by a pump. Cells will stay inside the separation chamber if the centrifugal force, which is a result of their size and density, is larger or identical to the counteracting force on them caused by the pump flow; in case the latter prevails, i.e., cells are smaller and lighter, they will leave the chamber by moving to the immobile center of the rotor, where they are separately gated into the outward tubing. The lighter and smaller cells will come out first, if pump volume increases at constant rotor speed, while the larger cells stay inside; by gradually accelerating the pump flow, the remaining cells can be driven out in several consecutive fractions, consisting of cells with increasing size and density. (Basically the same effect is obtained if the pump volume is kept constant, and the rotor speed is gradually diminished).

Evaluation

1 Cell counting: Cell density in total MNC and in the separated fractions is tested in the usual way in a counting chamber under the microscope, or in a Coulter Counter (Coultronics, Mountain View, CA).

2 Cytology: Cytospin preparations are made from the original MNC and the elutriated fractions, and stained by Wright-Giemsa for microscopic analysis.

3 Cytofluorimetric analysis: For determination of $CD34^+$ cells in the original MNC and elutriated fractions, immunofluorescent labeling is done with either HPCA 2 (B-D, San José, CA; Evembodegem-Aalst, Belgium) or QBEND-10 (Immunotech, Marseille, France) being conjugated with phycoerythrin. Evaluation is done using a dot plot of fluorescence and side light scatter (see *Sovalat,* pp. 79-87).

4 Short-term colony assay: This assay is performed in methylcellulose (Terry Fox Laboratories, Canada[1]) dissolved in Iscove's minimal essential medium (MEM) (GIBCO) containing fetal calf serum (FCS) and BSA in the following way: 5×10^6 and 1×10^6 cells suspended in 0.5 ml of medium are added to 2.4 ml methylcellulose mix in sterile 5 ml plastic tubes with snap cap. After addition of 50 ng granulocyte-macrophage colony stimulating factor (GM-CSF) and 10 ng interleukin 3 (IL-3) in 0.15 ml Iscove's, the suspension is well mixed by several-fold inversion. Then twice 1 ml is aspirated in a 1 ml pipette, and each is transferred into a 3.4 cm plastic Petri dish. After incubation at 5% CO_2 and 37°C for 10 days, colonies are evaluated under an inverted microscope, counting agglomerations of more than approximately 40 cells as a colony.

Technical Details and Hints

Elutriator

A main concern for obtaining cell fractions that can be further studied by in vitro culture is their sterility. It is of importance that the whole circuit is tight; the bearings in the central part of the rotor, which stays stationary while the separation chambers spin, are closed by circular rubber fittings, which wear down rapidly and need to be changed frequently; putting the fitting in place with sharp instruments like screwdrivers, etc., should be avoided in order to avoid damaging them. It is best to try out the tightness of the whole circuit with a practice run of sterile water or buffer prior to injecting the cells; at the same time the temperature of the chamber and rotor can adapt, usually at 10°C. Elutriation buffer is also precooled in the refrigerator and kept cool during the run. It is best to install the elutriator next to a sterile hood and to lead tubing inside through a hole in the side wall.

For the buffer either a 5-10 l reservoir is applied, or, if smaller bottles are used, the tubing has to be switched from one bottle to the next skillfully, in order to avoid air aspiration during the run. For receiving elutriated fractions, sterile plastic bottles of 100 to 500 ml volume or sterile transfusion bags must be at hand; collecting a minimum of ten times the volume of the separation chamber per fraction is recommended, but for exhaustive removal of cells higher volumes are preferable (chamber volume is either 4 ml or 40 ml). For avoiding cell losses by adhesion to tubing and chambers, the system is siliconized every third or fourth run with a silicon spray (Baysilan, Bayer Leverkusen, Germany); this procedure is nontoxic to cells, and losses can thus be reduced to 1-2%. In addition, a fast flush of buffer at the end of the separation removes sticking cells efficiently and thus keeps the system tidy inside; after the separation a wash run is done with cleaning fluid (Beckman 555 solution) dissolved in demineralized sterile water 1:10.

An additional safeguard for ascertaining sterility is the use of closed systems with plastic bags (Maco-Pharma, France[2]). This is more expensive, but its safety is certainly welcome if elutriated cells are to be used for grafting. The central rotor part with mounted chamber(s) is autoclaved after loosening screws.

Pump

It is of utmost importance to use pumps with a very constant debit during the run. The pump is not part of the elutriator machine and has to be bought separately. Beckman recommends Master Flex pumps with exchangeable pump heads; the larger model has digital regulation, while the small one is regulated by turning a knob. Although the latter is considerably cheaper, the regulation is not precise enough for the small debits needed; it has to be modified by installation of an additional second potentiometer. Since the pump function is not exactly reproducible from one run to the other, it has to be calibrated afresh each time with a chronometer and a graduated measurement cylinder, or by monitoring the weight of fluid flowing out per minute on-line on a balance. A two-point calibration is done, using approximate lowest and highest settings; both values are plotted in a diagram, and a straight line is drawn. Exact pump settings for the desired debits can be obtained from this diagram by interpolation.

Tubing

Master Flex supplies silicon tubing of varying diameters. If the 4 ml chamber is used, gauge 14 is appropriate, (for the large 40 ml chamber, gauge 16 is better adapted to the approximately five times larger debit). In the pump head white rubber tubing is used, which is kept from sliding through the pump head by special clamps; all the other tubing is made of transparent silicon.

Pulsations of the buffer resulting from pump actions can be reduced by putting a closed glass bell into the circuit, which stays half-filled with the passing buffer solution and has its entrance above the level of liquid; the air above the changing level of liquid can buffer the unequal flux. For this purpose also the screwcap vial supplied by Beckman (conceived for cell injection) can be used, if it is installed upside-down.

For sterilizing the system, it is best to autoclave tubing, central rotor parts and separation chambers; this is cumbersome, but necessary if separated cells are to be used in patients. For experimental purposes, it is sufficient to wash with 70% alcohol and 10 U/ml Polymyxin B (Sigma, St. Louis, MO).

The cell suspension is injected with a standard 10 ml syringe through a three-way tap. Since injection is done into the circulating buffer flow while the rotor is spinning, it has to be done very slowly. Special care is needed for keeping the tap entrance sterile; remaining alcohol should be cleaned off prior to injecting cells. Air injection into the system should be avoided, but a few little bubbles are not critical for the separation.

Observation of Separation Chamber

Since the lid of the elutriator centrifuge has a hole, and a stroboscope light inside is synchronized with rotor movement, the behavior of cells in the transparent plexiglas separation chamber can be conveniently observed during the run. Slight pulsations can be seen, and ideally separation zones of white cells can be distinguished. Usually some residual erythrocytes remain in the MNC fraction, and this makes the flow of injected cells in the tubing and arrival at the separation chamber easily visible.

Elutriation of Human Peripheral Blood MNC (PBMNC)

The centrifuge is operated at 10°C and 2,500 rpm. The Master Flex pump is set to the starting flow rate of 16 ml/min of precooled buffer (Gray's solution or PBS without Ca^{++} and Mg^{++})-BSA 0.5%, and the cell suspension is slowly injected into the circuit; collection of the first fraction starts simultaneously with injection. The rate of cells leaving the system can be checked quickly in aliquots which are put into a Coulter Counter or similar automatic device. We usually collect 400 ml per fraction. After completion, the pump setting is changed for the next fraction; flow rates 21, 28 and 33 ml/min in the small (4 ml) separation chamber correspond to fraction 2-4. Residual cells are washed out with a flush of 130 ml/min ("wash-out" fraction). After elutriation, cells of all five fractions are pelleted, resuspended in colorless RPMI 1640 (GIBCO) with 5% heat inactivated FCS (Lab System, Helsinki, Finland), and adjusted to 1×10^7/ml for cytofluorimetric labeling and to 1 and 5×10^6/ml in Iscove's modified MEM for culture of colony forming

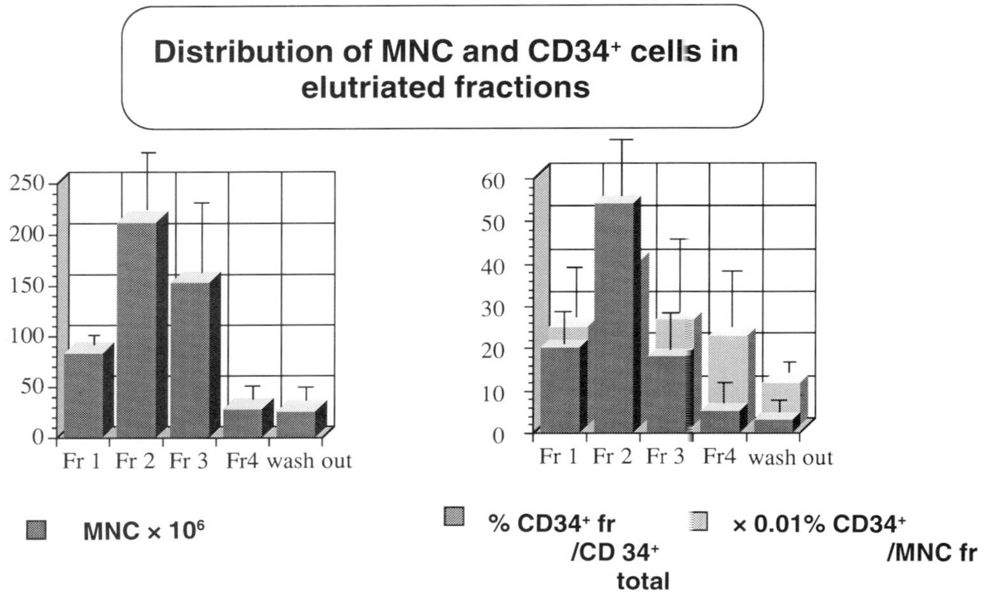

Fig. 1. Left: Distribution of MNC in elutriated fractions 1-4 and in the wash-out fraction; SD is indicated by bars. Right: anterior row. Content of $CD34^+$ cells in the elutriated and wash-out fractions, given as percentage of all recovered $CD34^+$ cells (=100%): SD is indicated by bars. Posterior row: Content of $CD34^+$ cells in elutriated fractions, given as percentage of MNC in the respective fraction × 0.01 ("purity").

units granulocyte-macrophage (CFU-GM) (see above). An aliquot is used from each fraction for cytofuge preparation and Wright-Giemsa staining.

Results and Discussion

In an unselected series of seven healthy adult blood donors the average yield of MNC after Ficoll-Hypaque fractionation was 497 (± 166 SD) × 10^6 cells containing an average of 0.15% (± 0.06 SD) $CD34^+$ cells. The distribution of absolute cell numbers in the elutriated fractions is given along with the content in $CD34^+$ cells in Figure 1.

The types of cells typically encountered in the different fractions are listed in Table I. As detailed elsewhere [3], with subsequent elutriation fractions forward and side light scatter also increases, showing that cell size and cytoplasmic density mounts.

The yield of CFU-GM relative to the number of $CD34^+$ cells in each fraction is shown in Figure 2. It is evident that in the $CD34^+$ cell subset in fraction 1,

Table I. Prevailing cell type in elutriated fractions

Cells typically encountered in elutriated fractions				
Total PBMNC:	lymphocytes	78.0	(9.6 SD)	
	monocytes	17.4	(6.9 SD)	
	granulocytes	4.6	(3.9 SD)	
				Diameter
Fr 1	small lymphocytes	98.4	(1.5 SD)	8.5 μm
Fr 2	large lymphocytes	91.6	(5.6 SD)	9.5 μm
Fr 3	monocytes	88.6	(6.3 SD)	10.5 μm
Fr 4	granulocytes	76.4	(10.5 SD)	12.0 μm

In the upper part cellular composition of total PBMNC is given. Below the content of the elutriated fractions in the characteristic cell type is given as percentage of all cells in the respective fraction; SD is indicated in parenthesis. The virtual average cell diameter in each fraction is shown in the last row.

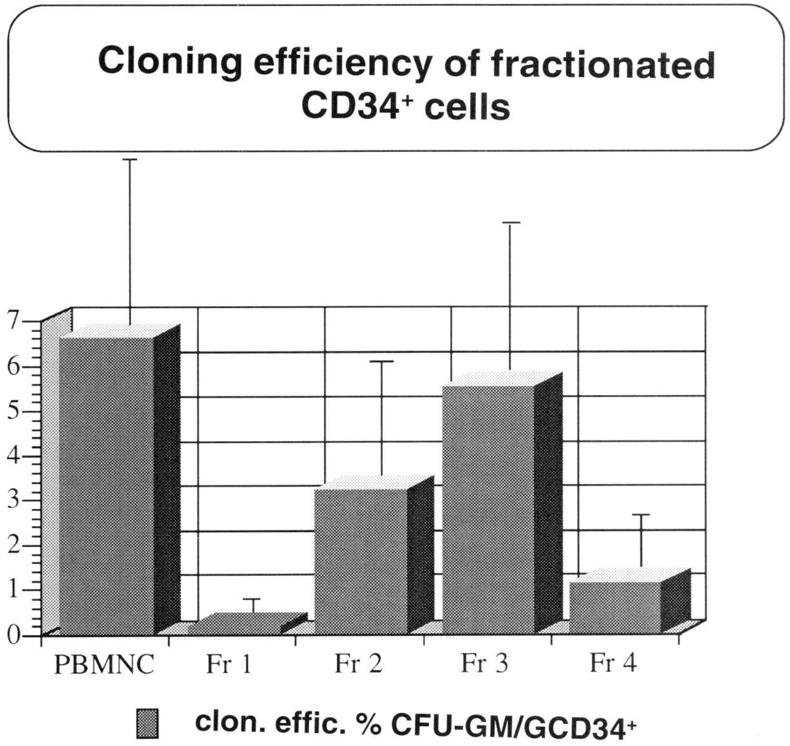

Fig. 2. Cloning efficiency of $CD34^+$ cells in the elutriated fractions after stimulation for granulo-monocytic colonies. The percentage of $CD34^+$ cells growing into a colony is given; SD indicated by bars.

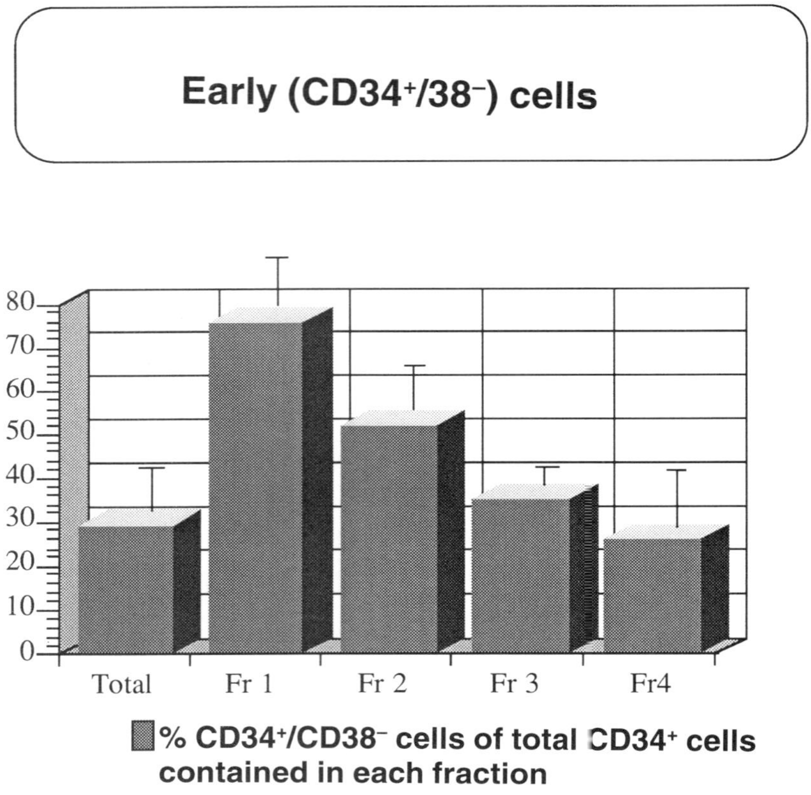

Fig. 3. Early CD34$^+$ cells as characterized by CD38$^-$ phenotype are given as a percentage of all CD34$^+$ cells in total MNC and in elutriated fractions; SD is indicated by bars.

which represents cells with the smallest size (around 8.5 μm) and lowest cytoplasmic density, only irrevelant numbers of GM-CFC are contained; at the same time, the lowest frequency of CD38 expression in hematopoietic cells is encountered here, which means that the majority of these small CD34$^+$ cells are highly immature (Fig. 3). This coincides with the highest mean CD34 expression as indicated by relative fluorescence intensity after specific immunofluorescent labeling [3]. In fraction 3, which is most clonogenic, fluorescent intensity is only two thirds of the former subset; coexpression of other differentiation markers, like CD13 and CD33 in the myeloid line, CD10 in the lymphoid line, and CD71 in the erythroid line increases with cell size, while CD19 seemingly, is mostly expressed in small cells [3].

In summary, it is evident that a subset of small and translucent CD34$^+$ cells is highly enriched in the first elutriated fraction, while most of the more mature committed progenitors are distributed in the following fractions, as was found independently by another group [4]. This is meaningful, since immature $CD34^+/CD38^-$ cells supposedly play a role in bone marrow repopulation for long-term multilineage recovery, while the advanced and committed progenitors are responsible for short-term recovery of white blood cells; functional dissection of both groups of $CD34^+$ cells has already been accomplished in mice, where repopulation experiments can be performed after ablative irradiation [5] . It can be reasonably assumed that the situation is analogous in man. Development of manipulated grafts thus could take advantage of elutriation by mixing these fractions in different proportions at will. Also, the early immature $CD34^+$ cells from fraction 1 can be expanded ex vivo and then be used for obtaining accelerated recovery. For experiments with pure stem cell subsets, the elutriated fractions can be subject to an adjacent second positive selection step.

Specific Materials

[1]HCC-4200's Iscove's Methylcellulose (Ref. No. HCC-4210) Terry Fox Laboratory, British Columbia Cancer Research Centre, 601 West 10th Avenue, Vancouver, B.C., Canada, V5Z 1L3. Phone + 1-604-877-0713, Fax + 1-604-877-0712.

[2]"Elutriation Kit" 1) Tubes for Elutriation (Ref. No. EEC 100A); 2) Kit of bags for elutriation (Ref. No. KUC 600K). Laboratoires Maco-Pharma, 96 rue du Pont Rompu, 59200 TOURCOING, France. Phone + 33-20234130, Fax + 33-20234174.

References

1 Noga SJ, Davis JM, Thoburn CJ, Donnenberg AD. Lymphocyte dose modification of the bone marrow allograft using elutriation. In: Gee A ed. Bone Marrow Processing and Purging. Boca Raton, Florida: CRC Press Inc., 1991:176-198.

2 Noga SJ, Wagner JE, Rowley S, Davis JM, Vogelsang GB, Hess AD. Using elutriation to engineer bone marrow allografts. In: Gross S ed. Bone Marrow Purging and Processing. New York: Alan R. Liss, 1990:345-361.

3 Herbein G, Sovalat H, Wunder E, Baerenzung M, Bachorz J, Lewandowsky H, Schweitzer C, Schmitt C, Kirn A, Hénon P. Isolation and identification of two $CD34^+$ cell subpopulations from normal human peripheral blood. (in press).

4 Almici C, Donnenberg AD, Rizzoli V. Counterflow centrifugal elutriation: experimental and clinical applications. J Hematoth 1992;1:279-288.

5 Jones RJ, Wagner JE, Celano P, Zicha MS, Sharkis SJ. Separation of pluripotent hematopoietic stem cells from spleen colony-forming cells. Nature 1990;347:188-189.

Common Problems Encountered in the Separation of CD34⁺ Cells Using Different Purification Systems

Erika de Wynter, Lucia H. Coutinho, Nydia G. Testa
Christie Hospital NHS Trust, Manchester, United Kingdom

Key Words. $CD34^+$ cells • Mononuclear cells (MNC) • Immunomagnetic beads • CELLector flasks • FACSorting • CFC assays • CD34 antibodies • Immunoaffinity columns • Cell separation

Introduction

In any cell separation or purification system the major objective should be recovery of a homogeneous and viable cell population with minimal loss of target cells. The separation of $CD34^+$ cells presents certain unique problems due to the fact that these cells are present in blood and normal bone marrow in extremely small numbers. Different approaches have been adopted to isolate these cells, most of which are outlined in the previous chapters. However, each method has its own intrinsic problems, and there is probably no "ideal" method for CD34 purification which optimizes for purity, recovery and viability simultaneously. The intention of this chapter is to follow a general procedure for purification from preparations of mononuclear cells (MNC) to analysis of purified $CD34^+$ cell populations. Throughout the chapter, common problems encountered at each stage with the different systems will be highlighted, and solutions or practical details which we have found useful in the laboratory are included.

Samples

Source

In the research laboratory little can be done about either the quality or "time in transit" of samples received, as this often rests with clinicians or other collaborators. Bone marrow samples contain on average about 2% $CD34^+$ cells while peripheral and cord blood generally contain a lower percentage. Leukapheresis harvests are abundant in platelets and monocytes and contain a variable percentage of $CD34^+$ cells. Therefore the purification method may have to be adjusted according to the source of the sample.

Storage

Samples can vary between a few hours and one or two days old; and, although most protocols stipulate fresh samples, clearly this is not always possible. In our laboratory samples arriving late in the evening have been maintained overnight at 4°C without any detrimental effect on progenitor cells.

Correspondence: Dr. Erika de Wynter, Christie Hospital NHS Trust, Wilmslow Road, Manchester M20 9BX, United Kingdom.

 ISBN 1-880854 17-1

Mononuclear Cells

These can be prepared using commercial solutions. Density of the solution varies with temperature making these gradient preparations one of the steps where cells may be lost. Preferably, one should give the density gradient solution sufficient time to equilibrate to room temperature as this allows optimal recovery of MNC. In using certain bead separation systems, specific instructions are provided for the isolation of MNC. These are designed to eliminate cell clumps and maintain single cell suspensions, so unless these guidelines are carefully followed, there is poor recovery of $CD34^+$ cells.

It is becoming increasingly apparent that separation of a light density fraction is not necessary for peripheral blood stem cells obtained by leukapheresis, and some $CD34^+$ cells may even be lost during centrifugation.

Storage

MNC can be stored at 4°C in 20% fetal calf serum (FCS) in Iscove's modified Dulbeccos medium (IMDM) at a concentration of not greater than 2-3 × 10^6/ml. The cell viability as determined by trypan blue exclusion is usually >95% after overnight storage under these conditions, although this may also depend on whether the sample had been stored before processing.

Cell numbers

Before deciding which separation system to use, the MNC numbers recommended for each system should be noted. For example, CellPro (avidin affinity columns) can process 25-500 × 10^6 MNC; Dynal (using Dynabeads) does not recommend less than 5 × 10^7 MNC in their procedures, while AIS (CELLector flasks) suggests a maximum of 2 × 10^7 cells per 25 cm^2 flask. The choice of a system may then be governed simply by the numbers of cells available.

Selection

Beads

Two types of positive selection are offered using beads [1]: either coating cells with a mouse CD34 antibody and selecting with beads coated with anti-mouse IgG (indirect), or binding the target cells directly to beads coated with CD34 antibodies (direct). Unlike both the flask and column systems, binding takes place at 4°C on a rotator, with a gentle tilt rotation to keep cells in suspension. When using Dynabeads it is absolutely essential to ensure that both beads and cells are well mixed and kept in suspension during the incubation period. This is a critical step in this method and it is worth investing in a tilt rotator if it should be the method of choice.

Note that unlike depletion methods, positive selection requires a relatively low bead:cell ratio, so ensure the bead:cell ratio is correct for your purposes and do not adjust this figure. Beads may have to be detached after selection.

CELLector Flasks

With the CELLector flasks, two binding steps are necessary [2]. The first is the soybean agglutinin coated flasks (SBA) to remove T, B, myeloid, fibroblast and stromal cells. On average, we found a minimum of 50% of bone marrow MNC remain bound to these flasks, but the percentage varies over a wide range and is reduced to only 20-30% if MNC from cord blood or leukapheresis harvests are used. The second binding step involves removal of the non-adherent cells from the SBA flask and introducing these cells into flasks coated with CD34 antibodies.

Fluorescent activated cell sorting (FACS)

Here, MNC are labeled with the appropriate CD34 antibody prior to sorting. To prevent the label being internalized and maintain viability of the cells, labeled cells must be kept cold. Cell viability after FACS sorting is usually >97% but if the sorting exceeds four hours the viability is reduced. (Sorting times can be reduced by using an enrichment step first—see chapter by *S. Miltenyi,* pp. 201-213). More importantly, cell concentrations should not exceed 5×10^6/ml if high purity is required and if cell clumping is to be avoided. In addition mixing the cell suspension from time to time during the sort will further prevent clumping of the cells and subsequent blockage of the sorting nozzle.

Affinity Columns

After a short incubation with a biotinylated CD34 antibody, the cells are overlaid onto the surface of the avidin column. As cells flow through the column, the antibody bound cells are trapped and retained. The flow rate must be adjusted so that there is a balance between binding the required cells and allowing unwanted cells to be washed through the column. Sometimes even separation under gravity can be too fast, and in this case the flow rate has to be reduced.

Detachment

Detachment is the next, critical and most problematic stage in separation procedures. Detachment methods including the use of enzymes, mechanical methods and competitive elution with polyclonal antibodies to Fab fragments are utilized in different systems.

Enzymatic Methods

Chymopapain is the enzyme most often cited for removing CD34$^+$ cells attached to beads [3]. Note that not all chymopapains work, and it is prudent to ask manufacturers for the details and source of the enzymes they use or suggest. Another point to remember when using chymopapain is that treating cells with this enzyme will perturb other surface antigens, and therefore cells may have to be given time to "recover" before analysis or any further manipulations. The recommendation is an overnight incubation at 37°C in medium containing 20% serum.

Recently, the enzyme glycoprotease from *Pasteurella haemolytica* was successfully used by *Sutherland et al.* [4] to examine the CD34 epitope. However, this is a crude preparation; and, to obtain an optimal concentration, the preparation has to be titrated against KG1a cells prior to use with CD34 cells.

Mechanical Methods

Cells are detached from CELLector flasks by hitting the flask two to three times with the hand or on any hard surface. However, as up to 10% FCS is present in the medium, this can cause excessive frothing resulting in loss of cells. It is advisable to reduce the percentage of FCS or substitute with 0.5% Gamimmune.

Detachment of bound cells from avidin columns is also accomplished mechanically by "vigorously squeezing" the column. Any difficulty experienced in removing the $CD34^+$ cells may be overcome by altering the flow rate through the column, (or by using a peristaltic pump) ensuring no bubbles are trapped in the system. Increasing the flow rate for detachment usually improves the yield of cells.

Polyclonal Antibodies

In this method cells are detached by competitive elution using a polyclonal antibody against a Fab fragment [5]. The product is prepared and distributed by Dynal (DETACHaBEAD). Use of this product has proved to be a major problem with many workers, including ourselves, who have experienced serious difficulties in removing the beads from cells. The degree of detachment is variable and complete detachment is rarely achieved for CD34 bound cells. DETACHaBEAD is said to be more effective with monoclonals of the IgM class since their interaction with CD34 antigen tends to be of a lower affinity than IgG, so one solution could be to use the indirect method with a CD34 antibody such as 12.8 (IgM). As DETACHaBEAD is a polyclonal antibody, there may be some batch to batch variation and possibly several batches may have to be tested to find one that is suitable for CD34 bound cells. A simple alternative, avoiding the use of enzymes or antibodies, is to incubate the bead/cell complexes overnight at 37°C in a high concentration of FCS.

General Comments

The above are the more common methods in use for removal of bound cells from the matrices. Some bead systems are designed solely for research purposes and do not require removal of the beads before analysis or colony assays (MACS, Immunotech). In contrast, other bead methods require the total removal of all beads once positive selection is complete, as any remaining beads can form new rosettes. We have found it extremely difficult to remove beads completely from positively selected cells, even after extensive washing. Possibly the best solution is just to remove as many beads as possible and rapidly analyze and plate the cells. Beads do not interfere with colony formation and will detach during the 10-14 day incubation period of the colony assays.

Analysis of Purification

Most analyses of purification are determined by flow cytometry using directly conjugated CD34 antibodies such as HPCA-2 (Becton Dickinson). It is essential to know which CD34 antibody has been used in the purification procedure as this will affect the choice of the antibody used in the analysis. The binding of one antibody to its epitope may block or inhibit subsequent binding of antibodies of the same class. For this reason it is not advisable to use the CD34 antibodies My10 or QBEND 10 to analyze CD34 cells recovered from CELLector flasks. Information on how to determine the $CD34^+$ cell content in a sample can be found in the preceding chapters. To monitor distribution of progenitors throughout the procedure, keep a record of volumes of all fractions, numbers of cells per milliliter at every stage and the percentage of $CD34^+$ cells determined for each fraction. Even cells removed by incubation on SBA flasks should be analyzed as some CD34 cells are lost at this stage. It is possible to detach and recover these bound cells by incubating in 0.1M N-acetyl galactosamine, the ligand for soybean agglutinin.

Generally, cells of lymphocyte size and morphologically recognized as small blasts stain brightly with CD34 monoclonal antibodies in the flow cytometer. Precursors of colony forming cells (CFC) with marrow repopulating ability are among this cell population. If the cell numbers are too low for cytofluorimetric determination, cytospins can be prepared (using about 2×10^4 cells for each slide) and stained with May-Grünwald Giemsa. $CD34^+$ cells are recognized by a blast-like morphology and a rough estimate of purity can be obtained by counting the numbers of blasts per 100 cells in several different fields.

After sorting by FACS, the cells obtained should be recounted. Again, this is a precaution as events recorded by FACS are not necessarily cells (they may be debris), and therefore do not always coincide with the number of cells separated. We have found routinely that our counts were 30-50% lower than those obtained by FACS.

Enrichment—Colony Assays

Although flow cytometry analysis can furnish information about purity of the separation, in order to determine viability and recovery of CFC, the cells must be assessed in colony assays. The essential requirement here is for reproducible in vitro assays which will reliably measure clonogenic potential. High purities are not necessarily coincident with high plating efficiency as some recovered cells may not grow. The failure of purified cells to generate colonies may be due to a number of factors including non-viable cells, poor initial samples, sub-optimal culture conditions, and source of stimulatory agents. Standardized media are now commercially available and should overcome some of these problems. It would also allow comparisons of colony numbers from one center to another. Ideally, clonal assays in both standardized media as well as your own assay system ought to be performed using at least two different cell concentrations per assay. Cells pre- and post-purification as well as all fractions obtained during the purification procedure should be analyzed to obtain a clear and informative picture of the distribution of CFC.

This is important and can be illustrated by using the Immunotech bead system as an example. $CD34^+$ cells isolated using the antibody Immu-133 did not give rise to burst forming units-erythroid (BFU-E) or colony forming units (CFU)-E. These erythroid progenitors apparently remain in the non-adherent $CD34^-$ fraction indicating a possible bias in the $CD34^+$ population selected (see chapter by *J. Hirn*, pp. 183-200).

Commercially available purification systems for $CD34^+$ cells employ a range of clonal assays for detection of progenitor cells to assess the systems. The figures quoted for enrichment of CFC may vary significantly from results obtained in the laboratory. This is generally due to the different assay systems used. The solution here is to either establish an "in house" baseline for assays commonly performed in the laboratory or obtain details from the manufacturers of the assays employed.

Long Term Bone Marrow Culture Assays of $CD34^+$ Cells

Pre-established irradiated bone marrow stroma can be used to test the long term hemopoietic potential of purified $CD34^+$ cells. After seeding the test cells on stroma, hemopoietic foci become apparent within 2-4 weeks and the kinetics of hemopoiesis proceeds in a similar manner to that observed in standard long-term bone marrow cultures (LTBMC) [6].

Discussion

We have focused on the more common problems encountered in purifying CD34$^+$ cells. The list is by no means exhaustive although certain essential points have been emphasized. Systems are constantly developing and others have been substantially modified, so much time can be saved by being aware of unnecessary steps and ensuring that the most up-to-date protocols are used (e.g., the one hour priming using the SBA CELLector flask is no longer required).

Some techniques may appear relatively straightforward and only after a series of disappointing attempts does it become clear that they require skillful technical application to achieve good results. The Dynabead system in particular is a meticulous technique, requiring numerous washing procedures and vigorous pipetting (avoiding frothing and loss of cells) with the emphasis on resuspension, mixing and selection. However, cells are available in 2-3 hours and sterility can be maintained if performed in a laminar flow cabinet.

CELLector flasks have the advantage that they are easy to manipulate and again sterility is easily maintained with cells being available for use in about two hours. Providing care is exercised in the choice of antibody for analysis of purified cells, this is a useful system. In general, the purity is not as high as FACS sorted cells. Also heat inactivated sera should be used throughout, particularly in the clonal assays.

Avidin affinity columns are now proving a suitable fast alternative to FACS sorting for bone marrow and leukapheresis harvests, giving high purity and good recovery. However, cord blood samples do not perform well with this system, and the column kits are rather expensive for the average research laboratory. The entire procedure can be completed in 1-2 hours and clearly this time factor is an advantage.

FACS is still the most popular method probably because cells are examined individually before selection. In the past, sorting was rather laborious, but with the FACS facilities now available, coupled with pre-enrichment techniques, it is possible to reduce the sorting time considerably. Sterility is perhaps the major problem but can be overcome by regularly checking and cleaning tubing and containment vessels.

No matter which system is chosen, some CD34$^+$ cells will be lost. The eventual choice may depend on the ultimate destiny of the purified cells but it will be based on a balance of factors: yield, purity, time and finance.

References

1 Hardwick RA, Kulcinski D, Mansour V, Ishizawa L, Law P, Gee AP. Design of large-scale separation systems for positive and negative immunomagnetic selection of cells using superparamagnetic microspheres. Journal of Hematotherapy 1992;1:379-386.

2 Miescher PA, Jaffe ER, eds. Symposium on harnessing the human immune response: advances in ex vivo cell therapy. Seminars in Haematology 1992;29(suppl 1):1-44.

3 Civin CI, Strauss LC, Trishmann MJ, Wiley JM, Loken MR. Progress in clinical and biological research. In: Gross S, Gee AP and Worthington White DA, eds. Bone Marrow Purging and Processing. New York: Wiley, 1990:387-402.

4 Sutherland DR, Marsh JCW, Davidson J, Baker MA, Keating A, Mellors A. Differential sensitivity of CD34 epitopes to cleavage by *Pasteurella haemolytica* glycoprotease: implications for purification of CD34 positive progenitor cells. Exp Hematol 1992;20:590-599.

5 Smeland EB, Funderud S, Kvalheim G, Gaudernack G, Rasmussen A-M, Rusten L, Wang MY, Tindle RW, Blomhoff HK, Egeland T. Isolation and characterization of human haemopoietic progenitor cells: an effective method for positive selection of CD34+ cells. Leukemia 1992;6:845-852.

6 Coutinho LH, Gilleece MH, de Wynter EA, Will A, Testa NG. Clonal and long-term cultures using human bone marrow. In: Testa NG and Molineux G, eds. Haemopoiesis (A Practical Approach). Oxford: IRL Press, 1993:75-106.

Selected Readings

Wunder E, Sovalat H, Fritsch G, Silvestri F, Hénon P, Serke S. Report on the European Workshop on Peripheral Blood Stem Cell Determination and Standardization. J Hematotherapy 1992:131-142.

Lord BI, Marsh JCW. Enrichment of progenitor cell populations from murine and human haemopoietic tissue. In: Testa NG and Molineux G, eds. Haemopoiesis (A Practical Approach). Oxford: IRL Press, 1993:21-36.

Stem Cell Differentiation and Expansion Ex Vivo

Ex Vivo Expansion of Purified Stem Cells

Stem Cell Differentiation Into Mature Lymphocytes Using the SCID Mouse Thymus Chimera Model

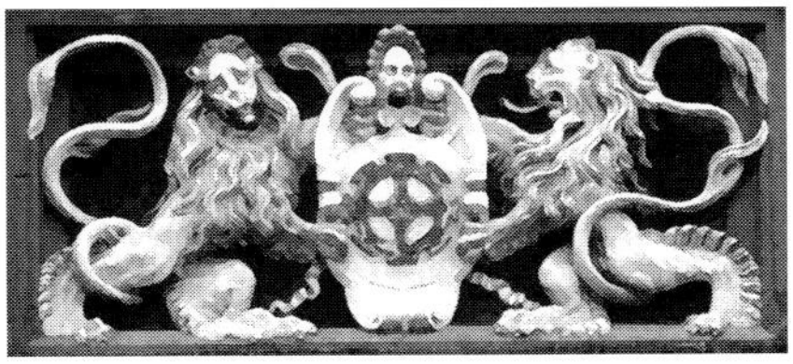

Ex Vivo Expansion of Purified Stem Cells

D. N. Haylock, L. B. To, T. L. Dowse, S. Makino, S. Trimboli, S. Niutta, C. A. Juttner, P. J. Simmons

Leukaemia Research Unit, Hanson Centre for Cancer Research, I.M.V.S., Adelaide, South Australia

Key Words. Ex vivo • Maturation • Enrichment • MACS • CEPRATE™ • Media • Hemopoietic growth factors • Hemopoietic reconstitution

Introduction

The use of peripheral blood stem cells (PBSC) for transplantation and administration of hemopoietic growth factors (HGF) such as granulocyte colony stimulating factor (G-CSF) has significantly reduced hemopoietic toxicity associated with aggressive chemotherapy regimes. It is now common for neutrophils and platelets to recover to safe levels within 8 to 12 days following PBSC rescue with or without administration of HGF postgraft. We and others [1, 2] have proposed that even earlier hemopoietic recovery may be possible if a greatly increased number of post-progenitor cells were added with the transplant. These cells could complete maturation and provide mature functional progeny within days of infusion. Such an approach may lead to the amelioration or abrogation of severe cytopenia after high-dose chemotherapy and allow the efficacy of aggressive treatment regimes to be tested in a safer, more widely applicable way.

Hemopoietic transplantation in human and nonhuman primates has clearly shown that the cells responsible for both early and sustained hemopoietic reconstitution reside within the $CD34^+$ population [3, 4]. The $CD34^+$ cells contain essentially all the unipotent and multipotent clonogenic cells [5, 6] as well as more primitive cells capable of sustaining hemopoiesis in long term culture systems or generating nascent myeloid progenitor cells (CFU-GM) in pre-CFU cultures [1, 7]. It follows then that ex vivo culture systems should be established with hemopoietic cells purified according to the expression of the CD34 antigen. A number of groups are working intensely on the laboratory aspects of ex vivo culture of $CD34^+$ cells, and the clinical use of these cells is imminent.

This report focuses on culture of $CD34^+$ cells specifically to generate myeloid progenitor and post-progenitor cells. The culture system is stroma-free, cytokine dependent and able to give an 800-1,000 fold increase in cell numbers within 14 days. Furthermore, while the system was established with small culture volumes (1.0 ml) it is easily scaled up to 500-1,000 ml without any reduction in cell generation capacity. The cells generated by this culture system

Correspondence: Dr. David N. Haylock, Leukaemia Research Unit, Hanson Centre for Cancer Research, Institute of Medical and Veterinary Science, P.O. Box 14, Rundle Mall, SA 5000, Adelaide, South Australia.

 ISBN 1-880854 17-1

progress through orderly myeloid maturation as assessed by morphology and immunophenotypic changes. The cells are functional in both superoxide anion production and transmigration assays.

Materials and Methodology

Source of Hemopoietic Progenitor Cells

Ex vivo culture can be performed on $CD34^+$ cells from either bone marrow or peripheral blood. Bone marrow collected by aspiration should be anticoagulated with preservative free heparin (20 units/ml). In steady state peripheral blood, $CD34^+$ cells are usually less than 0.1% of the mononuclear cells (MNC), and therefore it is difficult to obtain sufficient progenitors for large volume cultures [8]. The ideal source of $CD34^+$ cells for ex vivo culture is the peripheral blood or apheresis product from patients treated for mobilization of hemopoietic progenitor cells. A number of regimes—including high dose cyclophosphamide with or without HGF or HGF alone—produces increased levels of circulating myeloid progenitors (CFU-GM) and $CD34^-$ cells [9, 10]. Apheresis performed with either heparin or acid citrate dextrose anticoagulation is equally suitable for subsequent processing of cells.

Processing and Enrichment of $CD34^+$ Cells from Blood and Bone Marrow

A variety of methods (as detailed in other sections of this manual) can be used to enrich $CD34^+$ cells for ex vivo expansion/maturation culture. Our underlying aim is to obtain $CD34^+$ cells at high purity and to use methods with high recovery. While many methods are suitable for yielding sufficient high purity $CD34^+$ cells for laboratory scale experiments, only a few are practical for rapid and aseptic processing of an entire apheresis collection where the enriched and cultured cells are intended for therapeutic use.

In our laboratory we rely on magnetic cell sorting (MACS) [11] or the CEPRATE™ system [12] for CD34 enrichment from high numbers (5×10^8 – 1×10^{10}) of cells.

Collecting $CD34^+$ Cells by MACS

The MACS system (Miltenyi Biotec GmbH, Bergisch Gladbach 1, Germany) as described in detail by Miltenyi [11] relies on the capture of cells coated with magnetic microspheres. The cell suspension is labeled either directly with a biotinylated CD34 antibody or indirectly with a biotinylated anti-mouse second antibody (Caltag Laboratories, South San Francisco, CA). Streptavidin conjugated magnetic microspheres and streptavidin-fluorescein isothiocyanate (FITC) are added to coat the immunolabeled positive cells. The magnetic microspheres facilitate capture as the cell suspension flows through a magnetized mesh, while the streptavidin-FITC allows flow cytometric analysis of the starting, enriched and depleted cell populations.

The instructions for labeling cells and magnetic sorting as provided by the manufacturer are comprehensive and if followed strictly will ensure good recovery and purity. It is important not to lengthen the times for immunolabeling, to pre-chill the mesh columns and to use only ice cold buffers for the loading, washing and collection phases. Failure to adhere to these instructions will decrease purity. $CD34^+$ cells collected by MACS have magnetic microspheres on their surface which degenerate during culture without affecting growth.

Miltenyi Biotec has recently developed a two step isolation kit specifically for $CD34^+$ cells and claims 90-95% purity, even from low $CD34^+$ starting populations such as steady state peripheral blood. At present this system is only for small scale preparations although a clinical scale unit is being planned.

Collecting $CD34^+$ Cells by CEPRATE™

Enrichment of $CD34^+$ cells by the laboratory scale and clinical scale system (CEPRATE™; CellPro, Bothell, WA) is based on cellular affinity immunoadsorption. A comprehensive description of the separation principle and operation of the device are provided in an earlier section by *Dr. Heimfeld*, pp. 231-239. A major advantage of the CEPRATE™ is that it is a computer controlled, closed sterile system with the capacity to rapidly enrich $CD34^+$ cells from $1\text{-}2 \times 10^{10}$ MNC.

When selecting $CD34^+$ cells from apheresis collections, we routinely perform density gradient separation and at least two slow speed centrifugation steps in calcium/magnesium free Hank's balanced salt solution (CMF-HBSS) to remove platelets. Following immunolabeling with biotinylated 12.8 (anti-CD34 monoclonal antibody provided by CellPro), the MNC are washed then resuspended in CMF-HBSS. Washing and resuspension of cells in RPMI 1640 media as recommended by CellPro, in our experience, induces cell aggregation and activation of platelets. When assessing the recovery and purity of $CD34^+$ cells collected from the CEPRATE™ it is essential to immunolabel with a CD34 monoclonal antibody such as HPCA-2 (Becton Dickinson, Mountain View, CA) which recognizes sialic acid and carbohydrate independent epitopes.

The CEPRATE™ device performs well and can enrich $CD34^+$ cells 74-326 fold with good recovery (mean 74%, range 63-105%). Table I shows details of enrichment and recovery from four experiments including two on steady state peripheral blood where initially only 0.1% of MNC were $CD34^+$.

Table I. Enrichment of CD34⁺ cells from apheresis collections using the CEPRATE™ device (CellPro, Bothell, WA).

Cell fraction	Exp 1	Exp 2	Exp 3	Exp 4	Mean
Pre-enrichment					
Cells (× 10^9)	3.93	8.55	10.8	2.9	
%CD34$^+$	0.1	0.9	0.5	0.1	
Total CD34$^+$ (× 10^6)	3.93	76.9	54.0	2.9	
Adsorbed					
Cells (× 10^6)	7.5	80.0	79.6	7.25	
%CD34$^+$	32.6	66.7	71.3	23.2	48.4
Total CD34$^+$ (× 10^6)	2.45	53.4	57.0	1.68	
% Recovery CD34$^+$	63	69.4	105	58	73.4
Fold enrichment of CD34$^+$ cells	326	74	143	232	193.7
Unadsorbed					
Cells (× 10^9)	3.62	9.1	10.5	2.79	
%CD34$^+$	0.0	0.0	0.0	0.0	
Total CD34$^+$ (× 10^6)	0.0	0.0	0.0	0.0	

The apheresis product was washed with calcium and magnesium free Hank's balanced salt solution (CMF-HBSS); and immunolabeled with biotinylated anti-CD34 monoclonal (12.8); then, after washing with CMF-HBSS, it was processed on the CEPRATE™ avidin column according to the manufacturer's instructions. The total nucleated cells, percentage of CD34$^+$ cells and the total number of CD34$^+$ cells were assessed in cell suspension prior to separation (pre-enrichment) in the adsorbed and unadsorbed cell fractions. The fold enrichment of CD34$^+$ cells in the adsorbed fraction was calculated by dividing the %CD34$^+$ in the adsorbed fraction by the %CD34$^+$ in the pre-enrichment suspension.

CD34$^+$ Enrichment from Small Volumes of Blood and Bone Marrow

Small volumes (10-40 ml) of bone marrow, blood and aliquots from apheresis collections are first processed to reduce the number of mature end cells then immunolabeled with fluorochrome conjugated CD34 monoclonal antibodies (e.g., HPCA-1 or HPCA-2: Becton Dickinson). CD34$^+$ cells are collected by fluorescence activated cell sorting (FACS).

Bone marrow is separated over a Lymphoprep density gradient (1.077 g/ml; Nycomed Pharma As, Oslo, Norway) then treated with soybean agglutinin (SBA, Vector Laboratories, Burlingame, CA) according to previously published methods [13]. The SBA negative or unagglutinated fraction usually contains 8-15% CD34$^+$ cells which reduces the FACS time considerably. Peripheral blood and apheresis samples are also separated over a Lymphoprep density gradient. A further enrichment of CD34$^+$ cells can be obtained by combining plastic adherence followed by removal of T lymphocytes, granulocytes and residual monocytes. The cells are incubated with a combination of CD2, CD3,

CD8, CD19, CD14 and CD11b monoclonal antibodies of immunoglobulin (Ig)G isotype. After washing, the cells can be mixed with sheep anti-mouse (SAM) magnetic beads (Dynal A.S. Skoyen, Oslo, Norway) or alternatively incubated with a biotinylated SAM antibody to facilitate subsequent binding of streptavidin magnetic microspheres (MACS system). Both methods rely on capture of the mature cells by their retention within a strong magnetic field. A 10-50 fold enrichment of $CD34^+$ cells can be achieved if the manufacturer's methods are followed carefully. Immunolabeling of $CD34^+$ cells is then achieved by using 12.8 (IgM anti-CD34: gift from *Dr. R. Andrews,* Fred Hutchinson Cancer Centre, Seattle, WA) and phycoerythrin conjugated sheep anti-mouse IgM (Caltag Laboratories).

Collecting CD34⁺ Cells by FACS

During and after immunolabeling the cell suspension should be kept on melting ice. The flow cytometer should be aligned, calibrated, and operated to ensure the highest possible purity and recovery. A small diameter 0.22 μ filter should be placed in the sheath fluid line, and the sheath and sample tubing should be flushed with 70% alcohol immediately prior to sorting to ensure sterility. It is advisable for investigators to perform their own cell sorting, but where this is not practical they should be intimately involved in setting sort regions and confirming the purity of sorted populations.

Aggregates and clumps of cells should be removed from the suspension and $CD34^+$ cells deposited into a complete medium (e.g., Iscove's modified Dulbecco's medium (IMDM)) containing 5% fetal calf serum (FCS). The sample and collection tubes should be maintained at 4°C to ensure high viability. On completion of the sort, a purity check is performed. The cells are centrifuged at 300 *g* for 10 minutes and resuspended in 250-500 μl. A trypan blue viability and cell count is performed so that accurate numbers of $CD34^+$ cells can be placed into the relevant culture system. It is not advisable to rely on electronic counts given by the cell sorter as these only indicate the number of events that fulfill the sort criteria and not the number of cells actually collected.

Irrespective of the methods used for enrichment, the $CD34^+$ cells collected by FACS show similar growth in our ex vivo cultures and hemopoietic clonogenic assays. In addition, cryopreserved mononuclear cells, immunolabeled and sorted for $CD34^+$ cells, have identical growth potential compared to fresh cells.

Culture System

The culture of $CD34^+$ cells is performed in a stroma-free, cytokine dependent suspension system similar to that first reported by Iscove [14]. The detailed method for myeloid cell expansion and maturation has been described previously [1]. Briefly, FACS-sorted or positive selected $CD34^+$ cells are resuspended in IMDM (Cytosystems, Castle Hill, NSW, Australia; cat #50-016-PA) supplemented with 30% FCS (PA Biologicals, Sydney, Australia; lot #06353), 1% bovine serum albumin (BSA: Fraction V lot #2153; Sigma-Aldrich, Castle Hill, NSW, Australia), 3 mMol/l l-glutamine and 5×10^{-5} mol/l β-mercaptoethanol. A combination of six HGF (all supplied by Amgen, Thousand Oaks, CA) namely interleukin 1 (IL-1), IL-3, IL-6, G-CSF, GM-CSF and Stem Cell Factor (SCF or kit ligand) are each added at a concentration of 10 ng/ml and the culture incubated at 37°C in 5% CO_2. A sterile working solution of each HGF is prepared at 1 μg/ml in IMDM/1% BSA so that 10 μl of each is added to a 1.0 ml culture, or alternatively a large volume of the six HGF mixture can be prepared and sterile filtered immediately prior to use. Additional HGF may be provided during culture at days 7 and 14. $CD34^+$ cells can be cultured in Terasaki wells (1-10 cells in 10 μl), 96 well plates (100-500 cells in 200 μl), 24 well plates (1,000-3,000 cells in 1.0 ml), tissue culture flasks or bags using this media and HGF combination. We routinely use sterile individually wrapped wells or plates manufactured by either Costar (Cambridge, MA) or Nunc (Denmark).

Factors Influencing Cell Growth

Hemopoietic Growth Factors

As shown in Figure 1 and previously reported [1] the choice of HGF is critical for optimization of the myeloid progenitor cell and nucleated cell generation capacity of this system. The $CD34^+$ cell population is heterogeneous as it contains primitive and committed hemopoietic progenitor cells. The combination of IL-1, IL-3, IL-6, G-CSF, GM-CSF and SCF is an excellent synergistic combination of HGF with the ability to stimulate proliferation and differentiation of both primitive and committed cells, both those present initially and those generated in culture. Omission of G-CSF or SCF from this combination results in significant decreases in production of nucleated cells and CFU-GM (unpublished observation). Omission of other single HGF also decreases cell production albeit to a lesser extent but nevertheless indicates that all HGF are required for optimal growth.

The system has been improved by dose titration of each HGF. We now recommend using G-CSF and SCF at 100 ng/ml rather than 10 ng/ml. Also a more frequent addition of fresh HGF, particularly SCF, may be beneficial. Clearly there remains great scope for examining the interaction between these and other HGF and for further improvement in expansion and/or differentiation of stem and progenitor cells.

Erythropoietin (EPO) has been suggested by other investigators to improve growth of myeloid cells in similar stroma-free suspension cultures. We have

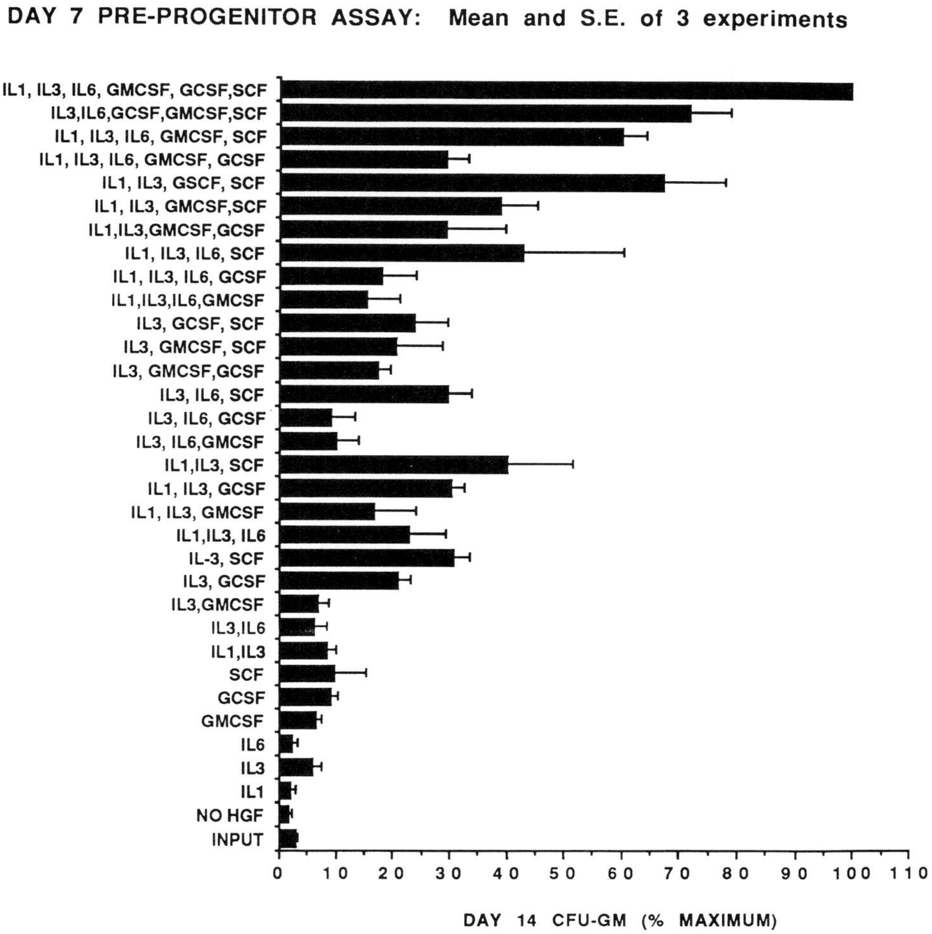

Fig. 1. The effect of single hemopoietic growth factors (HGF) or combinations of HGF on the generation of nascent CFU-GM after seven days of suspension culture of peripheral blood CD34+ cells. Triplicate 1.0 ml cultures were initiated with 1×10^3 FACS-sorted CD34+ in 24 well plates. The following HGF were used at 10 ng/ml either alone or in the combinations shown: IL-1 beta, IL-3, IL-6, G-CSF, GM-CSF and SCF. On day 7, the contents of each well were cultured to determine the number of CFU-GM present. The data from each experiment were first normalized by expressing CFU-GM output for each HGF combination as a percentage of the maximum, which in each case occurred with the six factor combination. The mean ± SEM of the three experiments is shown.

not found an increase in myeloid cell production by the addition of EPO. However we are able to generate significant numbers of nucleated erythroid cells (70,000 cells from 1,000 CD34+ cells in seven days) by adding four units/ml of EPO (Eprex, 2,000 U/ml; Janssen Cilag, Auckland, New Zealand) to the six HGF combination.

Media and Supplements

The choice of basal media for culture is probably not critical provided sufficient essential and non-essential amino acids, vitamins, inorganic salts, trace elements and sources of energy are provided. Iscove's modification of Dulbecco's minimal essential medium is adequate, and as such we have not tested any alternatives. The media supplements are however critical for supporting growth. When fetal calf serum or human serum is used as a source of lipid, protein and undefined mitogens, it is essential to screen batches for activity and to titrate the serum concentration.

We prepare all media and BSA solutions with endotoxin free water generated from a MilliQ UF Plus water system (Millipore: MA). Prior to use, the BSA is deionized with at least three exchanges of mixed resin beads (Duolite BM6113 beads, BDH, Poole, England). After preparation the complete medium containing 30% FCS and 1% BSA is sterile filtered through 0.22 μ filters (Costar, Cambridge, MA or Gelman Sciences, Ann Arbor, MI) and then aliquoted into 30 ml lots. The sterile media can be stored at –20°C for at least two months.

In serum free or serum deprived media it is necessary to provide insulin, transferrin and appropriate lipid sources. A great deal of experimentation may be required to optimize these media. A number of biotechnology companies (e.g., GIBCO, BioWhittaker) now manufacture completely defined media for culture of hemopoietic cells. These need to be tested with $CD34^+$ cells and appropriate HGF under the incubation conditions in individual laboratories to confirm their usefulness.

Large Volume Maturation Cultures

The main objective of clinical scale expansion/maturation cultures is to generate sufficient post-progenitor cells for transplantation. The $CD34^+$ cells need to be cultured in a system that supports continued cell proliferation and high viability. Two approaches can be taken: static culture or perfusion culture.

In static culture systems the cell concentration should be kept below 2×10^6 cells/ml otherwise cell viability is reduced significantly (unpublished observation). Thus if an ex vivo culture is started with 2×10^7 $CD34^+$ cells and a 500 fold expansion of nucleated cells is required to generate an estimated target number of post-progenitor myeloid cells for infusion, a five liter culture is required. We have successfully used Fenwal life cell tissue culture flasks (Baxter Healthcare Corporation, Deerfield, IL) for this type of culture. Two types of flasks/bags are manufactured: a) PL269 is a transparent bag designed for cryopreservation of bone marrow or PBSC, and b) PL732 was specifically designed for cell culture and has better gas exchange characteristics but is opaque, thus preventing microscopic examination of cells during culture. Either bag is suitable for culture of CD34+ cells despite allowing monocytes and macrophages to adhere during the latter stages of culture. The bags have two ports for introduction of cells and culture media and collection during the culture period. Each time the sampling port is used, a new sterile three-way tap is connected to prevent contamination.

It is important to consider the volume cultured in bags as this will affect gas exchange and buffering capacity of the system. Other variables likely to influence the growth of cells include the concentration of CD34+ cells at the start of culture and incubation at low oxygen tension.

Perfusion culture offers the potential advantage of being able to grow cells at much higher density than static cultures [15]. The system provides a continuous supply of culture medium and HGF and should be able to remove toxic metabolites and inhibitors. We have performed some preliminary testing of the CELLMAX Quad artificial capillary cell culture system (Cellco, Germantown, MD) for culture of CD34+ cells. This system does support expansion and maturation of CD34+ cells, although from our limited experience it seems no better than large volume cultures in flasks. However fully optimized perfusion culture of CD34+ cells may be better than static cultures, given the excellent results achieved by other investigators for the culture of T lymphocytes.

Assessing Ex Vivo Cultures

It is essential that ex vivo cultures of CD34+ cells be monitored to completely describe the type of cells produced and to assess the safety of the product prior to infusion. Such assessment should include:

- Total viable nucleated cell counts. Examination of trypan blue stained cells under phase contrast is adequate.
- Clonogenic assays to determine the number of myeloid CFU, megakaryocytic-CFU and erythroid burst forming units.
- Flow cytometric analysis to document cell differentiation by the loss or acquisition of specific antigens (e.g., CD34, CD33, CD11b, glycophorin A, etc.).
- Cell morphology from Romanovsky or esterase stained cytospin preparations.
- Alkaline phosphatase anti-alkaline phosphatase (APAAP) staining of cytospins specifically for megakaryocytic cells.
- Bacteriological culture and Gram stains.
- Endotoxin levels by limulus amebocyte lysate testing.
- Transmigration and superoxide anion assays to assess the function of cells.

Discussion

This section describes the ex vivo culture of $CD34^+$ cells with the specific aim of driving myeloid maturation rather than expanding primitive hemopoietic progenitor cells. The culture system is cytokine dependent and a specific six HGF combination has been identified that generates significant numbers of post-progenitor myeloid cells. Importantly there are also many nascent CFU-GM generated under the same conditions. It is feasible that a 14 day ex vivo clinical scale culture initiated from 200 ml of leukapheresis product could contain more CFU-GM than normally infused for a PBSC autograft. Erythropoietin does not increase the number of myeloid cells generated in cultures but generates large numbers of nucleated erythroid cells.

The culture system also supports growth of megakaryocytic precursors and progenitors (CFU-Meg) suggesting that infusion of ex vivo expanded cells may hasten platelet recovery. Further work in our laboratory is aimed at defining HGF combinations that preferentially expand megakaryocytic cells.

It is essential that any system for ex vivo culture of hemopoietic progenitor cells be reproducible both in terms of the cell generation capacity and the rate of cell proliferation. Therefore initiating cultures with pure $CD34^+$ cells is preferable, especially as contaminating $CD34^-$ cells such as T lymphocytes and monocytes could effect cell growth either directly by cell-cell contact or indirectly by production of other cytokines and inhibitors. We suggest that at a minimum the cell population cultured should comprise 50-75% $CD34^+$ cells so as to minimize the unpredictable influence of $CD34^-$ cells.

We have previously postulated that ex vivo cultured cells need to be capable of maintaining a neutrophil count of greater than 0.5×10^9/l for 10 days after infusion and should contain enough progenitors and post-progenitors to maintain a steady supply of granulocytes from one to three days of infusion. Assuming a neutrophil half-life of six hours, a blood volume of five liters and increased neutrophil consumption in the neutropenic state, then approximately 2×10^{11} neutrophils would be required over 10 days. Furthermore, if we assume that one promyelocyte is capable of generating 32 neutrophils, as suggested by previous studies on the kinetics of myelopoiesis, then at least 6.25×10^9 promyelocytes would be required over 10 days to produce 2×10^{11} neutrophils. The culture system described herein is capable of generating this number of promyelocytes from 2×10^7 $CD34^+$ cells after 14 days when a 500-600 fold increase in cell numbers is routinely obtained. A five liter culture is required to achieve this yield.

It is essential in all ex vivo cultures of $CD34^+$ cells to characterize the cells produced. At a minimum, cell viability, morphology and lineage should be defined by examination of appropriately stained cytospin preparations and immunophenotypic analysis.

References

1 Haylock DN, To LB, Dowse TL, Juttner CA, Simmons PJ. Ex vivo expansion and maturation of peripheral blood CD34+ cells into the myeloid lineage. Blood 1992:80;1405-1412.

2 Meunch MO, Moore MAS. Accelerated recovery of peripheral blood cell counts in mice transplanted with in vitro cytokine – expanded hematopoietic progenitors. Exp Hematol 1992:20;611-618.

3 Berenson RJ, Besinger WI, Hill RS, Andrews RG, Garcia-Lopez J, Kalamosz DF, Still BS, Spitzer G, Buckner CD, Beinstein ID, Thomas ED. Engraftment after infusion of CD34+ marrow cells in patients with breast cancer or neuroblastoma. Blood 1991:77;1717-1722.

4 Wagemaker G, van Gils FCJM, Bart-Baumeister JAK, Weilenger JJ, Levinsky RJ. Sustained engraftment of allogeneic CD34 positive hemopoietic stem cells in rhesus monkeys. Exp Hematol 1990:18;704-709.

5 Civin CI, Strauss LC, Brovall C, Fackler MJ, Schwartz JF, Shaper JH. Antigenic analysis of hematopoiesis III. A hematopoietic progenitor cell surface antigen defined by a monoclonal antibody raised against KG1a cells. J Immunol 1984:133;157-165.

6 Andrews RG, Singer JW, Beinstein ID. Monoclonal antibody 12.8 recognizes a 115-kd molecule present on both unipotent and multipotent colony-forming cells and their precursors. Blood 1986:67;842-845.

7 Sutherland HJ, Eaves CJ, Eaves AC, Dragowska W, Lansdorp PM. Characterization and partial purification of human marrow cells capable of initiating long-term hematopoiesis in vitro. Blood 1989:74;1563-1570.

8 Bender JG, Unverzagt KL, Walker DE, Lee W, Van Epps DE, Smith DH, Stewart CC, To LB. Identification and comparison of CD34 positive cells from normal peripheral blood and bone marrow using multiflow cytometry. Blood 1991:17;2591-2596.

9 Siena S, Bregni M, Brando B, Ravagnani F, Bonadonna G, Gianni AM. Circulation of CD34+ hematopoietic stem cells in the peripheral blood of high-dose cyclophosphamide-treated patients: Enhancement by intravenous recombinant human granulocyte-macrophage colony-stimulating factor. Blood 1989:74;1904-1914.

10 Sheridan WP, Begley CG, Juttner CA, Szer J, To LB, Maher D, McGrath K, Morstyn G, Fox RM. Effect of peripheral-blood progenitor cells mobilized by filgrastim (G-CSF) on platelet recovery after high-dose chemotherapy. Lancet 1992:339;640-644.

11 Miltenyi S, Meuller W, Weichel W, Radbruch A. High gradient magnetic cell separation with MACS. Cytometry 1990:11;231-238.

12 Heimfeld S, Andrews R, Zsebo K, Fogarty B, McGuire K, Williams S, Berenson R. Peripheral blood stem cell mobilization after stem cell factor (SCF) or G-CSF treatment: Rapid enrichment for stem and progenitor cells using the CEPRATE immuno-affinity separation system. Exp Hematol 1992:22;748a.

13 Simmons PJ, Torok-Storb B. Identification of stromal cell precursors in human bone marrow by a novel monoclonal antibody, STRO-1. Blood 1991:78;55-62.

14 Iscove NN, Shaw AR, Keller G. Net increase of pluripotential hematopoietic precursors in suspension culture to IL-1 and IL-3. J Immunol 1989:142;2332-2337.

15 Knight P. Hollow fiber bioreactors for mammalian cell culture. Biotechnology 1989:7;459-466.

Stem Cell Differentiation Into Mature Lymphocytes Using the SCID Mouse Thymus Chimera Model

Magda De Smedt, Georges Leclercq, Bart Vandekerckhove, Jean Plum
Department of Clinical Chemistry, Microbiology and Immunology, University of Ghent, University Hospital, Ghent, Belgium

Key Words. Hematopoietic stem cell • CD34 • Fetal liver cell • Fetal thymus organ culture • In vitro human T cell differentiation • Thymus • SCID mice

Introduction

Whereas in vitro stem cell assays are available for human myelopoiesis and B lymphocyte development, this is not the case for T cells. For T cell development, the three dimensional structure of the thymus seems to be indispensable. In the murine system, the fetal thymic organ culture (FTOC), originally described by *Jenkinson et al.,* is an excellent method to study thymocyte development. In addition, it allows several manipulations that are difficult or impossible to do in vivo.

Here we describe a method in which human fetal liver precursor cells are transferred to murine severe combined immunodeficient (SCID) fetal thymic lobes. The thymic lobes are cultured in a classical FTOC afterwards. A complete human T cell differentiation is achieved with this in vitro method.

Materials and Methodology

Human fetal liver cells: preparation, freezing and thawing

We obtain fetal liver tissues from fetuses after legal termination of pregnancy (gestational age ranges from week 18 to 22) and they are used following the guidelines of the medical ethical commission of the University Hospital of Ghent, Belgium. To have easy access to human fetal liver cells, we prefer to freeze them in liquid nitrogen. This has the additional advantage that several experiments can be done with the cells from one donor. The tissue is placed in Iscove's Modified Dulbecco's Medium (IMDM) with 10% heat inactivated (30 min at 56°C) fetal calf serum (FCS), 0.03% glutamine, penicillin (100 IU/ml) and streptomycin (100 μg/ml) (all from GIBCO). This medium will be further referred to as "complete medium". With scissors, the tissue is cut in small pieces, which are pushed through a cell strainer (Falcon). After centrifugation (5 min, 200 *g*, 4°C), cells are washed once in complete medium. Afterwards, cells are resuspended in complete medium and layered over Lymphoprep

Correspondence: Dr. Jean Plum, Department of Clinical Chemistry, Microbiology and Immunology, University of Ghent, University Hospital, Blok A, De Pintelaan 185, B-9000 Ghent, Belgium.

(density 1.077 g/cm^3) (Nycomed Pharma). After centrifugation (30 min, 800 *g*, 20°C), cells at the interface are aspirated and washed twice in complete medium. Cells are resuspended in ice cold FCS/dimethyl sulfoxide (DMSO) (90%/10%) at a cell density of 10^7 cells/ml. Cells are frozen overnight at –70°C, afterwards they are transferred to liquid nitrogen. For each experiment, one or more vials are thawed. This is done as quickly as possible. One, two and four ml of cold complete medium is added dropwise after one, two and three min respectively. After centrifugation (5 min, 200 *g*, 4°C), cells are washed twice.

Immunomagnetic depletion of fetal liver cells

After thawing, the human fetal liver cells are transferred as such to SCID fetal thymic lobes, or they are depleted of mature T cells by immunomagnetic depletion. For this purpose, cells are resuspended in cold PBS/2% FCS and labeled with biotinylated anti-CD3, anti-CD4 and anti-CD8 (all from Becton Dickinson Immunology System [BDIS]). One μg of each MAb is added per 10^6 cells. After incubation (30 min at 4°C), cells are washed twice in cold PBS/2% FCS. Afterwards, the cells are resuspended in 100 μl PBS/FCS, and 100 μl pre-washed (to remove the preservative) anti-streptavidin coated Dynabeads (Dynal) are added (ratio of cells/Dynabeads = 1/3). After 20 min at 4°C, 2 ml of PBS/2% FCS is carefully added and the rosettes of Dynabeads-cells are removed by placing the tube on a magnetic particle concentrator (Dynal). The supernatant containing the $CD3^-CD4^-CD8^-$ cells is decanted, centrifuged and the cells are washed once with complete medium. Figure 1 shows the phenotype of the remaining cells after immunomagnetic depletion of CD3, CD4, and CD8 cells from human fetal liver cells.

Transfer of human fetal liver cells to SCID thymic lobes by hanging drop

Timed pregnant SCID mice (C.B-17 scid/scid) are obtained by mating them overnight in our animal breeding facility. Embryos are used at fetal day 14-15 (plug date = day 0). Thymic lobes are removed and placed in tris buffer. Residual tissue surrounding the thymic lobes is carefully removed. Twenty μl of complete medium containing 10^5 undepleted or 10^5 $CD3^-CD4^-CD8^-$ human fetal liver cells are added to each well of a Terasaki plate (Nunc). One thymic lobe is added to each well and the plate (without the lid) is inverted to form hanging drops. This will result in contact between the cells and the thymic lobe and in an adequate gas exchange. To prevent excessive evaporation, each Terasaki plate is placed in a 150 × 20 mm petri dish containing three to four 35 × 10 mm petri dishes (Falcon) filled with water (without the lid). The plates are incubated in a humidified incubator at 37°C with 7.5% CO_2 for 48 h.

Fetal thymic organ culture (FTOC)

Gelfoam gelatin sponges (Upjohn) (20 × 60 × 7 mm) are cut into 20 × 20 mm squares. One square is placed in a 35 × 10 mm petri dish, 3.5 ml complete

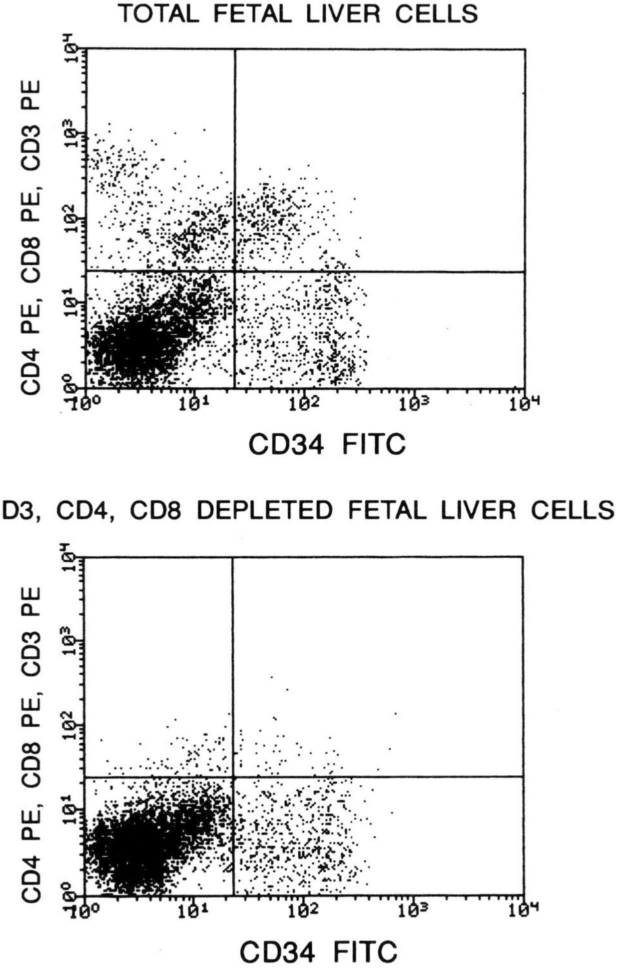

Fig. 1. Flow cytometric analysis of human fetal liver cells before and after immunomagnetic depletion of mature T cells. Human fetal liver cells were thawed and used as such or they were depleted of CD3, CD4, CD8 positive cells with Dynabeads. Cells were labeled with anti-CD34 FITC and with biotinylated CD3, CD4, CD8 and streptavidin PE.

medium is added and the petri dish is incubated in an incubator (37°C, 7.5% CO_2) for 2-3 h to saturate the sponges with medium. Afterwards, residual air bubbles in the Gelfoam are removed by squeezing the Gelfoam with sterile tweezers. A Nuclepore polycarbonate filter (Costar) (13 mm, 0.8 μm) (autoclaved before use) is placed on top of the Gelfoam sponge. The thymic lobes are removed from the Terasaki plates and washed in complete medium to remove liver cells that did not migrate into the thymic lobe. Four to six lobes are placed on the Nuclepore filters. We prefer to put the lobes 3-4 mm apart from each other rather than putting them together. This allows one to easily see if all the thymic lobes contain developing human cells as the lobes that were not seeded with human T cell precursors will remain small. The petri dishes are incubated at 37°C and 7.5% CO_2. For long-time cultures (>1 week), 1.5 ml medium is removed from each petri dish once a week and replaced by 1.5 ml fresh, prewarmed, complete medium.

Flow cytometric analysis of developing human T cells

At different time points, the thymic lobes are analyzed for the presence of the different maturational stages of human T cell development. The thymic lobes are carefully removed from the Nuclepore filters and placed in tris buffer without FCS. With a 2 ml tissue grinder (Kontes Glass) a cell suspension is made from the thymic lobes. Care should be taken that no thymic lobes or fragments from them are left. The cell suspension is removed from the tissue grinder and FCS is added to achieve a final concentration of 5%; this is done to prevent sticking of the cells to the tube. The cells are centrifuged and resuspended in PBS/1% bovine serum albumin (BSA)/0.1% NaN_3. Eosine is added to a small volume of the cell suspension and the cells are counted with a hematocytometer. More than 80% of the cells should be viable. Usually, we recover 50×10^3, 80×10^3 and 150×10^3 cells per lobe after one, two and three weeks of culture respectively. As the murine Fc receptor, that is abundant on SCID thymocytes, has the potential to bind added antibodies in an aspecific way, the Fc receptor should be blocked by addition of a saturating amount of anti-FcγRII MAb (clone 2.4.G2). We add 1 μg to 10^5 cells in 50 μl. Fifteen minutes later, without washing the cells, the antibodies of interest are added. We usually stain the cells with anti-CD1a, anti-CD3, anti-CD4, anti-CD8 and anti-TCRαβ (all from BDIS). Isotype controls are included in all staining series. After labeling, cells are washed twice with PBS/BSA/NaN_3. Biotinylated antibodies are revealed with streptavidin-PE or streptavidin-cychrome (BDIS). Anti-mouse CD45 (clone MI-9.3 HL) (GIBCO) and anti-human CD45 (clone HLe-1) (BDIS) are used to discriminate between murine and human cells. Figure 2 shows the dot plot analysis of anti-human CD45 fluorescein isothiocyanate (FITC) and anti-mouse CD45 phycoerythrin (PE) labeled cells from a chimeric FTOC. Figure 3 shows CD3, CD4 and CD8 expression of the human cells in the chimeric FTOC as a function of duration of the culture. Usually, we obtain human $CD4^{low}$ $CD3^{-}$ cells after 10-14 days of FTOC, the first CD4-CD8 double positive cells after 2-3 weeks and CD4 and CD8 single positive $CD3^{high}$ cells after 3-4 weeks.

Discussion

In our hands, the chimeric FTOC is a reproducible method to achieve the full differentiation of human thymocytes starting from human fetal liver precursors. Up to now, we have used four different sources of fetal liver cells and 98% of the cultures were successful (more than 300 lobes examined).

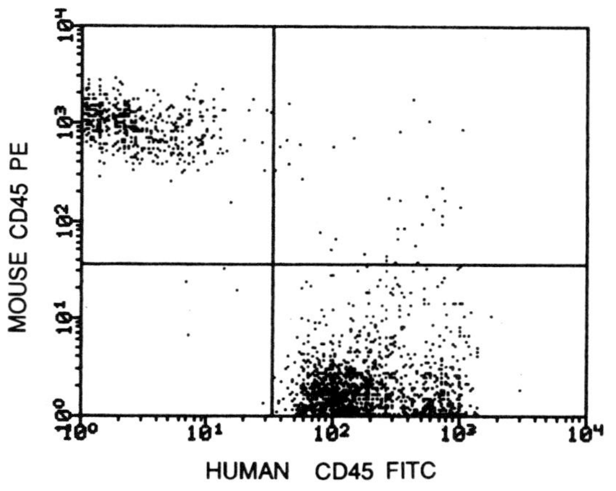

Fig. 2. Discrimination of murine and human cells after chimeric FTOC. CD3⁻CD4⁻CD8⁻ human fetal liver cells were transferred to fetal murine SCID thymic lobes. After 20 days of FTOC, cells were stained with anti-human CD45 FITC and anti-mouse CD45 PE.

Several parameters are important to obtain a successful experiment. First of all, the fetal liver cells should be frozen as quickly as possible after removal from the embryo, normally the same day. The way of freezing and thawing the human fetal liver cells is of crucial importance as a wrong manipulation will result in excessive cell death and eventual loss of the precursor activity. Also the cell density seems to be important for freezing the cells; we obtain good results with 10^7 cells per ml, a higher cell density should be avoided.

The removal of thymic lobes from fetal day 14 embryos requires practice. When doing it for the first time, it is easiest to have it demonstrated. If this is not possible, it is probably better to start with fetal day 16, and later with fetal day 15 embryos. It is important to work as quickly as possible, because the pH of the buffer and the medium in which the thymic lobes are placed changes gradually. This is certainly the case when placing the cells and the thymic lobes in the Terasaki plates, as only a very small volume of medium is present in each well. When one has no experience with FTOC, it is better to start with the classical FTOC in which fetal day 14 thymic lobes from *normal* murine embryos (instead of SCID mice) are cultured in FTOC, without the initial hanging drop culture and without transferring human cells. When the classical FTOC goes well (2-3 × 10^5 cells and 60-70% CD4-CD8 double positive cells after seven days of culture), one can shift to the chimeric human-murine FTOC. An important parameter in the FTOC method is the FCS batch as a variety of factors present in the FCS can affect the culture. Therefore, several batches of FCS should be tested in advance. The cell number obtained and the CD4-CD8 pattern can be used as a guideline for choosing the right FCS batch.

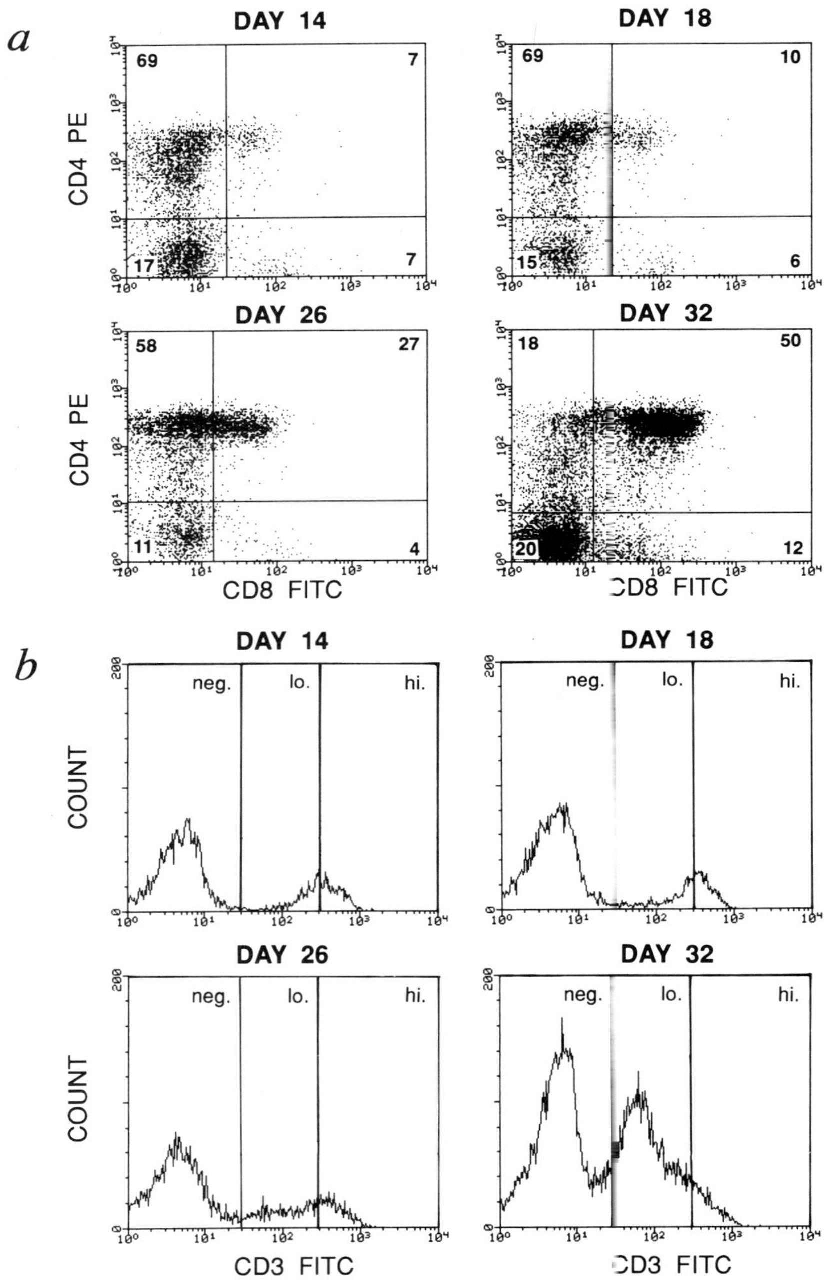

Fig. 3. Kinetic analysis of CD4, CD8 and CD3 expression on human cells in chimeric FTOC. $CD3^{-}CD4^{-}CD8^{-}$ human fetal liver cells were transferred to fetal murine SCID thymic lobes. At the indicated days of FTOC, cells were labeled with anti-human CD8 FITC and anti-human CD4 PE, or with anti-human CD3 FITC. Dot plots are shown for CD4-CD8 expression (a), histograms for CD3 expression (b).

We have always worked with thymic lobes from SCID mice. As a result of a defective recombination of the genes coding for the antigen receptor, these mice have an impaired thymocyte maturation: it is blocked before the CD4-CD8 double positive stage. This gives space for concurrent maturation of xenogeneic cells. When timed pregnant SCID mice are not easily available, one can also use fetal thymic lobes from normal mice. However, in this case the hematopoietic cells have to be removed from the murine thymic lobe. This can easily be done by treatment with 2-deoxyguanosine (1.35 mM) for five days. Afterwards, the lobes should be extensively washed to remove residual 2-deoxyguanosine as this would prevent any maturation of subsequently seeded human fetal liver cells.

During the hanging drop culture, the humidity is especially important. The Terasaki plate should be surrounded with petri dishes filled with water. For the same reason, we also never add thymic lobes in the outer wells of the plate. In the FTOC, the number of lobes should not be lower than three and not higher than 6-8 lobes per 13 mm polycarbonate filter. As there is sometimes some variability in the thickness of the Gelfoam sponge (normally seven mm), one should adjust the volume of the medium added to the petri dish when the sponge is considerably thinner: the lobes always have to be cultured at the liquid-air interface. When the cells are analyzed after FTOC, one should be aware that murine thymocytes are still present. Approximately 20,000 murine cells per lobe are present during the first three weeks of culture; their number drops afterwards. A discrimination between murine and human cells can be made by labeling the cells with anti-mouse and anti-human CD45. Another fact is that a high percentage of SCID thymocytes express the Fc receptor. As this could result in nonspecific binding of antibodies during the labeling procedure, the Fc receptor should be blocked with anti-Fc receptor antibody prior to adding the other antibodies.

In conclusion, full human T cell development can be achieved starting from fetal liver precursor cells with the method described here. The in vitro character of the method offers a number of advantages, such as the possibility to better define human stem cell populations and to study and manipulate various growth and differentiation factors in the thymus.

Acknowledgments

We thank *C. De Boever* for artwork. This work was supported by grants from National Fund for Scientific Research (NFWO), Fund for Concerned Research Program (OOA) and Flemish Action Program from Biotechnology (VLAB).

Selected Readings

Jenkinson EJ, Franchi LL, Kingston R, Owen JJT. Effect of deoxyguanosine on lymphopoiesis in the developing thymus rudiment in vitro: application in the production of chimeric thymus rudiments. Eur J Immunol 1982;12:583-587.

Ready AR, Jenkinson EJ, Kingston R, Owen JJT. Successful transplantation across major histocompatibility barrier of deoxyguanosine-treated embryonic thymus expressing class II antigens. Nature 1984;310:231-233.

Kingston R, Jenkinson EJ, Owen JJT. A single stem cell can recolonize an embryonic thymus, producing phenotypically distinct T cell populations. Nature 1985;317:811-813.

Ceredig R. Differentiation potential of 14-day fetal mouse thymocytes in organ culture: analysis of CD4/CD8-defined single-positive and double-negative cells. J Immunol 1988;141:355-362.

Watanabe Y, Gyotoku J-I, Katsura Y. Analysis of the development of T cells by transferring precursors into cultured fetal thymus with a microinjector. Thymus 1989;13:57-71.

Plum J, De Smedt M, Leclercq G. Exogenous IL-7 promotes the growth of $CD3^{-}CD4^{-}CD8^{-}CD44^{+}CD25^{\pm}$ precursor cells and blocks the differentiation pathway of TCR-αβ cells in fetal thymus organ culture. J Immunol 1992;150:2706-2716.

Fisher AG, Larsson L, Goff LK, Restall DE, Happerfield L, Merkenschlager M. Human thymocyte development in mouse organ cultures. Int Immunol 1990;2:571-578.

Merkenschlager M, Fisher AG. Human postnatal thymocytes generate phenotypically immature $CD3^{dim}$, $CD5^{dim}$, $CD1a^{bright}$ progeny in organ culture. J Immunol 1992;148:1012-1015.

Ramsdell F. Fetal thymus organ culture for T cell development studies. In: Coligan JE, Kruisbeek AM, Margulies DH, Shevach EM, Strober W, eds. Current protocols in Immunology. New York: John Wiley & Sons, 1991;3.18:1-10.

Companies

Becton Dickinson Immunocytometry Systems, 2350 Qume Drive, San José, CA 95131, USA, 800-223-8226 FAX: 408-954-2009

Dynal, 457 Northern Boulevard, Great Neck, NY 11021, 516-829-0039 FAX: 516-829-0045

Becton Dickinson Labware (Falcon products), 2 Bridgewater Lane, Lincoln, NJ 07035, USA, 800-235-5953 FAX: 201-628-1533

Life Technologies (GIBCO), P.O. Box 68, Grand Island, NY 14072-0068, 800-828-6686 FAX: 800-331-2286

Kontes Glass, P.O. Box 729, Vineland, NJ 08360, 800-223-7150 FAX: 609-692-3242

Costar, 1 Alewife Center, Cambridge, MA 02140, 800-492-1110 FAX: 617-868-2076

Nunc, 2000 North Aurora Road, Naperville, IL 60563, 800-288-6862 FAX: 708-416-2556

Nycomed Pharma As, P. O. Box 5012 Majorstua, N-0301 Oslo, Norway, 47-22-96-36-36 FAX: 47-22-96-35-30

Upjohn, 7000 Portage Road, Kalamazoo, MI 49001, 616-323-4000 FAX: 616-323-7034

Author Index

Subject Index

Suppliers

Amgen Biologicals, Amgen Center, 12301 Parklawn Dr., Rockville, MD 20852, USA, Tel: 800-638-6597.

Applied Immune Sciences, Inc., 200 Constitution Drive, Menlo Park, CA 94025-1109, USA, Tel: 415-326-7302; **Applied Immune Sciences, Inc.,** 5301 Patrick Henry Drive, Santa Clara, CA 95054-1114, USA, Tel: 408-492-9200, Fax: 408-980-5888.

Baxter Deutschland GmbH, Bibliotek Postfach 1165, 85701 Unterschleissheim, The Netherlands.

Baxter Healthcare Corporation, Fenwal Biomedical Therapy Systems, 3015 South Daimler, Santa Ana, CA 92705, USA.

Baxter-Hyland, Glendale, CA, USA.

Baysilan, Bayer Leverkusen, Germany.

BDH Ltd., Broom Road, Poole, Dorset BH12 4NN, United Kingdom, Tel: 44-202-745520, Fax: 44-202-738299.

Beckman Instruments Inc., 2500 Harbor Blvd., Fullerton, CA, 92634 USA, Tel: 800-742-2345, Fax: 714-773-8898 and Gagny, France.

Becton Dickinson Immunocytometry Systems, 2350 Qume Drive, San José, CA 95131-1807, USA, Tel: 800-223-8226 or 800-448-BDIS, Fax: 408-954-2009; **European HQ:** Denderstraat 24, B-9320 Erembodegem-Aalst, Belgium, Tel: 32-53-720211, Fax: 32-53-720450.

Becton Dickinson Labware (Falcon Products), 2 Bridgewater Lane, Lincoln, NH 07035, USA, Tel: 800-235-5953, Fax: 201-628-1533.

Behringwerke Ag, Emil-von-Behring-Strasse 76, Marburg, Lahn 3350, Germany, Tel: 49-6421-39-0, Fax: 49-6421-39-31388.

Biocytex, 140 Chemin de l'Armèe d'Afrique, 13000 Marseille, France, Tel: 33-91-94-29-39, Fax: 33-91-47-24-71.

Bio-Rad Chemical Division, 1414 Harbor Way South, Richmond, CA 94804, USA, Tel: 415-232-7000, and Munich, Germany.

Bio-Whittaker, P.O. Box 127, Biggs Ford Road, Walkersville, MD 21793-0127, USA, Tel: 301-898-7025.

Boehringer-Mannheim Biochemicals, P.O. Box 50816, Indianapolis, IN 46250-0414, USA, Tel: 800-428-5433.

Boots Pharmaceuticals Inc., 300 Tri State International Center, Lincolnshire, IL 60069, USA, Tel: 708-405-7400, Fax: 708-405-7505.

Calbiochem-Novabiochem Corp., 10933 N. Torrey Pines Road, P.O. Box 12087, La Jolla, CA 92039-2087, USA, Tel: 800-854-3417, Fax: 619-453-3552.

Caltag Laboratories, 436 Rozzi Place, South San Francisco, CA 94080, USA, Tel: 800-874-4007 or 415-873-6106, Fax: 415-873-2113.

Cellco, Inc., 12331 Middlebrook Road, Germantown, MD 20874, USA, Tel: 800-253-1803 or 301-916-1000, Fax: 301-916-1010.

CellPro, Inc., 22322 - 20th Avenue SE, Suite #100, Bothell, WA 98021, USA, Tel: 800-221-2778, Fax: 206-485-4787.

Clay Adams.

Cobe Laboratories, Inc., 1185 Oak St., Lakewood, CO 80215, USA, Tel: 302-232-6800.

Coherent/Coherent, Inc., Laser Products Div., 3210 Porter Drive, P.O. Box 10321, Palo Alto, CA 94303, USA, Tel: 415-93-2111, Fax: 415-858-7631, and France.

©AlphaMed Press ISBN 1-880854 17-1

Computer Associates International, One Computer Associates Plaza, Islandia, NY 11788-7000, USA, Tel: 800-531-5236.

Connaught, Willowdale, Ontario, Canada.

Consul T. S., Bruimo, Italy.

Corning Glass Works, Corning, NY 14831, USA, Tel: 607-737-1640, and Avon, France.

Costar, 1 Alewife Center, Cambridge, MA 02140, USA, Tel: 800-492-1110 Fax: 617-868-2076.

Coulter Corp., 601 W. 20th St., Hialeah, FL 33012, USA, Tel: 305-885-0131, Fax: 305-883-6820.

Coulter Electronics, Inc., P.O. Box 4486, Hialeah, FL 33014, USA, Tel: 800-633-7427 ext. 4866, Fax: 305-883-6805.

Coulter Immunology, Hialeah, FL, USA.

Coultronics, Mountain View, CA, USA.

Cricket Software, *See* Computer Associates International.

Cryoson Deutschland GmbH.

Cutter Biological, Fourth & Parker Sts., P.O. Box 1986, Berkeley, CA 94701, USA, Tel: 800-227-1762.

Cytosystems, Castle Hill, NSW, Australia.

Delmed Inc., New Brunswick, NJ, USA.

Dianova, Postfach 101705, D-20011, Hamburg, Germany, Tel: 40-32-30-74, Fax: 40-32-21-90.

Dynal International, Dynal AS, P.O. Box 158, Skoyen, N-0212 Oslo, Norway, Tel: +47-22-529450, Fax: +47-22-507015, Tlx: 79133; ***USA/Canada:*** Dynal Inc., 5 Delaware Drive, Lake Success, NY 11042 USA, Tel: 800-638-9416, Fax: 516-326-3298; Dynal, 475 Northern Boulevard, Great Neck, NY 10021, Tel: 516-829-0039 or 800-638-9416, Fax: 516-829-0045; ***UK/Ireland:*** Dynal UK, 26 Grove Street, New Ferry, Wirral, L62 5AZ UK, Tel: 051-644-6555, Fax: 051-645-2094; ***Germany/Austria:*** Deutsche Dynal GmbH, Postfach 11 19 65, D-20419 Hamburg, Germany, Tel: 040-366811, Fax: 040-366040; ***France:*** Dynal France S.A., Contre de Transfort de, 1 U.T.C., 66 Av. de Londshut, 60200 Compeigne, France, Tel: 44-23-45-95, Fax: 44-23-16-14; ***Japan:*** Nihon Dynal K.K., Champion Bldg., 1-1-9, Atago, Minato-Ku, Tokyo 105, Japan, Tel: 03-3435-1558, Fax: 03-3435-1526.

Eastman Kodak. 343 State St., Rochester, NY 14650, USA, Tel: 800-242-2424.

Elkins-Sinn, Inc., Cherry Hill, NJ, USA.

Esquire Chemic AG, Obere Zaune 12, P.O. Box 315-CH-8025 Zurich, Switzerland, Tel: 41-1-259-82-96, Fax: 41-1-259-21-77.

Eurobio, 7 Avenue de Scandinavie, Z.A. de Courtaboeuf, F-91953 Les Ulis, Cedex, France, Tel: 33-1-69-07-94-77, Fax: 33-69-07-95-34.

Exciton Chemical, 400 Linden Ave., Dayton, OH, USA, Tel: 513-252-2989.

Falcon Products (Becton Dickinson Labware), 2 Bridgewater Lane, Lincoln, NJ 07035, USA, Tel: 800-235-5953, Fax: 201-628-1533.

Fenwal. *See* Baxter Healthcare Corporation.

Flobio, 31, 33 rue de Lambrechts, F-92400 Courbevoie, France, Tel: 33-1-47-88-84-76, Fax: 33-47-68-57-67.

Flow Cytometry Standards Corporation, P.O. Box 12621, Research Triangle Park, NC 27709, USA, Tel: 800-227-8143, Fax: 919-967-7325.

Flow Laboratories Inc., 7655 Old Springhouse Road, McLean, VA 22102, USA, Tel: 703-893-5925, Fax: 703-356-0774.

Terry Fox Laboratory, British Columbia Cancer Research Centre, 601 West 10th Ave., Vancouver, BC V5Z IL3, Canada, Tel: 604-877-0713, Fax: 604-877-0712.

Fresenius A.G., D-61343 Bad Homburg, Germany, Tel: 61-71-600, Fax: 61-71-77-40.

Fresenius USA, 4090 Pike Lane, Concord, CA, USA, Tel: 800-227-2572.

Gelman Sciences, 600 S. Wagner Road, Ann Arbor, MI 48106, USA, Tel: 313-665-0651, Fax: 313-761-1208.

GIBCO, Life Technologies, Inc., P.O. Box 68, Grand Island, NY 14072-0068, USA, Tel: 800-828-6686, Fax: 800-331-2286.

Haemonetics Corporation, 400 Wood Rd., Braintree, MA 02184, USA, Tel: 617-848-7100.

Heidolph-Elektro, Starenstrasse 23, Postfach 1240, D-8420 Kelheim, Germany, Tel: 49-9441-707-0, Fax: 49-9441-707.

IEC Centrifuges, B.P. 56, F-95612 Cergy Pontoise, Cedex, France, Tel: 33-1-30-37-12-00.

Immunotech S.A., 130 av. J. de Lattre de Tassigny, F-13009 Marseille, Cedex 9, France, Tel: 33-91-172700, Fax: 33-91-412794.

Janssen Cilag, Auckland, New Zealand.

Kanoldt Arzneimittel GmbH, Hoechstaedt, Germany.

Kontes Glass, P.O. Box 729, Vineland, NJ 08360, USA, Tel: 800-223-7150, Fax: 609-692-3242.

Lab System, Helsinki, Finland.

Labindustries, Inc., 620 Hearst Avenue, Berkeley, CA 94710-1814, USA, Tel: 800-227-0128 or 415-843-0220, Fax: 415-843-1814.

Labo Industries, BP 5965, F-37059 Tours, Cedex, France.

Laboratoires Maco-Pharma, 96 rue du Pont Rompu, 59200 Tourcoing, France, Tel: 33-20-23-4130, Fax: 33-20-23-4174.

Labsystems OY, Pulttitie 8, P.O. Box 8, SF-00881 Helsinki, Finland, Tel: 358-0-75821, Fax: 358-0-789469.

Mallinckrodt Specialty Chemicals Co., Science Prods., Division, 675 McDonnell Blvd., P.O. Box 5840, St. Louis, MO 63134, USA, Tel: 314-895-2221, Fax: 314-895-2328; **Sales/Distributor Offices:** Paris, KY 40362, USA, Tel: 800-354-2050 or 606-987-7000, Fax: 606-987-3456.

E. Merck, Frankfurter Strasse 250, Postfach 4119, D-6100 Darmstadt, Germany, Tel: 49-6151-72-0, Fax: 49-6151-72-2000.

Millipore Corporation, 397 Williams St., Marlborough, MA 01752, USA, Tel: 800-225-1380.

Miltenyi Biotec GmbH, Friedrich-Ebert-Strasse 68, D-5060 Bergisch Gladbach 1, Germany, Tel: +49-2204-8096, Fax: +49-2204-85197.

Molecular Probes, Inc., P.O. Box 22010, 4849 Pitchford Avenue, Eugene, OR 97402-0414, USA, Tel: 503-465-8300, Fax: 503-344-6504.

Nunc, 2000 North Aurora Rd., Naperville, IL 60563, USA, Tel: 800-288-6862, Fax: 708-416-2556, and Denmark.

Nycomed Pharma AS, P. O. Box 5012 Majorstua, N-0301 Oslo, Norway, Tel: 47-22-96-36-36, Fax: 47-22-96-35-30.

Nyegaard Diagnostics & Co. AS Oslo, Postboks 4220 Torshov, Oslo 4, Norway, Tel: 47-22-96-36-36, Fax: 47-22-96-35-30.

Organon Teknika Corporation, 100 Akzo Ave., Durham, NC 27704, USA, Tel: 800-682-2666.

Ortho Diagnostics, Route 202, Raritan, NJ 08869, USA, Tel: 800-322-6374.

PA Biologicals, Sydney, Australia.

Paar Scientific Ltd., 594 Kingston Road, Raynes Park, London SW20 8DN, United Kingdom, Tel: 44-81-540-8553, Fax: 44-81-543-8727.

Paesel, Frankfurt, Germany.

Partec GmbH, Otto-Hahn-Strasse 32, D-4400 Münster, Germany, Tel: +49-2534-5270, Fax: +49-2534-8588.

Pharmacia Biosystems, Ges.m.b.H., Munzinger Strasse 9, Postfach 5480, D-7800 Freiburg 1, Germany, Fax: 49-761-490-3159.

Pharmacia Biotech SpA, via Alessandro Volta 16, 20093 Cologno Monzese (MI), Italy, Tel: 02-273221, Fax: 02-27302212.

Pharmacia LKB Biotechnology, Box 175, S-75182 Uppsala, Sweden, Tel: 46-18-16-3000, Fax: 46-18-143820.

Pharmacia LKB Biotechnology, Inc. 800 Centennial Avenue, Box 1327, Piscataway, NJ 08855-1327, USA, Tel: 201-457-8000, Fax: 201-457-0557.

Polysciences, Inc., 400 Valley Road, Warrington, PA 18976-2590, USA, Tel: 215-343-6484 or 800-523-2575, Fax: 215-343-0214.

Quantum Analytics 363-D Vintage Park Drive, Foster City, CA 94404, USA, Tel: 800-992-4199 or 415-570-5656, Fax: 415-570-6087.

Quantum Instruments, Inc. 1075 Stewart Avenue, Garden City, NY 11530, USA, Tel: 516-222-0611, Fax: 516-222-0569.

Quantum Logic Corp. 25 Van Zant St., East Norwalk, CT 06855, USA, Tel: 203-838-4008, Fax: 203-838-3690.

Quantum Technol. Corp. 250 H. St., P.O. Box 8110-183, Blaine, WA 98230, USA, Tel: 206-647-9211, Fax: 206-671-2955.

Quantum Technology Corp. 6237 148th St., Surrey, British Columbia V3S 3C3, Canada, Tel: 604-594-6170.

Sacco Srl, via Manzoni 29/A, 22071 Cadorago (Como), Italy, Tel: 031-904443, Fax: 031-904596.

Sandoz Pharmaceuticals, Route 10, East Hanover, NJ 07936, USA, Tel: 201-503-7500, and Nurnberg, Germany.

Seromed, Berlin, Germany.

Serva Feinbiochemica GmbH, Carl-Benz-Strasse 7, D-6900 Heidelberg, Germany, Tel: 49-6221-502-0, Fax: 49-6221-502-113.

Sigma-Aldrich, Castle Hill, NSW, Australia.

Sigma Chemical Company, P.O. Box 14508, Saint Louis, MO 63178, USA, Tel: 800-325-3010, Fax: 800-325-5052.

Sigma Chimica, via Gallarate 154, 20151, Milano, Italy, Tel: 02-334317310 or 1678-27018, Fax: 02-38010737.

Streck Laboratories.

Unipath SpA, via Montenero 180, 20024 Garbagnate Milanese (MI), Italy, Tel: 02-9955651, Fax: 02-9958260.

Upjohn, 7000 Portage Road, Kalamazoo, MI 49001, USA, Tel: 616-323-4000, Fax: 616-323-7034.

Vector Laboratories, 30 Ingold Road, Burlingame, CA 94010, USA, Tel: 800-227-6666, Fax: 415-697-0339.

Zynaxis Cell Science, Malvern, PA, USA.